# THE
# MEDITERRANEAN DIET
## GUIDE *and* COOKBOOK

# THE
# MEDITERRANEAN DIET
## GUIDE *and* COOKBOOK

**Kimberly A. Tessmer, RDN, LD, and
Chef Stephanie Green, RDN**

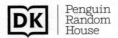

**Publisher** Mike Sanders
**Editorial Assistant** Kylie McNutt
**Art & Design Director** William Thomas
**Cover Designer** Laura Merriman
**Book Designer** Ayanna Lacey
**Proofreader** Lisa Starnes
**Indexer** Johnna VanHoose Dinse

First American Edition, 2023
Published in the United States by DK Publishing
1745 Broadway, 20th Floor, New York, NY 10019

Published in the United States by Dorling Kindersley Limited.

Library of Congress Catalog Number: 2023901512
ISBN: 978-0-7440-7659-2

DK books are available at special discounts when purchased
in bulk for sales promotions, premiums, fundraising,
or educational use. For details, contact:
SpecialSales@dk.com

Printed and bound in China

For the curious
www.dk.com

Reprinted from *The Complete Idiot's Guide® to the Mediterranean Diet*

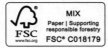

This book was made with Forest
Stewardship Council™ certified
paper—one small step in DK's
commitment to a sustainable future.
**For more information go to**
www.dk.com/our-green-pledge

# Contents

Introduction ................................................................................................................ 14

## Part 1: Eating the Mediterranean Way ................................................. 17

### Chapter 1: What Makes It Mediterranean? ................................................. 19

A Little Background on the Mediterranean Diet ............................................. 20

Key Components of the Mediterranean Diet .................................................. 22

Adopting the Mediterranean Way of Life ...................................................... 23

Other Lifestyle Factors .................................................................................. 25

A Common Mediterranean Diet Myth Debunked ........................................... 28

A Whole-Life Approach .................................................................................. 28

### Chapter 2: The Good Health Diet ................................................................ 31

Improve Cardiovascular Health ...................................................................... 32

Aid in Weight Management ............................................................................. 34

Cancer Protection ........................................................................................... 36

Prevent Depression ........................................................................................ 37

Take Control of Diabetes ................................................................................ 38

Connection to Other Health Issues ................................................................ 39

### Chapter 3: Components of the Mediterranean Diet ................................... 43

The Mediterranean Diet Pyramid .................................................................... 44

Dietary Guidelines for Americans/MyPlate ................................................... 51

Comparing the Symbols .................................................................................. 51

Making Your Choice ......................................................................................... 52

### Chapter 4: How Other Diets Stack Up ......................................................... 55

The American Heart Association's Heart-Healthy Diet ................................... 56

The Atkins Diet ............................................................................................... 58

The South Beach Diet.................................................................59

The Ornish Diet.......................................................................60

The Zone Diet..........................................................................61

The Sonoma Diet ....................................................................62

How to Lose Weight on the Mediterranean Diet ...................63

## Part 2: Basics of the Mediterranean Diet ............................... 67

### Chapter 5: Transitioning Your Diet .........................................69

Foods to Reduce and Foods to Add.......................................70

Changing Your Approach ........................................................ 71

Essential Mediterranean Diet Foods List ..............................72

What About Sweets?................................................................74

Reading Food Labels ..............................................................75

The Mediterranean Foods Alliance ........................................79

### Chapter 6: Olive Oil..................................................................81

The History and Production of Olive Oil.................................82

Olive Oil and the Mediterranean Diet ...................................83

Olive Oil, Every Day................................................................83

Olive Oil's Health Benefits......................................................84

Olive Oil's Nutritional Properties............................................85

Storing Olive Oil......................................................................88

Cooking with Olive Oil ............................................................89

Baking with Olive Oil ..............................................................90

### Chapter 7: Whole Grains..........................................................93

What Are Whole Grains? .........................................................94

Whole Grains and the Mediterranean Diet ...........................96

Whole Grains' Health Benefits ...............................................96

Whole Grains' Nutritional Properties .....................................97

Choosing Whole Grains ........................................................................................97

Popular Grains of the Mediterranean...............................................................99

Flours to Discover ...............................................................................................101

Cooking Whole Grains........................................................................................103

Tips for Going Whole Grain................................................................................104

**Chapter 8: Fruit**.............................................................................................107

Fruit and the Mediterranean Diet....................................................................108

Fruit's Health Benefits .......................................................................................108

Fruit's Nutritional Properties............................................................................108

Popular Fruits of the Mediterranean ..............................................................109

More Popular Fruits.............................................................................................113

Fruit for Dessert ..................................................................................................115

Fresh Isn't the Only Option ..............................................................................115

Tips for Eating More Fruit..................................................................................117

**Chapter 9: Vegetables**.................................................................................119

Vegetables and the Mediterranean Diet........................................................120

Vegetables' Health Benefits.............................................................................120

Vegetables' Nutritional Properties .................................................................121

Popular Vegetables of the Mediterranean ...................................................121

More Popular Vegetables ..................................................................................124

Going for the Super Greens ..............................................................................126

Tips for Vegging Out...........................................................................................128

**Chapter 10: Seafood**....................................................................................131

Seafood and the Mediterranean Diet.............................................................132

Seafood's Health Benefits.................................................................................132

The Experts Agree ..............................................................................................133

Seafood's Nutritional Properties ....................................................................133

Selecting Seafood...............................................................................134

Popular Seafood Choices of the Mediterranean................................135

Cooking Seafood................................................................................139

A Few Issues......................................................................................140

Tips for Eating More Seafood.............................................................142

**Chapter 11: Nuts, Seeds, and Legumes**...........................................**145**

Nuts, Seeds, and Legumes and the Mediterranean Diet......................146

Nuts' and Seeds' Health Benefits.......................................................146

Legumes' Health Benefits..................................................................147

Nuts' and Seeds' Nutritional Properties.............................................147

Legumes' Nutritional Properties........................................................148

Storing and Preparing Nuts, Seeds, and Legumes..............................149

Popular Nuts and Seeds of the Mediterranean...................................149

Popular Legumes of the Mediterranean.............................................151

Nuts for Desserts..............................................................................154

Tips for Eating More Nuts, Seeds, and Legumes................................154

**Chapter 12: Other Proteins**.............................................................**157**

Meat and Poultry...............................................................................158

Eggs..................................................................................................162

Dairy.................................................................................................163

**Chapter 13: Herbs and Spices**.........................................................**167**

Getting to Know Herbs and Spices.....................................................168

Herbs and Spices and the Mediterranean Diet...................................169

Herbs and Spices' Nutritional Properties...........................................169

Popular Herbs and Spices of the Mediterranean................................169

Flavoring with Herbs and Spices.......................................................171

**Chapter 14: Wine** ................................................................................**173**

Why Is Wine Heart Healthy?...........................................................174

Wine and the Mediterranean Diet.................................................174

Wine's Nutritional Properties.........................................................175

Which Wines Are Best for Heart Health? ......................................176

Pairing Red Wine with Food..........................................................178

Everything in Moderation...............................................................179

What If You Don't Drink?.................................................................179

**Part 3: Treasures of the Mediterranean Diet.....................181**

**Chapter 15: Fat**....................................................................................**183**

Fats Matter.....................................................................................184

How the Mediterranean Diet Delivers Healthy Fats.....................184

What Are Fats?................................................................................185

The Good Fats.................................................................................186

The Bad Fats...................................................................................189

Replacing Unhealthy Fats with Healthy Ones...............................192

**Chapter 16: Fiber**................................................................................**195**

What Is Fiber?.................................................................................196

Types of Fiber.................................................................................196

Fiber's Health Benefits...................................................................197

How Much Fiber Do You Need?......................................................200

How the Mediterranean Diet Delivers High Fiber.........................202

**Chapter 17: Nutrients** ........................................................................**207**

Nutrients of Mediterranean Foods.................................................208

Vitamins..........................................................................................208

Minerals..........................................................................................211

Antioxidants ........................................................................212

Phytonutrients ....................................................................213

Protein ...............................................................................214

Energy-Boosting Mediterranean Carbohydrates .................216

**Part 4: Flavors of the Mediterranean.........................219**

**Chapter 18: Appetizers and Snacks ..............................221**

Roasted Red Pepper Tapenade ...........................................222

Pesto .................................................................................223

Melon, Figs, and Prosciutto................................................224

Stuffed Dates .....................................................................225

Mushroom Crostini .............................................................226

Lemon Cannellini Spread .....................................................227

Hummus .............................................................................228

Eggplant Rolls.....................................................................229

Baked Vegetable Omelet......................................................230

Crab Cakes .........................................................................231

Tomato Basil Bocconcini......................................................232

Lamb Pesto Crostini............................................................233

Lemon Minted Melon ...........................................................234

Onion Apple Marmalade ......................................................235

Parmesan Pepper Crisps .....................................................236

Smoked Salmon Bites ..........................................................237

**Chapter 19: Soups and Salads ....................................239**

Tomato Basil Soup...............................................................240

Lemon Lentil Soup...............................................................241

Butternut Squash Soup........................................................242

Vegetable Orzo Soup...........................................................243

Split Pea Soup.................................................................................244

Gazpacho.........................................................................................245

Mixed Bean Soup...........................................................................246

Marinated Artichoke Salad..........................................................247

Roasted Beet Salad.......................................................................248

Golden Couscous Salad...............................................................249

Tuna Salad with Capers and Potatoes.......................................250

Fennel and Apple Salad...............................................................251

Shrimp and Melon Salad..............................................................252

Minted Cucumber Salad..............................................................253

Spinach, Orange, and Feta Salad...............................................254

Classic Mixed Greens Salad with Balsamic Vinaigrette.........255

Tabbouleh Salad...........................................................................256

**Chapter 20: Flatbreads, Pizza, Wraps, and More.................... 257**

Caramelized Onion Flatbread......................................................258

Pear, Provolone, Asiago, and Balsamic Flatbread...................259

Mushroom, Artichoke, and Arugula Flatbread.........................260

Tomato Basil Pizza.......................................................................261

Butternut Squash and Goat Cheese Pizza................................262

Veggie Wrap..................................................................................263

Chicken Almond Wrap..................................................................264

Chicken Tzatziki Pita....................................................................265

Prosciutto and Roasted Vegetable Panini................................266

**Chapter 21: Main Dishes .......................................................... 267**

Seafood Stew................................................................................268

Pan-Seared Orange Scallops......................................................269

Sole Florentine.............................................................................271

Almond-Crusted Barramundi......................................................272

*Salmon Fennel Bundles*.................................................................273

*Spicy Tomato Sauce with Linguine*.................................................274

*Angel Hair Pasta with Pesto, Mushrooms, and Arugula*.................275

*Lamb Patties and Pasta*...............................................................276

*Lamb Shanks*...............................................................................278

*Crispy Turkey Cutlets*..................................................................279

*Chicken Piccata*...........................................................................280

**Chapter 22: Side Dishes**.................................................................**281**

*Zucchini and Walnuts*...................................................................282

*Two-Cheese Risotto*......................................................................283

*Sautéed Spinach and Mushrooms*.................................................285

*Rosemary Garlic Potatoes*............................................................286

*Curried Cauliflower*......................................................................287

*Lemon Kale Ribbons*.....................................................................288

*Minted Peas with Pancetta*...........................................................289

*Pickled Asparagus*........................................................................290

*Bean and Vegetable Patties*..........................................................291

*Panzanella*...................................................................................293

*Golden Chard*...............................................................................294

*Sweet Polenta with Sun-Dried Tomatoes*.......................................295

*Quinoa Pilaf*.................................................................................297

*Barley and Vegetable Sauté*.........................................................298

**Chapter 23: Desserts**.....................................................................**299**

*Cinnamon Apple and Nut Phyllo Rolls*...........................................300

*Vanilla Panna Cotta*.....................................................................301

*Poached Summer Fruit*..................................................................302

*Mixed Berry Torte*.........................................................................303

*Berry Sorbet*.................................................................................304

*Fruit and Cheese Plate* .................................................................*305*

*Baked Stuffed Peaches* ...............................................................*306*

*Lemon Ricotta Muffins* ................................................................ *307*

*Baklava* ........................................................................................ *308*

*Almond Cookies* ..........................................................................*310*

*Walnut Cake* ................................................................................. *311*

*Orange Rice Pudding* .................................................................. *312*

*Fig and Apricot Compote* ............................................................*313*

**Chapter 24: Seasonal Menu Plans** ................................................**315**

Seven-Day Summer Menu Plan ...................................................*316*

Seven-Day Fall Menu Plan ........................................................... 318

Seven-Day Winter Menu Plan .....................................................*321*

Seven-Day Spring Menu Plan .....................................................*323*

**Appendixes**

**Appendix A: Glossary** ..................................................................... 327

**Appendix B: Resources** ................................................................. 333

**Index** .................................................................................................337

# Introduction

The Mediterranean diet is consistently shown to be a way of eating—and, as you will learn, a whole way of *living*—that is beneficial for the heart, for those living with diabetes, for weight loss, and for overall health. It's been the traditional style of eating, and living, for so many people in the countries surrounding the Mediterranean Sea, but anyone, anywhere can adopt it and enjoy the benefits.

*The Mediterranean Diet Guide and Cookbook* explains the details of this popular heart-healthy diet in terms that are easy to understand and, most importantly, easy to implement in your everyday life. It shares loads of fascinating nutritional information, practical shopping and cooking tips, and simple advice on making the Mediterranean diet your own. To that end, 80 mouthwatering recipes are also included, from snacks, to salads and soups, to main dishes and sides, to desserts, plus nearly a month's worth of Mediterranean diet meal plans that help get you started.

After reading this book, it is our hope that you will have a clear understanding of what the Mediterranean diet is all about and how to follow it. As importantly, we hope you have a much stronger understanding of what "good nutrition" means and how it relates to your health.

This book is written for the person who wants to live a longer, healthier, happier life—and we would guess that's most of us. If you are ready to make some relatively simple changes and take control of your life and your health, we invite you to give the Mediterranean diet a try.

## How We've Organized This Book

We divided this book into four parts. Each part offers unique information and helps guide you through the Mediterranean diet.

**Part 1, Eating the Mediterranean Way,** explores the background of the Mediterranean diet and what makes it "Mediterranean." We share all the health benefits this diet has to offer and review the food groups that make up the Mediterranean Diet Pyramid, along with their Mediterranean guidelines—all the aspects important to this style of eating, from food to lifestyle. We also show you how the Mediterranean diet stacks up against other popular diets.

**Part 2, Basics of the Mediterranean Diet,** provides you with the tools and knowledge you need to make this diet your own. Helpful tips get you started transitioning your current diet to more of a Mediterranean style. We take a comprehensive look at all the foods and beverages associated with the Mediterranean diet, including olive oil, whole grains, fruits, vegetables, fish, seafood, herbs, spices, nuts, seeds, legumes, meats, eggs, dairy products, and red wine.

**Part 3, Treasures of the Mediterranean Diet,** explores the components of Mediterranean foods that make them so health promoting. This part reviews the facts on the macronutrients, including fats, carbohydrates, and protein; it also takes a look at fiber. You become very familiar with the micronutrients, including vitamins, minerals, antioxidants, and phytonutrients—all the nutrients you know are healthy but maybe weren't sure why. This part helps you make the food-nutrition connection and explains how it all relates back to the health benefits of the Mediterranean diet.

**Part 4, Flavors of the Mediterranean,** is home to 80 tasty recipes that incorporate many of the foods, beverages, herbs, and spices we discuss in the book. These recipes help bring it all together, giving you the ability to create healthy dishes that incorporate Mediterranean diet benefits. We then use these recipes to create nearly a month of seasonal meal plans that will help inspire you to begin this heart-healthy diet right away and make it a fixed part of your life.

## Acknowledgments

*From Kimberly:* I want to extend a special thank you to Chef Stephanie Green, RDN, who developed the wonderful and delicious recipes in this book. Thank you for your hard work and expertise! It was a complete pleasure to work with you.

A special thanks to my literary agent, Jessica Faust, and her crew at BookEnds, LLC, for making this project happen.

Many thanks to people who lent their expertise: Nour El-Zibdeh, RD; Aphrodite Dikeakos, MS, RD; and Jo Ann Hattner, MPH, RD.

I am grateful to Oldways Preservation Trust (oldwayspt.org) for granting us permission to use the Mediterranean Diet Pyramid and Whole Grain Stamps images in the book.

On a personal note, I want to dedicate this book to my husband, Greg, and my daughter, Tori, who encourage and support me in everything I do, both professionally and personally. I love you both dearly. This book was written in loving memory of my parents, Donald and Nancy Bradford, who passed on to me their incredible passion for helping others. They were two incredibly special people I was lucky enough to call *Dad* and *Mom*.

*From Stephanie:* Much appreciation and thanks to my co-author Kimberly Tessmer, RDN, LD, for holding my hand during the process of this book and offering guidance and support.

Big heartfelt thanks to all my assistants who worked alongside me on the recipes and shopped, chopped, washed, and ate! Joanna Burnett, Linnea Caldeen, Joey Morgan, Lindsay L'vova, and Elizabeth Milburn.

I want to dedicate this book to my husband, Duane, for his gracious support.

## Special Thanks to the Technical Reviewer

The recipes in this book were reviewed by an expert who double-checked the accuracy of what you'll learn here to help us ensure that this book gives you everything you need to know about the Mediterranean diet. Special thanks are extended to Rowann Gilman, a freelance New York City–based food magazine and cookbook editor and writer.

## About the Authors

**Kimberly A. Tessmer, RDN, LD,** is a registered and licensed dietitian nutritionist, digital health coach, freelance writer, and published author. She holds a BS in technology (dietetics) from Bowling State University. Kim's expertise is in the fields of weight loss and health coaching, and nothing gives her greater satisfaction than helping and educating people to achieve their overall health goals. As a digital health coach, Kim guides people of all ages to transform themselves through healthy eating and lifestyle changes.

**Chef Stephanie Green, RDN,** is a registered dietitian nutritionist, chef, author, and professional speaker. She's the owner of Green's Cookery (greenscookery.com), specializing in nutrition and culinary education, recipe development, food demonstrations, and food styling. She teaches hands-on food demo workshops to community educators and has appeared nationally on television and radio.

# EATING THE MEDITERRANEAN WAY

Part 1 begins with the first steps you should take before starting any type of new eating style: learning all you can about the plan's background and the components that make up the diet. If you are wondering why you should eat the Mediterranean way and how it can help your health, this part helps answer those questions by explaining all the benefits currently attributable to this way of eating and this way of life. We explain both the food groups that make up the Mediterranean diet and also why they are essential to this way of eating.

You might be wondering how the Mediterranean diet compares with other types of diets. The last chapter in Part 1 gives you a good idea of how the Mediterranean diet stacks up against some popular diets, including the Atkins diet and the South Beach diet.

# CHAPTER 1

# What Makes It Mediterranean?

The Mediterranean diet is a traditional style of eating that continually ranks at the top of the charts as one of the best diets for heart health, diabetes, weight loss, and overall healthy eating.

Before embarking on any diet plan or new eating pattern, you should have a good understanding of its history, including what it entails and where it came from. If you are going to trust your health to a new way of life, you need to learn all you can, starting at the beginning.

# A Little Background on the Mediterranean Diet

When you think of the Mediterranean, you may picture blue water, pristine coastlines, spectacular scenery, and a rich culture. Experts see something very different in this area, and they appreciate more and more the eating style of the people who inhabit the region around the Mediterranean Sea. A growing body of scientific evidence confirms that the Mediterranean diet not only is heart healthy but also can help improve health and protect against chronic health conditions.

The Mediterranean diet was actually first developed in the 1970s but didn't gain real recognition until the 1990s. Known for its heart-healthy eating style, the Mediterranean diet is a permanent way of life. Once you embrace this lifestyle, you will experience a way of eating—and living—that people throughout the Mediterranean regions have practiced for centuries. The results will be an everyday way of living that helps you feel your best.

## Where the Mediterranean Diet Came From

There is no single Mediterranean diet; in fact, there are close to 18 countries in the region around the Mediterranean Sea. Diet preferences can vary depending on each country's ethnic background, religion, culture, economy, and agricultural differences. However, even with the slight differences among them, the eating patterns of these countries all have a great deal in common.

For our purposes we will discuss the most common Mediterranean diet, which is based on the traditional eating style of people within the Mediterranean region such as Crete, Greece, and southern Italy. By "traditional," we refer to a time, around the 1960s, when rates of chronic diseases in these areas were among the lowest in the world and the life expectancy of adults was at its highest.

## Whom the Mediterranean Diet Came From

Dr. Ancel Keys, an American physiologist, nutritionist, and researcher who lived in Italy, developed the original idea for the Mediterranean diet and discovered the health benefits that accompany it. In 1958, he began his 20-year landmark study (popularly known as the Seven Countries Study) that analyzed the role of diet in heart disease throughout seven countries: the United States, Italy, Greece, Spain, South Africa, Japan, and Finland. In 1970, he published the results of this study, establishing the basis of what would eventually be known as the Mediterranean diet.

In general, the study revealed that people in these areas who followed a Mediterranean-style eating pattern had lower percentages of death due to cardiovascular disease. Dr. Keys discovered that people in the Mediterranean region consumed fewer saturated fats and trans fats; more healthy fats—monounsaturated, polyunsaturated, and omega-3 fatty acids—especially monounsaturated fats; less dairy; and more fruits, vegetables, nuts, legumes, and whole grains than in other diets around the world. One of the strongest conclusions from this study was that a higher intake of saturated fat put one at risk for cardiovascular disease.

Although it was Dr. Keys who first developed the idea behind the Mediterranean diet, it was another group of professionals that introduced the concept as a whole. In 1993, the Oldways Preservation and Exchange Trust, along with the Harvard School of Public Health and the World Health Organization, first introduced the total concept of the Mediterranean diet at a conference in Cambridge, Massachusetts. The Mediterranean diet, along with the Mediterranean Diet Pyramid (which we discuss in Chapter 3), has become known worldwide as the gold standard for dietary patterns that promote heart health and long life. As time goes by, researchers are discovering even more proven effects of sticking to this diet, including healthy weight loss and maintenance; a lower risk of certain cancers; improved cognitive function, including helping prevent Alzheimer's disease; improvement for those with depression; lower risk of type 2 diabetes; relief from inflammation, including rheumatoid arthritis symptoms; and lowering a woman's risk for stroke.

## A Healthier Approach to Eating

The irony of this diet is that the people of the Mediterranean consume more fat overall than what is recommended for a typical Western diet, yet they have lower mortality rates from cardiovascular disease. The reason? They eat much less saturated fats (or "bad" fats) and much more unsaturated fats (or "good" fats).

Keep in mind that even though including healthier fats is key, it is not the only factor that results in lower mortality rates. It is also the many other healthful foods that make up a healthy eating pattern, as well as overall lifestyle habits, such as increased physical activity and lower stress levels, that make this lifestyle a healthier approach. It is no one food but rather a combination that appears to be responsible for the positive health benefits of this style of eating. In addition, people from the Mediterranean regions tend to eat slowly, use smaller plates, eat rich foods sparingly, and eat food that's in season. It's all about the diet as a whole—the way foods are prepared and the recipes used on a day-to-day basis that is the foundation of this healthy approach to eating.

This follows closely the position of the American Dietetic Association, which emphasizes that it is not individual foods that are key to good health but rather the total diet or overall eating pattern that is the most important focus of a healthful eating style. Many experts seem to agree on this approach.

# Key Components of the Mediterranean Diet

The Mediterranean diet is not complicated; however, it relies on several key components to work its magic. When you become familiar with all the basic components of the Mediterranean diet, you can begin to set realistic goals for yourself to slowly make the necessary changes.

To make this diet a permanent part of your life, it's essential that you adapt it to your own personal lifestyle and preferences. The more components you are able to incorporate into your life, the better your body will function and the more health benefits you will reap. The more this diet becomes your own, the more successful you will be at sticking with it—and the more it will become second nature.

Key components of the Mediterranean diet include the following:

- Minimally processed foods.

- Lots of fruits and vegetables that are fresh and preferably locally grown.

- Whole grains such as pastas, cereals, breads, and other grain products.

- Legumes (dried beans), nuts, and seeds.

- Moderate amounts of fish and shellfish (at least twice per week) with low to moderate amounts of poultry, eggs, and other lean meats to help meet protein needs. Red meats are used very little, if at all.

- Moderate amounts of dairy products (preferably fat-free or low-fat).

- Healthy, unsaturated fats from fish, avocados, olive oil, and canola oil. Butter, margarine, and other saturated and trans fats are avoided.

- Herbs and spices to flavor foods instead of salt.

- Sugars that come from natural sources such as fruit and honey.

• Red wine consumed in small amounts with meals (in moderation, of course). If you don't drink, don't start. You can always use purple grape juice as an alternative.

# Adopting the Mediterranean Way of Life

Although a move to the Mediterranean might sound inviting, it isn't necessary to reap the benefits of this region's healthy eating habits and lifestyle. You can adapt your behavior to incorporate this way of life by learning the ins and out of the lifestyle and then making smarter food choices.

## What Makes the Mediterranean Diet So Healthy?

As you begin to adopt this way of life, it is important to know exactly why the Mediterranean diet is said to be so healthy. Many factors contribute to the health benefits, and it has been proven in numerous studies that people of the Mediterranean are indeed healthy.

It is the multiple factors at work that provide the health benefits of the Mediterranean diet. It incorporates an abundance of nutritional-powerhouse foods working together that cannot be replaced by a supplement. This translates into a diet that is rich in unprocessed foods, lean protein, essential vitamins and minerals, whole grains, fiber, antioxidants, and healthy fats. It is the whole nutritional package and doesn't leave out any part of a well-balanced, healthy diet. Add the other aspects of this healthy lifestyle, and you get something so powerful, it can reduce your risk for many chronic and fatal health conditions.

Keep in mind, though, that a diet can only be as healthy as you allow it to be. In other words, the more closely you follow it, the more benefits you reap. If you decide this diet is for you and you are counting on its health benefits, you need to ensure you have the knowledge and the motivation to adopt this new way of life to its fullest. Commitment and consistency are key!

## Helpful Tips for Getting Started

Now that you're aware of the key components of this diet, it's time to start making some changes. However, making changes all at once can be overwhelming and often can undermine your best intentions. The most important concept is to gradually implement new changes while continuing to work the ones you've already made. If it seems overwhelming, try writing down your goals weekly to keep track of your action plans and successes.

Here are some tips for beginning the shift to the Mediterranean diet:

- Substitute and/or replace foods slowly. You don't want to jump in all at once, especially if your diet needs a lot of help. A good way to start is to replace side dishes and then move on from there.

- Start by using extra-virgin olive oil, avocado oil, and/or canola oil as your main fat source instead of unhealthy fats such as margarine or butter. Consider using it in cooking, sautéing, and/or as a replacement for your favorite salad dressing.

- Begin to make fruits and vegetables the bulk of your meals. Fill at least half of your plate with vegetables. Leave the rest for whole grains, lean meat, fish, or beans. Sneak fruit and vegetables in wherever you can, like adding spinach to eggs; loading sandwiches with tomato, avocado, and/or cucumber; or having an apple with almond butter for a snack.

- Visit your local farmers or produce markets to buy fruits and vegetables. (Or start your own garden!)

- Introduce a new fruit and/or vegetable each week to your meal plans to include variety in your diet. Don't be afraid to experience the taste of new foods.

- Substitute grilled, broiled, or steamed fish instead of red meat or other high-fat meats at least twice a week. Each week, reduce the number of meals in which red meat (or other high-fat meat) is served—and decrease portion sizes as well.

- Begin to replace refined grains (such as white bread, white rice, or white pasta) for whole grains (such as whole-wheat bread, brown rice, and whole-wheat pasta).

- Try out whole grains common to the Mediterranean, such as barley, bulgur, and couscous, by using some in new recipes.

- Snack on nuts. Don't be afraid of the fat content. The fat in nuts is a healthy fat, not to mention that nuts contain protein and fiber. Watch your portions, though. A quarter cup will do.

- Plan a few meatless meals each week. Make legumes or beans the main focus of those meals.

- Rethink your dairy choices. Switch to soft or semisoft cheeses that are low in fat (such as low-fat goat cheese, part-skim mozzarella, or Parmesan), and skip the processed cheeses. Use cheese in moderation—a smaller amount will do. Enjoy fat-free milk and fat-free or low-fat plain Greek yogurt. Skip the high-sugar flavored yogurts, and flavor your yogurt yourself by topping it with fruit and nuts.

- Season your foods and recipes with herbs and spices instead of table salt. It may take some practice and experimentation to get good at it!

- Begin cooking more of your meals from scratch and using whole foods, cutting back on processed foods. Invest in a few good Mediterranean cookbooks to help get you started and get those creative juices flowing.

- Limit much of your sugar intake. Replace sweets, baked goods, and other fat- and sugar-laden desserts and treats with fresh fruit, fruit-based desserts, and/or nuts. Indulge in sweets only occasionally.

- Work on making mealtime a special time of the day. Eat at the table with the family, and set aside enough time to slow down and enjoy your meal.

- Accept the fact that it is okay to revert to your traditional diet once in a while. If you don't have control of a meal—say you're at a friend's house—do the best you can. Don't beat yourself up.

- If it is approved by your doctor, have a glass of red wine with dinner. If you don't drink, try substituting purple grape juice to reap some of the health benefits.

These are all simple suggestions to help get you started, but remember that you don't have to tackle them all at once. You will read many tips and much helpful advice throughout this book that can assist you in transitioning your eating style. When you begin to incorporate some of these suggestions into your daily life, you will begin to realize how simple, healthful, and tasty eating this way can be. It should become a permanent way of life!

# Other Lifestyle Factors

The Mediterranean lifestyle is not only about its tasty foods and red wine. (Wouldn't that be nice!) You need to incorporate all the lifestyle factors to derive all the potential health benefits. Making these types of lifestyle changes can help change you in mind, body, and spirit.

Incorporating these types of changes means breaking a few bad habits and replacing them with good ones. How long do you let those bad habits go on before admitting to them, taking responsibility for them, and doing something about them? Is it time to quit smoking, get moving, reduce your stress, and generally take better care of yourself? There is no time like the present!

And the good news is that it's never too late to get started on the Mediterranean way of life to help increase longevity and reduce risk for chronic diseases. In fact, the sooner you begin, the better chance you have to begin reversing some of the damage that may have already been done. Your efforts will be well rewarded.

## Physical Activity

Although people of the Mediterranean consume plenty of healthy fats and a bit of red wine with their meals, they do not seem to be plagued with weight problems. They are able to balance the amount of food they consume with regular physical activity. This is an extremely important part of what makes the Mediterranean way of life a healthy one. The key is that these people make activity part of their everyday lifestyle instead of considering it something they have to do.

No matter how you include physical activity in your life, the key is to just do it. Physical activity can take many forms, and it is important to choose an activity you enjoy. Being physically active needs to be a habit that you adopt for the rest of your life. Just like any other habit, it takes time, perseverance, and commitment to get that habit to stick. You don't have to join the nearest gym and work out for two hours a day—unless you want to, of course—but you do need to be active on a daily basis to get any type of health benefit from it.

The Dietary Guidelines for Americans recommend at least 150 minutes per week of moderate-intensity physical activity and 2 days of muscle strength training activity. Increasing the time or intensity of your physical activity provides even more health benefits. Walking in your neighborhood or on your lunch break at work can be a great start. You can look into dancing, yoga, walking groups, swimming, or whatever activity you enjoy.

The keys are to get started, do something you enjoy, vary your exercise, challenge yourself along the way, and stick to it! Be more physically active in every way. Walk into stores or restaurants instead of using the convenient drive-thru, park farther away from buildings to get extra steps, take the stairs instead of the elevator, or play outside with your kids instead of just watching them. There are plenty of ways to get active and stay active. Your job is to implement those methods and get moving. Be sure to check with your physician before starting any type of exercise program.

And if you need further motivation: the World Health Organization (WHO) states that physical inactivity is the fourth leading risk factor for mortality. Inactive people have a 20 to 30 percent increased risk of all-cause mortality compared to those people who engage in at least 30 minutes of moderate-intensity activity most days of the week.

## Less Stress

The people of the Mediterranean are much more geared to a lower-stress lifestyle than we are in the United States. With our fast-paced lifestyle of parenting, working, managing our finances, and daily chores, we often become much more stressed than we would like to admit. This can add to a whole host of health issues, whether you realize it is happening or not.

It may be time to slow down, decrease the stress, and enjoy life a bit more. Staying physically active is one factor that can help alleviate some of the stress in your life. Other strategies might include meditation, breathing exercises, reading a good book, listening to soothing music, doing yoga, or better managing your time. The possibilities are endless. The key is to find what works for *you*.

## Slow Down

Our fast-paced lifestyle often means eating meals on the run. For many, that involves the drive-thru at the nearest fast-food joint, resulting in unhealthy choices. The people of the Mediterranean tend to enjoy leisurely dining and take pleasure in all the wonderful flavors and aromas. A lesson in slowing down and enjoying your meals should be on your list.

Slowing down when it comes to your meals can help you plan and choose your meals more wisely. You can take the time to prepare meals at home, making better choices and eating as a family. Plus, you give yourself time to think and consider not just what you are eating but also how much you are eating. Did you know that slowing down can actually help satisfy your hunger at the end of the meal? You eat much less and are much more satisfied when you eat at a slower pace.

## Good Hydration

The people of the Mediterranean don't live on wine alone. Water is one of the most essential substances we can give our body. In fact, water is present in almost every cell and every part of our body. Staying properly hydrated helps your body regulate its temperature, transport nutrients and oxygen, carry waste products, cushion joints, protect body organs; assists in the digestive process; and helps prevent constipation. The Mediterranean diet is one that is high in fiber, which means it is even more important to drink the water your body needs to keep that fiber moving in the right direction. (You can read more on fiber in Chapter 16.)

Being properly hydrated also can help provide more energy, an improved sense of well-being, and greater endurance and stamina during physical activity. Water is essential to life, and our bodies need a sufficient amount to function properly. The best part is that water has no calories. All that water may just be the reason for the beautiful skin the people of the Mediterranean have.

Because your body cannot store water, you must continually replace the water your body loses naturally through perspiration, breathing, urination, and bowel movements. Keep in mind you do get water through foods and other beverages, but it's important to be aware of how much water you are actually drinking each day. Many factors impact how much water every individual needs, including age, gender, activity level, and overall health. We normally get about 20 percent of the water we need from the foods we eat. Taking that into account, women should drink about 9 cups of water per day, and men should drink about 13 cups per day to replenish what's lost. Drink water throughout the day, keep a water bottle at your desk or in your car, drink plenty of water while exercising, and drink water at most meals.

# A Common Mediterranean Diet Myth Debunked

Every diet out there has its doubters. There are always people who don't believe that a diet stands up to its claims. Even with all the research and scientific studies that prove that the principles underlying the Mediterranean style of eating are sound, you can still find a common myth: the Mediterranean diet contains a high percentage of fat and, therefore, can be hazardous to your waistline and can contribute to obesity.

Although the Mediterranean diet is a healthy diet, calories and portion size still matter. The fats included in this diet are heart healthy, but keep in mind that fat in general—whether healthy or not—is still high in calories.

Low-fat diets are not always the answer to permanent weight loss and good health because it's the *type* of fat you eat that matters most. Just because someone follows a low-fat diet doesn't mean they are eating healthy fats. A diet can be higher in healthy fats and still be a healthy way of eating.

As long as you keep your portion sizes in check—not just with healthy fats and oils, but with all the foods included in the diet—your waistline shouldn't have anything to worry about. If you consider all the healthy foods you'll be eating, the decrease in unhealthy fats and foods, and the addition of more physical activity, you'll probably even lose a few pounds.

# A Whole-Life Approach

This diet does not entail making drastic changes to your present eating style. In fact, what makes the Mediterranean diet so unique and so impressive is how practical it is in real life. It is a realistic way of life and one that you can incorporate and feel good about for a lifetime.

The health differences between people of the Mediterranean and people who consume the typical Western diet are due to their lifestyles as a whole. The Mediterranean way of life is unique in that it focuses not only on what you eat but also on overall lifestyle—it's a whole-life approach to good health. It's a permanent solution as opposed to changes one might make for a temporary period of time simply to lose weight.

## Not Just a "Diet"

The Mediterranean diet is not really a "diet" at all. When we think of the word *diet,* thoughts of fad diets gone wrong, expensive weight-loss schemes, and days of deprivation often come to mind.

This way of life focuses on what you *can* have instead of what you *cannot.* And what you can have are the very best, healthiest, freshest whole foods. That doesn't sound like the typical "diet," does it? We're not saying that one of the health benefits of a Mediterranean diet can't be shedding a few pounds, but that is not the main purpose of this so-called "diet." It's intended to be a lifestyle change.

## Making It Mainstream

You don't need to live in the Mediterranean or be of Mediterranean descent to enjoy this diet and lifestyle and reap its benefits. However, for the Mediterranean diet to be effective, you do need to make a commitment to making this diet a permanent way of life. The Mediterranean diet is sensible and realistic, both of which are essential when it comes to something you follow for life.

The components of this diet work like the wheels on a car. They all need to be present to make the car go. However, the tires don't all need to match for the car to go. In other words, you don't always have to eat the traditional foods of the Mediterranean to get the most from this diet. Throughout this book, we will help you incorporate this diet and realistically fit it into your lifestyle while still reaping all the important health benefits.

## In This Chapter

The Mediterranean diet originates from 18 different countries around this region. The key components of this whole-life approach include healthy fats, fresh whole foods, an abundance of plant foods, physical activity, and lower stress levels. The Mediterranean diet incorporates many nutritional powerhouse foods that can fit realistically into anyone's life.

# CHAPTER 2

# The Good Health Diet

If you are looking for a heart-healthy eating plan, the Mediterranean diet might just be for you. However, that is far from the only health benefit this diet can provide. The Mediterranean diet boasts an impressive list of health benefits countless people can relate to.

You can improve your heart health, manage your weight, lower your risk for some cancers, reduce your risk for cognitive decline, and even improve blood sugar control by making some realistic lifestyle changes. Soon you will see how.

# Improve Cardiovascular Health

Who says eating a heart-healthy diet has to be tasteless? Incorporating some recommendations from the Mediterranean diet into your everyday life can be something you can actually enjoy. The days of bland, low-fat, incredibly restrictive diets that were once recommended for heart disease prevention are gone, replaced by a colorful, fresh, and flavorful diet that amps up the healthy fats, seasonal produce, whole grains, legumes, seafood, and wonderful herbs and spices.

The Mediterranean diet is known as the gold standard for a heart-healthy approach. It has been researched, studied, and proven that this type of diet has a strong correlation to improved cardiovascular health. Ever since Dr. Ancel Key's famous Seven Countries Study, research supporting a Mediterranean eating pattern has been flowing in.

A 2018 study published in the *New England Journal of Medicine* featured almost 7,500 people between the ages of 55 and 80 who were at high cardiovascular risk. Participants were enrolled in either a Mediterranean diet supplemented with extra olive oil or mixed nuts, or a traditional low-fat diet. Results concluded that the people on the Mediterranean diet, the one supplemented with either extra olive or mixed nuts, had a much lower incidence of major cardiovascular events compared to those participants on the traditional low-fat diet.

In addition, a large clinical study sponsored by the National Institutes of Health (NIH) and the American Association of Retired Persons (AARP) published results in the *Archives of Internal Medicine* in 2007 suggesting that there is strong evidence that implementing a Mediterranean dietary pattern lowers the risk for death from all causes, including deaths due to cardiovascular disease and cancer in the U.S. population.

Need more proof? How about results from a study published in the *American Journal of Clinical Nutrition* in 2007, which concluded that frequent consumption of foods from the Mediterranean pattern may reduce cardiovascular disease as well as ischemic heart disease risks? Or a 2018 cohort study, published on the JAMA Network, of close to 26,000 U.S. women who had a higher baseline Mediterranean diet intake that was associated with up to 28 percent relative risk reduction in cardiovascular events?

## What Is Cardiovascular Disease?

The terms *cardiovascular disease* and *heart disease* are often used interchangeably. Both generally describe several health issues that relate to the heart and the blood vessels, including heart disease, heart attack, stroke, heart failure, arrhythmia, and heart valve issues.

Heart disease is the leading cause of death for both men and women in the United States. According to the American Heart Association, an estimated 121.5 million American adults— nearly half of all adults in the United States—have one or more forms of cardiovascular disease, including high blood pressure. Coronary heart disease, the most common type of heart disease, kills almost 400,000 Americans each year. It is estimated that heart disease costs the United States more than $300 billion (£2.5 billion) each year through health-care services, medications, and loss of productivity.

Do these statistics startle you? They should! The good news is there *is* something you can do to avoid becoming one of these statistics. Making smarter dietary and lifestyle choices can put you on the road to better heart health.

## Are You at Risk?

Two risk factors for heart disease that we don't have any control over are age and genetics. Your risk increases as you get older, and a strong family history can put you at risk. Other risk factors include a high level of low-density lipoprotein (LDL) or "bad" cholesterol, a low level of high-density lipoprotein (HDL) or "good" cholesterol, high triglycerides, and/or high blood pressure. A normal and healthy blood pressure should read less than 120 systolic over 80 diastolic or 120/80 millimeters of mercury (mmHg) consistently.

In addition, you could be putting yourself at risk if you are sedentary, are overweight or obese, have uncontrolled diabetes, have uncontrolled high blood pressure, drink alcohol excessively, consume a poor diet, and/or deal with high stress levels consistently. If any of these apply to you, it may be time to take a serious look at your diet and lifestyle.

## How Does the Mediterranean Diet Help?

The good news is that, even with most risk factors, many forms of heart disease can be prevented and possibly treated with both proper diet and exercise. That is where the Mediterranean diet comes in. Key components of this diet make it possible to help prevent and even reverse some major health problems.

## The Cholesterol Connection

Blood cholesterol levels are a significant risk factor for heart disease. The higher your cholesterol levels, both total and LDL, the higher your risk for heart disease. Therefore, it is vital to have your cholesterol tested on a regular basis. You should know what your personal numbers are so you understand this vital risk factor. Knowing your levels for total cholesterol, as well as LDL and HDL, discloses whether your blood cholesterol is putting you at risk for heart disease and/or stroke.

As we have mentioned, cholesterol comes in two basic forms: LDL (or bad) cholesterol and HDL (or good) cholesterol. When LDL, or low-density lipoprotein, and total cholesterol are too high, it causes cholesterol (or plaque) to build up in the walls of your arteries. This condition is known as atherosclerosis, or hardening of the arteries, and it puts you at higher risk for heart disease. HDL, or high-density lipoprotein, rids your body of cholesterol by taking it from the artery walls and sending it to the liver for removal from the body, giving your heart some protection. Your total cholesterol level should be less than 200 milligrams per deciliter (mg/dL) to be at a desirable level. LDL cholesterol should be less than 100 mg/dL, with HDL being above 60 mg/dL to offer any heart protection. Cholesterol testing should be done after fasting for at least 12 hours. Your doctor can determine how often you should get your cholesterol tested.

It has been concluded that with the Mediterranean diet's combination of a high amount of fiber (especially soluble fiber), low amounts of saturated and trans fats, high consumption of unsaturated fats (especially monounsaturated fats), and physical activity, this diet can modestly lower LDL and raise HDL cholesterol. In addition, it has been shown to decrease triglyceride levels, another possible risk factor for heart disease.

Triglycerides are the main form of fat in foods. Excess calories from any type of food source are processed in the body and changed to triglycerides for storage as fat in the body. Normal triglyceride levels should be less than 150 mg/dL.

# Aid in Weight Management

We have all heard the debate about which is the best way to lose weight. Is it low fat, high fat, no carbs, high protein, low protein, no sugar, good fat? There is no one "best way" to lose weight. However, the eating in the style of the Mediterranean region is catching on as a realistic and healthy way to shed some pounds.

Most of us know that to lose weight and keep it off you need to permanently change your lifestyle. The Mediterranean diet encompasses this whole-life approach. A change to this type of lifestyle, with its healthy food choices, moderate consumption of foods, and physical activity, can help you to maintain a healthier weight.

A study published in the *New England Journal of Medicine* revealed that a calorie-controlled Mediterranean diet could be more effective for weight loss than a low-fat diet, while offering additional health benefits. The Mediterranean diet is not a quick fix for your weight problems; however, by conforming to this type of lifestyle, you may see your waistline begin to slowly shrink. With the good habits you establish, and the bad ones you throw away, it is bound to happen. And it can be empowering to make positive changes in your life and have control over the way you are living it. That is a great motivator!

## The Dangers of Obesity

The prevalence of obesity in the United States is truly staggering. A study done by the U.S. Centers for Disease Control and Prevention (CDC) showed that a whopping 41.9 percent of American adults are obese. Being overweight or obese carries many risk factors. Research has shown that being overweight or obese increases one's risk for the following conditions:

- Coronary heart disease

- Type 2 diabetes

- Breast cancer

- Colon cancer

- Endometrial cancer

- High blood pressure (hypertension)

- High cholesterol and/or triglyceride levels

- Stroke

- Liver disease

- Gallbladder disease

- Sleep apnea and other respiratory problems

- Osteoarthritis

- Gynecological problems

There are countless reasons to choose a lifestyle that will not only increase your health but also help you shed excess weight. Given the statistics, it is obvious that the traditional Western diet leaves much to be desired. Not only can the Mediterranean diet help you manage your weight, but many of the health problems associated with obesity are the exact problems that can be treated, prevented, or reversed by following the Mediterranean diet.

## What Should You Weigh?

Are you are obese, overweight, or at a normal weight? Does your weight put you greater risk for health problems? Do you even know what you should weigh? Now is the time to find out.

Body mass index, or BMI, is used to screen adults for weight categories that may lead to health risks. BMI is determined by using weight and height to calculate a number, or index. You can easily calculate your BMI by visiting nhlbi.nih.gov/health/educational/lose_wt/BMI /bmicalc.htm, or you can use the following formula:

> Weight in pounds ÷ height in inches$^2$ × 703

> (Or weight in kilograms ÷ height in meters$^2$ if using metric.)

For example, if you weigh 160 pounds and have a height of 5 feet 7 inches (67 inches), you would calculate your BMI this way:

> $160 \div 67^2 \times 703 = 25.05$

When you know your BMI, you can determine your weight category:

> Underweight = BMI of less than 18.5

> Normal weight = BMI of 18.5 to 24.9

> Overweight = BMI of 25 to 29.9

> Obese = BMI of 30 or greater

Calculating your BMI is not a direct measure of body fat. Some folks, such as athletes or body builders, who carry extra weight due to more muscle may be classified as overweight or obese even though they do not have excess body fat.

# Cancer Protection

Cancer is the second leading cause of death in the United States behind heart disease, so it's no surprise that many of us will take note when we hear that something may help lower our risk for this disease.

Recent studies suggest that a strict adherence to the Mediterranean diet is associated with a reduced risk of overall cancer mortality as well as a reduced risk of several types of cancers, including breast, gastric, colon, esophageal, and liver.

In 2008, the *British Journal of Cancer* concluded from a general population investigation that adherence to the traditional Mediterranean diet is associated with markedly and significantly reduced incidence of overall cancer, and this reduced incidence was appreciably larger than predicted from examining individual Mediterranean diet components. This is evidence that it's the diet as a whole, and the many cancer-fighting foods included in the diet, working to provide protection.

The NIH-AARP Diet and Health Study, developed by the National Cancer Institute and in collaboration with AARP, found a 12 percent decreased cancer mortality in women and a 17 percent decreased mortality in men who were following the Mediterranean diet after a 5-year follow-up.

All the practices of the Mediterranean diet are realistic lifestyle changes that can arm you with one more weapon in the battle against cancer.

# Prevent Depression

Depressive disorders are serious and affect almost 10 percent of the U.S. population. Recent research is beginning to suggest that people who follow a traditional Mediterranean diet may be less likely to develop depression. And at the 2019 American Psychiatric Association's Annual meeting, a conclusion was reached that a Mediterranean-type diet may protect against symptoms of depression in later life and older adults. Researchers believe these findings are based on the foods and the components of those foods, including vitamins, minerals, antioxidants, and phytonutrients.

Although researchers aren't exactly clear yet on how the foods of the Mediterranean diet actually help fight depression, they do believe that individual components of the diet may help improve blood vessel function, fight inflammation, reduce the risk for heart disease, and repair oxygen-related cell damage—all of which may affect a person's (especially an older person's) risk for developing depression. It could be many components of the diet working together synergistically to add a degree of protection. These components may include omega-3 fatty acids; other unsaturated fatty acids; antioxidants from olive oil and nuts; large amounts of natural folates and other B vitamins; and flavonoids and other phytochemicals from fruits, vegetables, and other plant foods. The research continues on the diet's connection to depression, so stay tuned.

# Take Control of Diabetes

Type 2 diabetes has become very prevalent in the United States, with more than 37 million Americans having diabetes and approximately 90 to 95 percent of those cases as type 2 diabetes. Most research reports that a Mediterranean diet and lifestyle can help improve glycemic control and cardiovascular risk factors that are so common in people with diabetes. Even for those people who are at risk for type 2 diabetes, the diet can provide a protective effect.

Benefits of lifestyle interventions, including diet, are essential and should not be overlooked for diabetes intervention. Although a Mediterranean diet is not the magic cure, it has plenty of features that may help control diabetes and help people possibly avoid or reduce medication use.

Always check with your doctor before stopping or reducing any type of medication for diabetes. Diet and lifestyle changes can help, but your doctor should decide whether diet alone is enough to control your diabetes. Keeping blood sugar in check can mean the difference between a healthy life and one with serious health issues.

## Types of Diabetes

The term *diabetes* refers to a group of diseases that are marked by high levels of blood glucose or blood sugar due to defects in the production or action of insulin, a hormone produced in the pancreas. There are three basic forms of diabetes: type 1, type 2, and gestational (during pregnancy). Type 2 diabetes is the most common form.

With type 2 diabetes, the body does not produce enough insulin and/or utilize it effectively enough. When we eat food, our body breaks down sugars and starches into glucose, which is the main fuel for our body's cells. It is the job of insulin to take the sugar from the blood into the cells. When there is not enough insulin or the insulin isn't working effectively, glucose builds up in the blood instead of entering the cells, causing high blood sugar levels. This can lead to complications if not treated properly. Treatment can include diet and exercise modifications, oral medications, and/or insulin injections. Treatment is modified for each individual and their own personal needs in order to manage their blood sugars.

Diabetes can lead to a host of serious health complications, especially if it is not controlled. These include heart disease, stroke, high blood pressure, blindness, kidney disease, diseases of the nervous system, amputation, and even death.

Unlike type 2 diabetes, when the body doesn't produce enough or effectively utilize insulin, type 1 diabetes is caused when the body produces *no* insulin. People with type 1 diabetes need insulin injections to survive. Type 1 diabetes is much less common than type 2 diabetes and cannot be treated with diet and lifestyle changes alone.

## Are You at Risk?

People with uncontrolled diabetes can be at risk for serious health conditions. Therefore it is important to know if you have diabetes or are at risk for it, so you can take the proper precautions.

Type 2 diabetes most often occurs in middle-aged and older people. People who are overweight or obese, have a family history of type 2 diabetes, and/or are physically inactive and sedentary have a higher risk for developing type 2 diabetes. Other risk factors include a diagnosis of prediabetes, a history of gestational diabetes, and high blood pressure. Clinical studies have shown that high cholesterol levels may be a risk factor for insulin resistance, which also can be a risk factor in developing type 2 diabetes. Ethnicity can play a role in determining your risk as well.

Having diabetes tends to lower HDL, or "good," cholesterol levels and increase triglycerides and LDL, or "bad," cholesterol levels. This puts people with diabetes at a higher risk for heart disease, heart attacks, and strokes. It is vital that their treatment and lifestyle be aimed at not only stringent blood sugar control but also other health aspects. Following the Mediterranean diet has been shown to possibly help control blood sugar, but for people with diabetes, it can be even more important because it is also a heart-healthy way of life.

# Connection to Other Health Issues

To really soak up all the Mediterranean diet has to offer, it's essential to look at all its benefits. As more research is done, more health benefits are being revealed about the Mediterranean way of life.

## Hypertension

In today's hectic and chaotic society, it is not surprising that hypertension, or high blood pressure, is becoming more and more common. With the number of Americans who are overweight or obese, eat unhealthy diets, are physically inactive, and experience high stress levels, problems with high blood pressure will likely continue to be a reality.

Blood pressure is the force of blood against the walls of your arteries. When your blood pressure is elevated over time, it is diagnosed as hypertension. Hypertension makes your heart work too hard and can increase your risk for a host of serious health issues, including heart and artery damage, stroke, kidney disease, and vision loss. These are not symptoms of high blood pressure because this disease really has no symptoms or warning signs. Your risk for health issues increases even more if, along with high blood pressure, you smoke, are overweight or obese, have high cholesterol, have type 2 diabetes, are physically inactive, are male, are an older adult, or have a genetic predisposition. Anyone can develop high blood pressure, and it's estimated that one in every four Americans has high blood pressure.

Even though hypertension does have strong genetic links, plenty of evidence confirms that good nutrition and a healthy lifestyle can delay or prevent the onset of hypertension as well as treat it. When it comes to both preventing and treating hypertension, many people today look to natural alternatives. Could the Mediterranean diet be the answer for so many?

According to a 2020 study published in the journal *Nutrient,* promoting adherence to the Mediterranean diet can significantly decrease the likelihood of hypertension in all participants, including overweight/obese individuals. A 2019 study published in *Hypertension Journal* concluded that a Mediterranean-style diet is effective in improving cardiovascular health with relevant reduction in blood pressure and arterial stiffness.

The bottom line is that even though a Mediterranean eating style may not be effective for all people, especially those at high risk of hypertension due to family history, the diet could help delay the onset of hypertension and possibly reduce the amount of medication needed for treatment.

## Alzheimer's Disease

Alzheimer's disease is the most common type of dementia and is defined as a progressive neurologic disorder that ultimately causes the brain to shrink and atrophy. This causes a continuous decline in memory, intellectual thinking, behavioral and social skills, and eventually a person's ability to live and function independently. It is estimated that 5.8 million Americans are living with Alzheimer's disease. This progressive disease is eventually fatal, and currently there is no cure.

Studies suggest that following a Mediterranean diet may lower the risk for mental decline. A 2021 study in *Neurology* found the Mediterranean diet regimen to be a protective factor against memory decline and brain atrophy. They suggest that eating this way may protect the brain from the protein buildup that can lead to memory loss and dementia. Continuing studies are showing that what you eat may influence your memory skills later in life.

It's important to remember that the Mediterranean diet may not completely protect a person against Alzheimer's disease and cognitive decline, but it may help lower one's risk.

## Parkinson's Disease

Parkinson's disease is a degenerative disorder that affects the central nervous system, often impairing motor skills, speech, and other functions. It is a chronic and progressive disease, meaning it persists for a lifetime and symptoms become worse with time. There is presently no cure for Parkinson's disease, but medications can help dramatically relieve symptoms for many sufferers.

Through the many studies done on the Mediterranean diet, it has become evident that the incidence of Parkinson's disease is lower in people who adhere to a Mediterranean eating style. In 2007, a study published in the *American Journal of Clinical Nutrition* concluded that dietary patterns with a high intake of fruits, vegetables, legumes, whole grains, nuts, fish, and poultry, combined with a low intake of saturated fat and a moderate intake of alcohol, may help protect against Parkinson's disease. Does that diet sound familiar? It should—that's the Mediterranean diet in a nutshell.

## Rheumatoid Arthritis

People diagnosed with rheumatoid arthritis (RA) suffer from painful swelling, mostly in the joints of the hands and feet. Rheumatoid arthritis is an autoimmune disorder, meaning it occurs because your immune system mistakenly attacks your own body's tissues. There is currently no cure for this type of inflammatory arthritis, but advances in treatment options have been made in the past few decades.

The Mediterranean diet has been shown to positively benefit people with arthritis by reducing inflammation and improving function. Due to its anti-inflammatory properties, the diet is highly recommended by health professionals to help fight the inflammation associated with RA. A 2018 study published in the journal *Rheumatology International* concluded that the Mediterranean diet can reduce pain and increase physical function in people living with RA.

This is not to say that the diet will cure or dramatically improve a person's symptoms, but it does seem that there is a modest benefit for arthritis sufferers.

## In This Chapter

The Mediterranean diet has been a proven ally in helping lower the risk for cardiovascular disease and heart disease. In addition, the Mediterranean eating plan can help lower the risk of some types of cancer, help with weight loss, and be a tool in managing type 2 diabetes and blood sugar. Studies show that the Mediterranean diet may be beneficial for other medical conditions, such as depression, hypertension, Alzheimer's disease, Parkinson's disease, and rheumatoid arthritis.

# CHAPTER 3

# Components of the Mediterranean Diet

The Mediterranean diet encapsulates an entire eating pattern. It is much more than any one single food that generates health benefits and longevity. Instead, the diet revolves around how particular healthy cuisine involving all the food groups and a healthier lifestyle work cohesively to construct the diet and make it what it is. The Mediterranean Diet Pyramid puts this all together in one neat, visual package.

# The Mediterranean Diet Pyramid

Since the Mediterranean Diet Pyramid was first introduced, many people have taken notice. Restaurants, chefs, cookbooks, weight-loss companies, and health professionals have willingly embraced this way of eating and meal planning.

The Oldways Preservation and Exchange Trust, along with the Harvard School of Public Health and the World Health Organization, introduced the diet and the pyramid at a conference in Cambridge, Massachusetts, in 1993, and since then, it has remained a universally recognized guide to the Mediterranean style of eating.

The pyramid, developed as a graphic to help people better visualize the diet, was created using the most current science-based research to symbolize the traditional Mediterranean diet. The pyramid not only represents the foods of the Mediterranean but also takes into account other factors that come highly recommended as part of the lifestyle, including physical activity, the enjoyment of meals with others, and the appreciation for the pleasure of eating these tasty and healthy foods.

## A Few Changes

Since its initial development, the pyramid has undergone some renovations to reflect the latest research findings and ongoing studies. During the fifteenth anniversary of the Mediterranean Diet Conference (where the diet and pyramid were first introduced), updates were made by the Scientific Advisory Board to provide some beneficial improvements. The major changes made to the pyramid included the following:

- The grouping of all plant foods, including fruits, vegetables, grains, nuts, legumes, seeds, olives, and olive oil. This group now encompasses the largest section of the pyramid. This change was made to draw direct attention to the key role plant foods play in good health.

- The addition of herbs and spices to the pyramid. These enhance flavor and aroma and reduce the need for fat and salt in cooking.

- The emphasis on eating more fish and shellfish. Consuming these foods at least twice per week is recommended to obtain their unique health benefits.

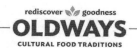

# Mediterranean Diet Pyramid

*A contemporary approach to delicious, healthy eating*

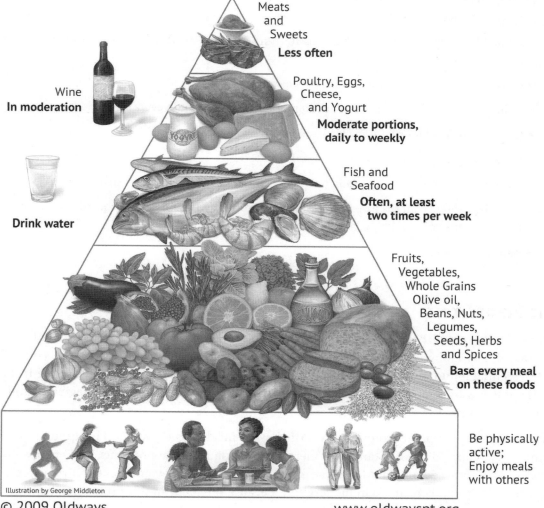

Meats and Sweets
**Less often**

Wine
**In moderation**

Poultry, Eggs, Cheese, and Yogurt
**Moderate portions, daily to weekly**

**Drink water**

Fish and Seafood
**Often, at least two times per week**

Fruits, Vegetables, Whole Grains Olive oil, Beans, Nuts, Legumes, Seeds, Herbs and Spices
**Base every meal on these foods**

Be physically active; Enjoy meals with others

Illustration by George Middleton

© 2009 Oldways

www.oldwayspt.org

*(Used by permission. © 2009 Oldways, www.oldwayspt.org.)*

## Explaining the Pyramid

The Mediterranean Diet Pyramid is an easy-to-follow visual aid to help people implement the Mediterranean diet. The pyramid is arranged in a way that suggests how often certain types of foods should be consumed to get the most health benefits, so the base of the pyramid shows foods to consume more often, and as you move up the pyramid, it shows foods to eat less often. The pyramid does not get specific with serving sizes but instead displays how often certain foods should be consumed. Portion sizes are still important, and moderation should always be practiced. The pyramid emphasizes:

- Being physically active as much as possible and enjoying meals with others as the foundation of this type of healthy lifestyle.

- Choosing the least-processed forms of plant foods.

- Using olive oil for most cooking, baking, salad dressings, and vegetables.

- Consuming low-fat or fat-free cheeses and yogurts in moderation.

- Consuming poultry more often than red meats.

- Drinking red wine in moderation (or purple grape juice, if you do not drink wine).

- Drinking water. Water is essential for life and proper hydration, which contributes to good health, a sense of well-being, and higher energy levels.

- Eating in moderation.

## The Plant Group

The plant group is the largest in the pyramid. This food group sits near the bottom of the pyramid, above physical activity and enjoying meals with others, signifying that it is one of the essential foundations of this eating style. It incorporates *all* plant foods, including fruits, vegetables, grains (mostly whole), olives and olive oil, beans, nuts and seeds, legumes, and herbs and spices.

Guidelines for the plant group specify basing every meal on these foods. This group is an important source of fiber, vitamins, minerals, antioxidants, phytonutrients, and energy. An eating pattern based on plant foods promotes good health and even weight control when chosen wisely and consumed in moderation. Because the foods in this group are near the bottom of the pyramid and tend to be eaten in larger amounts and more frequently, moderate portion sizes are key.

## Fruits and Vegetables

A vast variety of produce is popular in the Mediterranean region, and because they are frequently eaten in season, these fruits and vegetables are commonly fresher and more nutritious. Locally, shop the perimeter of your grocery store, where most of the fresh foods are located, and consider local farmers markets in your area.

Although the pyramid does not specify serving sizes, it is recommended that you aim for at least 7 to 9 servings of a variety of high-fiber fruits and vegetables daily. You do not need to eat produce straight from the Mediterranean or even rely on only the most popular fruits and vegetables to reap the benefits. Finding produce that is in season in your area and that you enjoy is the most important point to remember.

You shouldn't rely on them exclusively for fruit intake, but dried fruits such as prunes, dates, cranberries, figs, raisins, and apricots are very high in fiber and can be easy to find and store all year long. Try them in salads, rice dishes, casseroles, and desserts or as a quick snack.

## Grains

Grains are chock-full of carbohydrates and are the body's main source of energy. They also include good-for-you fiber, vitamins, and minerals. The Mediterranean diet includes plenty of whole grains that are as minimally processed as possible. The less processed they are, the more nutrition they retain.

Whole grains include whole-wheat bread, whole-grain cereal, whole-wheat pasta, brown rice, couscous, bulgur, barley, oats, polenta, and quinoa (a seed but considered a whole grain for our purposes).

## Olives, Olive Oil, and Other Fats

When most people think of the Mediterranean diet, olives and olive oil usually come to mind first. Most foods are cooked with healthier oils such as olive oil (the most popular), and olives are served quite often at meals throughout the day. Olive oil is the chief source of dietary fat used for most cooking, baking, and salad dressings. Extra-virgin olive oil is highest in healthy monounsaturated fats, phytonutrients, and other essential nutrients.

To transform your diet, begin to use olive oil as a main source of fat. Replace butter, margarine, and/or salad dressings with olive oil. Rather than use margarine or butter on your bread, try dipping it in extra-virgin olive oil.

In addition to olive oil, nuts, seeds, fish, and foods such as avocados provide healthier fat options. Although avocados are not native to the Mediterranean, they have become a familiar food in Mediterranean dishes.

## Beans, Nuts, Legumes, and Seeds

Beans, nuts, legumes, and seeds are all good sources of healthy fats, fiber, and protein, and they add unique flavor and texture to popular Mediterranean dishes. You can add beans and legumes to all types of dishes, and in the Mediterranean, they are often the center of the daily main meal. In addition, nuts and seeds make great snacks and are often used in desserts.

Because nuts are high in fat—although healthy fat—they can be high in calories, so eat in moderation (as in a handful of nuts daily).

## Herbs and Spices

Herbs (fresh or dried) and spices have always been used abundantly throughout the Mediterranean; however, they are a more recent addition to the Mediterranean Diet Pyramid. Herbs and spices such as oregano, rosemary, red pepper, garlic, and mint add flavor and aroma to foods and can reduce or even eliminate the need to add salt or fat when cooking. They can help bring out the natural flavor of foods, and many are rich in health-promoting antioxidants. Herbs and spices directly contribute to the exclusive identity of various Mediterranean cuisine and dishes.

# Fish and Seafood

The next step up on the Mediterranean Diet Pyramid is the fish and seafood group. It is not surprising that fish and shellfish are so popular; the Mediterranean regions are surrounded by coastlines. Fish and shellfish are sources of healthy, lean protein and heart-healthy fats in the form of omega-3 fatty acids. Fish is not just heart healthy—recent research shows that eating fish can help reduce the cognitive decline that can come with aging.

The guiding principle for this food group is to consume seafood and/or fish at least twice a week. In the Mediterranean, fish and shellfish are commonly cooked in stews or steamed rather than battered or fried. Fish cooks quickly and can make for fast and easy meals. Many varieties are available to choose from, and they all have their own distinct flavors.

All types of fish and shellfish are included in this category, but the fattier fish, such as tuna, herring, sardines, and salmon, are most popular. The fattier the fish, the healthier they are because their fat source is heart healthy. (See Chapter 15 for more information on these fat sources and their health benefits.) Shellfish such as mussels, oysters, clams, and shrimp also have similar benefits and are quite popular.

## Cheese and Yogurt

As we continue up the Mediterranean Diet Pyramid, the cheese and yogurt group is the next stop. The calcium and vitamin D found in cheese and yogurt is essential for strong bones and a healthy heart. These dairy foods are also good sources of protein.

Cheese and yogurt are eaten often in the traditional Mediterranean diet, but you do not need to limit this group to these two foods. Low-fat or fat-free milk and other dairy products are also great sources of protein, calcium, and vitamin D and can definitely fit into this food group.

For a nondairy alternative, plant-based milks such as almond, oat, or soy can provide calcium and vitamin D as well without the lactose. Many plant-based milks are not quite as high in protein as cow's milk, so be sure to check labels. It's best to opt for the unsweetened versions to avoid too much added sugar.

The guidelines of the pyramid specifically state that moderate portions should be consumed on a daily or weekly basis and recommend capping your dairy intake to no more than 2 cups per day. Low-fat and nonfat dairy products are recommended. Avoid yogurts with too much added sugar, and choose Greek yogurts for a higher protein content. For a touch of sweetness, try adding a bit of honey and/or fresh fruit.

## Poultry and Eggs

One more step up the pyramid is poultry and eggs, which are another important source of high-quality protein. However, as we move up the pyramid, the sections become smaller, signifying the need for lower consumption. The pyramid guidelines state that poultry and eggs should be eaten in moderate portions every two days or weekly.

Eggs are used commonly in cooking and baking, and it is recommended to consume no more than one yolk per day or four yolks per week as a healthy alternative to fish or meat. However, there is no limit on egg whites.

When consuming poultry, choose the white meat portions, and remove the skin to lower unhealthy saturated fat and cholesterol content.

## Meats and Sweets

Meats and sweets top the pyramid, meaning these should be consumed the least. Sweets are not all that popular in the Mediterranean and are usually consumed only in small portions. Fresh fruit and/or nuts are commonly eaten to end a meal instead of a sugar-laden dessert. Gelato and sorbet in small portions are popular and sometimes consumed a few times per week.

When the pyramid refers to meats in this section, it is essentially singling out red meats such as beef and pork. There is not much room for red meats in this diet because they can be high in saturated fat and cholesterol and, therefore, are not heart healthy. Red meat is consumed only a few times per month, with a recommendation to eat no more than 7 ounces (200g) per week of unprocessed red meat. Lean and extra-lean cuts are preferred, and you should always trim away any visible fat. Still have a craving for a burger? Try a ground turkey breast patty or salmon patty, and add a slice of avocado, a slice of tomato, and a dab of olive oil.

## Red Wine

Red wine is a part of the pyramid because it is a normal part of the Mediterranean lifestyle. It is consumed quite regularly, but moderately, with meals in the Mediterranean. Red wine has more nutritional benefits than you might realize.

Women can include one 5-ounce (140g) serving per day, and men can include one or two 5-ounce (140g) servings daily. Of course, individuals should only drink wine if they are medically able to do so and are of age. Purple grape juice, made from Concord grapes, or eating purple grapes can be a great alternative.

# Dietary Guidelines for Americans/MyPlate

In 2011, the U.S. Department of Agriculture (USDA) unveiled MyPlate as a food group symbol to help consumers make healthy food choices consistent with the Dietary Guidelines for Americans. The Dietary Guidelines for Americans provide recommendations on what to eat and drink to meet general nutrition requirements, promote good health, and help prevent disease. The guidelines are updated every 5 years by the USDA and the U.S. Department of Health and Human Services (HHS). MyPlate took the place of the Food Guide Pyramid, which was more like the Mediterranean Diet Pyramid.

The 2020–2025 Dietary Guidelines for Americans were released in December 2020. In this newest version, the Healthy Mediterranean-Style Dietary Pattern is recognized as a dietary pattern that aligns with Dietary Guidelines recommendations.

Both the Mediterranean Diet Pyramid and MyPlate emphasize choosing from healthy food groups. However, they differ in the fact that the guidelines for the Mediterranean diet is not about measuring serving sizes but rather eating whole, nutrient-dense foods.

# Comparing the Symbols

The most basic difference between MyPlate and the Mediterranean Diet Pyramid is that one focuses on common foods in the United States and the other focuses on the more common cuisine of the Mediterranean regions. In addition, how foods are grouped together and recommended differ greatly in some aspects.

## Similarities

Several similarities can be found between the two symbols and styles of eating. Both eating patterns recommend consuming a variety of fruits, vegetables, and whole grains; choosing low-fat or fat-free dairy products; choosing lean proteins; eating sweets less often; and including physical activity.

## Differences

Let's look at some general differences.

MyPlate groups lean meats; seafood/fish; and other proteins such as eggs, beans, peas, lentils, nuts, seeds, and soy products. It includes beans, peas, and lentils as part of the vegetable group as well.

The Mediterranean Diet Pyramid separates red meats, fish/seafood, and poultry and eggs into three different sections. Red meat is at the very top of the Mediterranean Diet Pyramid, next to sweets, and is recommended much less than MyPlate, with fish/seafood being emphasized more and having a more specific recommendation.

MyPlate groups dairy products in a separate group, while the Mediterranean Diet Pyramid groups dairy products like cheese and yogurt along with poultry and eggs. The Mediterranean diet does not promote milk as an element of the pyramid. MyPlate emphasizes low-fat or fat-free milk as an important part of the dairy group.

MyPlate does not symbolize fats; the Mediterranean Diet Pyramid emphasizes the use of healthy fats—specifically olive oil, which is grouped with plant foods.

MyPlate divides fruits, vegetables, and grains into separate groups. On the Mediterranean Diet Pyramid, these foods are together in a plant food group, which includes fruits, vegetables, whole grains, olive oil, beans, nuts, legumes, and seeds as one large group.

The Mediterranean Diet Pyramid was designed to illustrate proportions rather than specific amounts or serving sizes of foods, recommending only how often to eat certain foods. Detailed information on serving sizes and number of servings are not provided as they are with MyPlate and the Dietary Guidelines for Americans.

# Making Your Choice

Even though there are several differences between the USDA's MyPlate and the Mediterranean Diet Pyramid, the one common goal they both share is guiding people to a healthier eating style and a more beneficial way of life. MyPlate is based on American eating patterns with flexibility in food choices but recommended daily servings being an important objective. A person can easily choose to eat a Mediterranean-style diet by choosing foods common to that region, within the framework of the USDA's MyPlate. If you are a die-hard Mediterranean fan, utilizing the Mediterranean Diet Pyramid can be highly beneficial in helping you reach your health goals. The choice is yours—whichever method helps you reach your goals and maintain a healthier lifestyle is the right choice.

Keep in mind that a healthy and balanced diet will accommodate most foods and drinks. As long as you practice moderation and make wise choices the majority of the time, you will do well. You can enjoy a steak or a piece of birthday cake occasionally. These are all parts of a realistic lifestyle and can be part of a healthy lifestyle as well.

## In This Chapter

Oldways, the Harvard School of Public Health, and the World Health Organization first introduced the Mediterranean Diet Pyramid, along with the actual Mediterranean diet concept, in 1993. The Mediterranean Diet Pyramid is a visualization of the Mediterranean diet and is intended to represent not only recommended foods but also what is suggested on a whole as part of a healthy lifestyle. In 2008, the Mediterranean Diet Pyramid was revised to reflect a few beneficial changes. Although there are more differences than similarities in the Mediterranean Diet Pyramid and the USDA's MyPlate, both promote a healthy diet and lifestyle.

# CHAPTER 4

# How Other Diets Stack Up

Being healthy and living longer interests most people. As luck would have it, scores of different diets out are out there for those seeking help, whether it is to become healthier or shed some unwanted pounds. The problem is that there are almost *too many* choices. Countless diets say they are the best and the most effective diet, and they all have their own health and weight-loss claims, but some are safer and more effective than others.

What do the experts say about the Mediterranean diet? According to years of studies and research, the Mediterranean diet is, without doubt, a healthy way of life. Renowned medical journals, professional health organizations, and doctors from all walks of life have agreed that the Mediterranean diet has what it takes to improve health for many.

Whatever your reason for adopting a new way of eating, you should always do your homework before making such an important decision.

# The American Heart Association's Heart-Healthy Diet

When you think of a heart-healthy diet, you might assume that the American Heart Association (AHA) is expert on the topic. The AHA is a national voluntary health agency whose mission is to help people lower their risk of cardiovascular diseases and stroke and live healthier lives. Like the Mediterranean diet, the recommendations and guidelines of the AHA's heart-healthy diet are proven through years of studies and research.

## AHA Guidelines

The Mediterranean style of eating closely resembles the AHA's dietary recommendations. The biggest difference is the higher percentage of healthy fat on the Mediterranean diet. The AHA diet recommends limiting total fat to about 25 to 35 percent of your total calories and is considered a low-fat diet. The Mediterranean diet is a bit higher in fat, with about 35 to 40 percent of total calories from fat. However, even though total fat differs slightly, both diets recommend a low intake of unhealthy fats, such as saturated fats and trans fats, and a higher intake of healthy fats, including monounsaturated and polyunsaturated fats.

When it comes down to it, the AHA actually recommends the Mediterranean-style diet as a way to help you achieve its dietary recommendations. If you take a close look at the guidelines, you can determine just how similar these two diets really are.

The AHA recommends limiting the amount of saturated fat (less than 6 percent of total daily calorie intake) and trans fat (less than 1 percent of total daily calorie intake) you consume daily. The Mediterranean diet is naturally low in these unhealthy fats because it recommends limiting whole-fat dairy products, red meats, eggs, processed foods, baked goods, and fried foods. The Mediterranean diet also eliminates butter and/or margarine, both of which can be high in saturated fats, trans fats, or cholesterol.

The AHA recommends cutting back on foods and beverages with high sugar content and added sugars. The Mediterranean diet is low in added sugars. People who follow this diet eat very few sweets and instead consume more foods that are naturally sweet, such as fruit.

The AHA recommends choosing and preparing foods with little to no salt. This helps lower the risk for high blood pressure and may help manage it. The Mediterranean diet is naturally low in sodium because it includes very few processed foods. Most foods are consumed in their natural, whole forms or made from scratch. In addition, in place of salt, herbs and spices are used abundantly in Mediterranean diet cooking.

The AHA recommends keeping your calorie intake in check, and for healthy adults, it suggests aiming for at least 30 minutes of moderate-intensity physical activity at least 5 days a week to help maintain a healthy weight and develop cardiovascular fitness. One of the main foundations of the Mediterranean diet is physical activity.

The AHA recommends eating at least 25 to 30 grams of dietary fiber every day, preferably from food sources such as whole grains, fruits, vegetables, and legumes as opposed to supplements. All these plant-based foods are included in the largest part of the Mediterranean Diet Pyramid (see Chapter 3).

Just like the Mediterranean diet guidelines, the AHA recommends eating a variety of *nutrient-dense* foods from all the food groups, including vegetables, fruits, whole grains, legumes, and fat-free or low-fat dairy products.

The AHA recommends eating 3½ ounces (100g) of fish at least twice a week, much like the recommendations of the Mediterranean diet.

To learn more about the guidelines of the AHA, check out its website at heart.org.

## The DASH Diet

The DASH diet, which stands for "Dietary Approaches to Stop Hypertension," was developed by the American Heart Association. This heart-healthy diet is meant to help people manage their high blood pressure and shares many of the same characteristics as the Mediterranean diet. The diet is easy to follow, tasty, and proven effective. It focuses on consuming foods that are rich in magnesium, potassium, calcium, protein, and fiber to help manage blood pressure.

The DASH diet emphasizes many of the same foods highlighted in the Mediterranean diet, including vegetables, fruits, fat-free or low-fat dairy products (it recommends a bit more dairy than what the Mediterranean diet recommends), whole grains and other high-fiber foods, fish at least twice weekly, skinless poultry, beans, seeds, and nuts. The DASH diet plan is low in red meats and emphasizes lean meats, whereas the Mediterranean diet is more restrictive when it comes to meat in general and focuses mainly on seafood. The DASH diet also severely limits foods like chocolate and wine, and the Mediterranean diet encourages those foods, just in moderation.

As with the AHA guidelines, the DASH diet limits fat intake a bit more than the Mediterranean diet. The Mediterranean diet focuses more on choosing fats wisely rather than limiting them.

Both diets are low in saturated fat, sodium, and added sugars and offer numerous health benefits, including managing blood pressure, improving insulin function, preventing blood clots, and improving heart health. Both are dietary approaches that can help support good health, just in slightly different ways.

All in all, the dietary guidelines of the AHA and the DASH diet are quite similar to the Mediterranean eating style. All are proven to be heart healthy and to decrease risk for some chronic diseases. Make room for the Mediterranean diet though, because the AHA's diets aren't the only reliable diets in town.

# The Atkins Diet

The Atkins diet is a well-known low-carbohydrate, high-protein diet. Developed by Dr. Robert Atkins, this diet promises that you will not only lose weight but that you also will be on the road to better heart health and memory function (along with other health benefits).

The Atkins diet works on the concept that people have gone "carb crazy," and that is the sole reason for the obesity problem. The diet works on the premise that consuming too many carbohydrates—especially sugar, white flour, and other refined carbs—increases insulin levels. This can lead to blood sugar imbalances, causing weight gain and other cardiovascular problems. The theory behind the weight loss is that by eating more protein (and there is no cap on how much protein you eat) and fat and fewer carbohydrates, the body will go into ketosis and turn to fat for fuel when its glucose stores from carbohydrates are depleted.

The Atkins diet revolves around four phases, which don't focus on calorie counting and/ or portion control but do require carb tracking. The diet drastically restricts carbohydrates, especially in the first phase. (Carbohydrates are reintroduced in later stages of the diet.) To ensure enough calories to keep your body functioning and to make up for the lack of calories from carbohydrates, protein and fat consumption are drastically increased.

Even though refined starches such as white bread, sugar, and white flours are limited, so are fruits, vegetables, whole grains, beans, and other nutritious foods that contain carbohydrates.

The plan allows for protein foods that are high in saturated fats, such as red meats, regular cheese, cream, butter, and more. It advocates eating a variety of fats but in limited amounts, from unhealthy saturated fats to healthy omega-3 fatty acids. On this diet, you can eat fish and olive oil, but you also can indulge in bacon, mayonnaise, and steak with béarnaise sauce.

This diet could not be more contradictory to the Mediterranean diet. The Atkins diet is about restriction, while the Mediterranean diet is focused on making good choices and healthy lifestyle changes. Many health experts question the Atkins diet, and it remains a controversial way of eating.

These types of diets are rarely successful in the long term for keeping the weight off, and they can have negative impacts on your health. Short-term effects can include headaches, muscle cramping, bad breath, diarrhea, constipation, and general fatigue. Long-term effects can include regaining weight, heart disease, certain cancers, kidney problems, diabetes complications, and osteoporosis. The Atkins theory remains unproven, unlike the proven benefits of the Mediterranean diet.

# The South Beach Diet

The South Beach diet was created by cardiologist Arthur Agatston, MD. Consisting of three phases, this is another type of low-carbohydrate eating regime that touts good heart health as a result.

Unlike the Atkins diet, the South Beach diet emphasizes foods that are somewhat more heart healthy by cutting out "bad" carbs, including "good" carbs, and emphasizing healthy fats. This diet is also based on the theory that people have gone "carb crazy"; however, the diet assumes that the main culprits are not *all* carbs but highly processed simple carbohydrates such as white flour and added sugars found in breads, snacks, sweets, and baked goods. The theory here is that consuming too many of these types of simple carbohydrates causes insulin resistance, which causes the body to store more fat, resulting in weight gain. The diet claims that the craving for carbs disappears once you go through phase 1 for two weeks. In addition, the diet explains that cutting out these processed, simple carbohydrates lowers one's triglyceride and cholesterol levels, resulting in better heart health.

Carbohydrates are basically prohibited during the initial restrictive phase of the diet and are then slowly reintroduced after two weeks. The diet stresses lean meats such as chicken, turkey, and fish as well as other protein sources, including nuts, eggs, and low-fat cheese. After carbohydrates are reintroduced, you can have fruits, vegetables, whole grains, legumes, and others; however, you must limit consumption to keep carbohydrates at or below a specified amount.

In addition, the diet relies heavily on the glycemic index (GI), putting a limit on some of the foods that are allowed. The glycemic index is a numerical scale that indicates how fast a single food raises blood glucose (blood sugar). The higher the GI, the quicker it will affect blood sugar. Foods that are higher in fiber and/or less processed tend to have a lower GI. There is much controversy over the GI because it is specific to individual foods. However, some factors can change the GI of foods, such as whether they are eaten in a certain combination of foods, how foods are cooked, and the protein and fat content. Just because a food has a high GI doesn't mean it isn't healthy—in fact, many fruits have a high GI.

The South Beach diet is similar to the Mediterranean diet in that both suggest reducing consumption of unhealthy saturated fats and promote consumption of healthy monounsaturated fats. They both emphasize "good" carbohydrates—those that are complex and less refined (such as whole grains). However, depending on which of the three phases of the South Beach diet you're in, the two diets can differ considerably. The Mediterranean diet is high in fiber and counts on healthy, carbohydrate-containing foods as its foundation, but the first phase of the South Beach diet is devoid of most of these foods. There are numerous reasons that don't make this diet as much of a lifestyle change or a way of eating for life as the Mediterranean diet.

# The Ornish Diet

The Ornish diet, developed by renowned doctor Dean Ornish, is yet another alternative lifestyle approach that may help prevent, or even reverse, heart disease. Experts believe it also aids in weight loss, establishes overall good health, lowers cancer risk, and can make diabetes and hypertension more manageable. The advice in this program is supported by three decades of research.

The Ornish diet not only focuses on food intake but also on other important issues such as stress reduction, exercise, and social support. Much like the Mediterranean diet, it focuses less on counting calories and more on choosing foods wisely.

Like the Mediterranean diet, the Ornish diet emphasizes complex carbohydrates such as fruits, vegetables, whole grains, and legumes as well as fat-free dairy products, egg whites, soy products, and some fish. Unlike the Mediterranean diet, it excludes all meat (any type), avocados, nuts, seeds, and any oil-containing food—basically nothing with fat. This diet plan is a low-fat lacto-ovo-vegetarian diet that focuses on consuming very little cholesterol or fat of any kind. Sugar and sodium are consumed very little, alcohol is prohibited, and one daily serving of soy is highly recommended. Ornish also recommends taking supplements of omega-3 fatty acids rather than getting them from foods. If you are trying to prevent heart disease, the diet affords more discretion; however, if you are trying to reverse heart disease, it takes an even more restrictive approach.

One of the biggest differences between this and the Mediterranean diet is that the Ornish diet is extremely low in fat. This diet recommends that no more than 10 percent of calories come from fat, while the Mediterranean diet recommends a moderate fat intake of 35 to 40 percent. You can't eat much good fat (such as olive oil) on the Ornish diet if you want to stick to only 10 percent of calories from fat.

Critics say the Ornish diet is difficult to follow and maintain due to its restrictive nature. It is said to be a healthful diet if you can live with it. The Mediterranean diet requires a less-drastic change in eating style to reap the health benefits.

# The Zone Diet

The Zone diet was developed by Dr. Barry Sears, a biochemist. The theory behind his diet again revolves around limited consumption of carbohydrates. His belief is that when you eat too many carbohydrates, a hormonal message is sent via insulin, telling the body to store fat. Dr. Sears claims that if you moderate your intake of carbohydrates and balance them with an equal proportion of fat and protein, you will enter the "zone" where you will burn fat more efficiently and revamp your metabolism, helping you lose weight. In addition, you will reduce stress, create mental clarity, improve your energy levels, and have better overall health. The Zone diet also claims that using food in this way will aid in the prevention and management of heart disease and diabetes.

What does it mean to be in the "zone"? According to Dr. Sears, it means that your meals and snacks are specifically divided:

- 40 percent of calories from carbohydrates

- 30 percent of calories from protein

- 30 percent of calories from fat

These proportions are the key to the entire diet. In addition, it's essential that meals and snacks are precisely timed: eating within 1 hour of waking up and then every 4 to 6 hours after a meal or 2 hours after a snack, even if you are not hungry. If you work the ratios and the timing the right way, the diet claims you will not be hungry, and at this point you are in the zone. Calories count in this diet plan: meals should not exceed 500 calories, and snacks should be no more than 100 calories.

The Zone diet may specify certain food choices, but it does not leave out any food groups. Carbohydrates come mostly from fresh fruits, fresh vegetables (ones low in starch), beans, lentils, and whole grains, and protein sources include lean meats. However, the diet specifies which carbs you can and cannot eat according to their glycemic index, whether they are healthy carbs or not. Recommended fats include nuts, avocados, olive oil, and canola oil. The diet is fairly low in saturated fats. Foods high in sugar and sodium, or foods that are highly processed, are discouraged. The diet encourages drinking water and getting regular exercise. Overall, the diet is much higher in protein and fat than traditional diets.

The Zone diet has received mixed reviews from nutrition experts. Some agree it includes all the foods necessary for a healthy diet, yet others question the diet's scientific proof of its claimed health benefits. Still others feel it is just another fad diet. The American Heart Association classifies it as a high-protein diet and not optimal for weight loss.

There are some definite similarities between the Zone diet and the Mediterranean diet: both have some common food choices, are well-balanced, and encourage physical activity. In addition, both are a bit higher in fat than traditional diets.

There are more differences than similarities, however. The Zone diet can be complicated to understand and follow because it takes some work to get your fat, protein, and carbohydrate ratios exactly balanced at each meal and snack. This makes you wonder how easily someone could live with this type of diet long term. The Zone diet also limits carbohydrates in quantity and through the glycemic index, which differs from the Mediterranean diet, which is based on these all-important plant foods.

# The Sonoma Diet

Inspired by the Mediterranean diet, the Sonoma diet was developed by dietitian Connie Guttersen and combines the major principles of the Mediterranean diet with a typical weight-loss diet. It emphasizes eating a generous variety of healthy foods that protect your heart and boost your health. It is low in saturated fats, high in fiber, and high in heart-healthy fats.

The Sonoma diet was designed to be simple and has very little counting or measuring to complicate matters. Portion control is emphasized using the size of your plates and bowls. The diet includes phases, with the first phase being extremely restrictive. However, the diet becomes much less restrictive as you move on to the second and third phases. This diet does include foods to avoid as well as power foods to consume.

Because this diet was designed with the Mediterranean diet in mind, there are some strong similarities, mostly with respect to the types of foods included. Like the Mediterranean diet, the Sonoma diet emphasizes eating slowly, savoring your meals, and having a glass of wine with dinner (after your initial phase, that is). However, because it is also a weight-loss diet, it has an extensive forbidden food list and very little flexibility. Even though it may seem to mimic the Mediterranean food choices, the initial phase is low in carbs and doesn't focus on as many healthy plant foods as the Mediterranean diet does.

The biggest difference between the Mediterranean diet and the Sonoma diet is that the goal of the Sonoma diet is to lose weight, while the Mediterranean diet is more of a lifestyle change and everyday way of eating. That being said, it doesn't mean you can't lose weight by simply following the Mediterranean diet.

# How to Lose Weight on the Mediterranean Diet

The diets discussed in this chapter have all been touted to improve heart health, although many of them are better known for their effects on weight loss. The Mediterranean diet is known first for its health benefits—especially heart health—but it also can have a positive impact on your weight. There is really no need to follow structured diets or fad diets; these are not your only means to lose weight. The Mediterranean diet certainly proves that permanent weight loss is a direct result of lifestyle change—and that is what this eating style is all about.

Every year people commit to new diet plans and then abandon them just as quickly because they are too restrictive with food choices and/or calories. Many have complex phases or steps to follow and are too complicated to fit into everyday life. None of these describe the Mediterranean diet. It is full of wonderfully tasty and healthy foods and does not restrict you from enjoying what you like. You don't start and end your day feeling hungry and deprived. So why not use this healthy diet to your advantage?

Losing weight isn't only about the foods you choose—there is so much more to consider. Here are some tips to make the Mediterranean diet work for your waistline as well as your health.

First, understand your true reasons, your "why"s for wanting to lose weight and improve your health. Knowing what will motivate you and keep you committed to your goals is what will ultimately make you successful. Consider your realistic short- and long-term goals. Short-term goals are essential to keep you going and reach your long-term goals. Goals need to be specific and measurable. Write them down so you know exactly what you are working toward.

Plan each day so you eat three balanced meals with healthy snacks in between. Familiarize yourself with the guidelines of the Mediterranean Diet Pyramid (see Chapter 3) so you can create a well-balanced menu. This will keep you from feeling hungry during the day and help you avoid eating too much at meals or snacks. Don't skip meals!

Plan your week's meals in advance so you have control over what is in the house and what you eat daily. When you've made your plan for the week, put it in writing in the form of your grocery list.

Keep a food journal until you become comfortable with your new way of eating. Write down everything you eat, no matter how big or small. This is for your eyes only, so don't hold back. Review your journal every few days to check your progress and/or problem areas. A food journal can help you stick with the commitments you have made.

Spend more time preparing your own meals so you know exactly what is going into the foods you are eating. The Mediterranean diet is all about eating more whole foods and fewer processed foods, so it's time to try out your culinary skills. Invest in some good cookbooks, look for recipes online, or share recipes with friends. And see Part 4 for some wonderful Mediterranean diet recipes!

Read food labels at the grocery store to choose foods that best fit into the guidelines of the Mediterranean diet. This also will give you a good idea of portion sizes and calorie intake.

Don't avoid your favorite foods. Deprivation can cause cravings that you just can't let go of. Eat the foods you love from time to time in moderation.

Pay attention to portion sizes, and only put small portions of food on your plate so you are not tempted to overeat. Use a smaller plate if needed. Portion your food before bringing your plate to the table, and refrain from eating while doing other tasks like watching television or working at the computer. Leave distractions behind when you eat.

Do as the people of the Mediterranean do: slow down your meals, and enjoy your foods. Eating too quickly can cause you to eat too much before you even realize you're full. Eating slower can result in eating less and enjoying more.

Think about the foods you put in your mouth each and every time you eat. Make a commitment to yourself to be accountable for what you eat and the way you live your life.

Experiment with new foods, and fill your plate with a rainbow of colors. The more colors you have on your plate, the more nutrition you have in your meal. The Mediterranean diet is full of a variety of tasty foods—use that to your advantage.

Follow the guidelines of the Mediterranean diet for all foods but especially for fruits, vegetables, whole grains, beans, and lentils. These foods are packed with fiber, which can be very filling and help you eat fewer calories.

Drink plenty of water throughout each day. Staying properly hydrated is essential to digestion and the fat-burning process. It also can help you with portion control at meals and/or with snacks.

Be physically active each and every day. Obesity can be a direct result of an imbalance between the calories you take in and the calories you burn. The more active you are, the more calories you burn. Something as basic as walking can be a great start.

These simple tips and changes can help you improve your health and reduce your waistline using the Mediterranean diet. Remember, it is all about lifestyle changes that you can live with. Losing weight slowly over time is more manageable and, experts agree, more permanent. Make changes to both your eating style and your lifestyle a little at a time—and most importantly, stick with your commitment to become a healthier person.

## In This Chapter

Experts agree that the Mediterranean diet is indeed a preferred way of life and favorably compares with the American Heart Association's recommendations and the DASH diet. The Mediterranean diet comes out on top compared to many of the diets that claim to be heart healthy. You can lose weight on the Mediterranean diet with the right motivation, commitment, and helpful tips.

# PART 2

# BASICS OF THE MEDITERRANEAN DIET

Now that you have learned about all the benefits of the Mediterranean diet in Part 1, in this part, we teach you how to fit this way of eating into your daily life.

The chapters in Part 2 take a closer look at the essential foods and food groups from the Mediterranean Diet Pyramid. We review all the foods and beverages you need to embrace on this diet, from extra-virgin olive oil, to fruits and vegetables, to whole grains—focusing on how, what, and why.

# CHAPTER 5

# Transitioning Your Diet

Moving from your current diet to the Mediterranean style of eating is a smart way to begin taking control of your health. Some aspects of the transition might be easier than others, but the key is to do it slowly. Don't be determined to change everything all at once. Make changes to your diet and lifestyle habits one step at a time, and before you know it, you will be fully living the Mediterranean way of life and reaping all the health benefits.

# Foods to Reduce and Foods to Add

As always, moderation is the key. Begin to reduce or replace the foods in your diet gradually. If your current diet needs a lot of help, the last thing you want to do is jump in with both feet. Instead, start slowly and progress steadily by gradually reducing the foods you don't need and replacing them with the foods you do.

The Mediterranean diet is not one of deprivation but rather one that focuses on eating a variety of healthy foods, so adding foods should be painless.

## Foods to Reduce

Start by reducing portions of the foods in your diet that are not part of the Mediterranean diet. These include red meats, whole-fat dairy products, fried foods, fast foods, processed foods, and foods with added sugar. The goal is to eat as little of them as possible, not necessarily eliminate them altogether. Remember to be realistic with yourself.

Replace portions of your diet with food from the Mediterranean. For example, instead of using ground beef, replace half or all with ground turkey breast.

Trade your full-fat dairy products for low-fat versions—or better yet, opt for fat-free products. Choose low-fat or nonfat yogurt and cheeses. Not quite at the point of drinking fat-free milk? Start by mixing equal amounts of fat-free and 2 percent milk. Or choose a plant-based milk such as almond or oat milk.

Prepare to eat fewer fatty foods such as animal products and especially red meat. This is eaten very rarely in the Mediterranean diet and is one of the first foods you need to begin reducing to make a successful transition. Start by reducing red meat to once or twice a week, and transition down to a few times a month.

Think fresh, and begin to reduce your consumption of processed foods. There is no room in the Mediterranean diet for white sugar, white flour, junk foods, and other foods that come neatly packaged and processed. Shopping the outside aisles of the grocery store will ensure you are choosing fresher foods.

Reduce your use of butter and margarine when cooking and preparing foods until you have completely replaced them with healthier fats such as olive oil.

## Foods to Add

Load up on fresh fruits and vegetables. Cook with them by trying out new recipes. Your daily diet should be packed with these foods because plant-based foods make up a good proportion of the Mediterranean diet.

Start to think of grains in a different way. Begin steering away from the refined grains you might be used to such as white breads, white rice, and regular pasta, and replace them with whole grains such as oatmeal, whole-grain bread, brown rice, whole-wheat pasta, bulgur, and couscous.

Use olive oil for cooking, as a replacement for butter or margarine on breads and vegetables, and as a salad dressing. Olive oil is the backbone of the Mediterranean diet.

Rely on leaner protein choices, such as fish and skinless white meat chicken or turkey, to replace red meat. Include fish at least a few times weekly in your meal plans.

Add a few meatless meals to your weekly meal plans. This will help you cut back on red meat and other saturated fats. Meat isn't the only way to get the protein you need. Try basing some meals on beans, legumes, lentils, low-fat cheeses, and nuts.

# Changing Your Approach

Adopting a new lifestyle means becoming more mindful about the foods you consume and the habits in which you engage. You need to move away from old habits and adopt new ones, and that can take some work and commitment. Think as the people of the Mediterranean do, and approach what you would normally eat with a new attitude.

Changing your approach to food isn't as hard as you might think. Take pasta, for example. In the typical Western diet, we might cover pasta with meaty spaghetti sauce or a creamy Alfredo sauce, both loaded with unhealthy fats. To make it Mediterranean, you simply could use whole-grain pasta and toss it with fresh-cut tomatoes, garlic, fresh basil, and olive oil. You could even throw in some fresh spinach, mushrooms, and peas to make it a filling, healthy meal.

Need another example? Sandwiches are not as popular in the Mediterranean as they are in the United States. So how do you update your sandwich to give it some Mediterranean flair? Instead of two pieces of white bread filled with high-fat deli meat, full-fat cheese, and mayonnaise, consider a vegetable sandwich: a whole-wheat pita stuffed with red peppers, eggplant, tomatoes, mushrooms, and/or zucchini topped with low-fat cheese and a touch of olive oil. If you like, add a few chunks of white meat chicken or broiled fish. You can even add a bit of brown rice. You've just changed your approach to the all-American sandwich.

It takes creativity to retrain your thought process and find a way to fit the foods you normally eat into the Mediterranean diet. That goes not only for meals and snacks but also for lifestyle habits like physical activity and drinking alcohol.

# Essential Mediterranean Diet Foods List

A huge variety of foods are included on the Mediterranean diet—it is not a diet of deprivation but one of healthy choices, remember. These might be foods you have never tried or foods you already incorporate into your current diet. If your pantry and kitchen are stocked with the foods you need to follow the Mediterranean diet, it will be easier for you to plan and prepare meals on a regular basis.

**Fruit**
Apricots
Avocados
Blueberries
Cherries
Dates
Dried fruit
Figs
Melons (cantaloupe, honeydew)
Olives
Pomegranates
Strawberries

**Vegetables**
Arugula
Artichoke hearts
Bell peppers (red, green)
Broccoli
Cabbage
Celery (celery leaves, celery root)
Dandelion greens
Eggplant
Grape leaves

**Vegetables (continued)**
Mushrooms
Mustard greens
Onions
Pepperoncinis
Spinach
Swiss chard
Tomatoes (fresh, canned, sun-dried)
Zucchini

**Breads, Grains, and Pastas**
Brown rice
Couscous
Oatmeal
Phyllo dough
Polenta
Quinoa
Rye bread
Wheat berries
Whole-grain bread
Whole-grain pita bread
Whole-wheat pasta (any kind)

**Flours**
Barley flour
Buckwheat flour
Bulgur flour
Farro (spelt) flour
Unbleached all-purpose flour
Whole-wheat flour

**Oils**
Avocado oil
Canola oil
Grapeseed oil
Olive oil (extra-virgin)

**Legumes**
Black beans
Black-eyed peas
Borlotti beans (cranberry beans)
Cannellini beans (white kidney beans)
Chickpeas (garbanzo beans)
Fava beans (broad beans)
Hummus
Lentils
Pinto beans
Split peas

**Nuts and Seeds**
Almonds
Cashews
Chestnuts
Flaxseeds
Hazelnuts
Peanuts
Pine nuts
Pistachios
Sesame seeds
Sunflower seeds
Walnuts

**Herbs, Spices, and Seasonings**
Balsamic vinegar
Basil
Garlic
Honey
Mint
Oregano
Paprika
Rosemary
Tahini
Tomato paste
Wine vinegar

**Fish and Seafood**
Clams
Crab
Halibut
Octopus
Salmon
Sardines
Shrimp
Squid
Swordfish
Tilapia
Tuna

**Dairy Products**
Asiago cheese
Cottage cheese (low-fat)
Cow's milk (fat-free or low-fat)
Unsweetened almond milk
Feta cheese
Goat cheese
Greek yogurt (plain or fruited, fat-free
  or low-fat)
Mozzarella cheese
Provolone cheese
Ricotta cheese

**Meat/Protein**

Chicken (white meat, skinless)

Eggs

Lamb

Turkey (white meat, skinless and/or
  breast, ground)

Veal

**Miscellaneous**

Eggs

Hummus

Phyllo dough

# What About Sweets?

The majority of us have a sweet tooth, so transitioning to the Mediterranean diet, where sweets are eaten only a few times a week and in small amounts, can be an immense change. Desserts are more of an afterthought as opposed to an expected ending to a meal in the Mediterranean lifestyle. Sometimes sweets accompany afternoon tea or coffee.

Remember that the Mediterranean diet is not about deprivation though. It is more realistic to consume sweets on occasion and in moderation instead of focusing on completely eliminating them.

In the Mediterranean, what follows a meal leans more toward fresh fruits and nuts instead of sweets with added sugar and fat. A fruity dessert makes the perfect end to a healthy meal, and fruit can be fresh, baked, stewed, or cooked into jams or tarts. (Check out the Mediterranean-style dessert recipes in Chapter 23.)

The Mediterranean diet embraces naturally sweetened foods rather than using added sugar. Honey, for example, is commonly used as a natural sweetener in many Mediterranean meals and desserts. It's widely used to sweeten plain yogurt and in place of sugar in coffee or tea. It makes a nice addition to toast and breads, and you can even drizzle it on your salad along with a little olive oil, lemon, and vinegar.

In addition to being a natural sweetener, honey also can be beneficial to your health and even help boost your immune system. It contains vitamins, minerals, antioxidants, enzymes, and even a few amino acids (the building blocks of protein). Honey's antibacterial and antioxidant properties can help aid in digestion, help keep you healthy, and fight disease. A wide assortment of floral honey varieties are made—23 to be exact—all with unique flavors. Honey contains about 64 calories per tablespoon, while refined table sugar contains about 46 calories per tablespoon. However, because honey is much sweeter than table sugar, you can use much less of it. As a result, you may consume fewer calories using honey versus table sugar. Leave it to the people of the Mediterranean to find a way to enjoy something sweet that is also good for you.

# Reading Food Labels

The Mediterranean diet is all about choosing healthier foods. We all can use a little help when it comes to choosing healthier foods, and that's where the Nutrition Facts label on food packaging can help.

People of the Mediterranean consume mostly fresh foods—in that area of the world, it is much more realistic—but the rest of us might need a little extra help weeding through the foods available at local supermarkets. Food labels help you decipher the nutrition facts about the foods you buy. Learning and understanding the differences in the types of fats and knowing how to interpret other parts of the food label can help you become a much smarter food shopper and more equipped to choose foods that fit into the Mediterranean way of life.

## The Nutrition Facts Label

You've probably seen a Nutrition Facts label on packaged foods, full of detailed nutrition information. This panel includes the nutrients that people often consume in excess—like total fat, saturated fat, trans fat, cholesterol, sodium, and added sugar—that should be limited because they may cause an increased risk for chronic diseases.

Other nutrients—such as dietary fiber, vitamin D, calcium, iron, and potassium—are also listed because they often come up short in the typical diet, and eating enough of these nutrients can help improve health and lower risk for some chronic health conditions.

Total carbohydrate, total sugars (including both naturally occurring and added sugars), and protein are also listed.

Some manufacturers may include additional nutrients, but all the above are required. In fact, the information on the panel is so important, it is required by the U.S. Food and Drug Administration (FDA) and the U.S. Department of Agriculture (USDA) to be on most packaged foods.

Food labels also include other helpful information, including an ingredient list and optional health and nutrient content claims. All this information is there to help consumers make healthier food choices.

When reading the Nutrition Facts label, start at the top. The first listings are the servings per container and serving size. All the information on the label pertains to that all-important serving size. Serving sizes on packaged foods are standardized to make it easier for consumers to compare nutritional facts on similar foods. For example, the standard serving size on salad dressing, no matter what the brand, is 2 tablespoons. That makes it easier to pick up two bottles of dressing and carefully compare their nutritional content.

Servings per container also are listed at the top of the panel. Be careful not to fall into the trap of assuming there is only one serving in a package. All the information on the label pertains to *one* serving—so if it states there are two servings per package, you need to double all the numbers if you plan to eat the whole thing.

As a general guide to calories:

- 40 to 99 calories per single serving of a food is considered low.

- 100 to 399 calories is considered moderate.

- 400 calories or more is considered high.

This universal guide provides a general reference and is based on an average 2,000-calorie diet. Eating too many high-calorie foods on a daily basis can cause you to take in more calories than your body needs, which can be directly linked to obesity-related health problems. By reading the food label and being aware of calories, you can balance your daily calories and better manage your weight.

## Key Nutrients

All nutrients listed on the Nutrition Facts label are important; however, when it comes to the Mediterranean diet, some are more crucial than others at helping you to stick with your new way of eating.

**Fat:** Look at not only total fat, but also what makes up that fat. Is it mostly saturated fats and trans fats, or is it mostly healthy fats of the Mediterranean diet, such as monounsaturated fat? The food label must list total fat, saturated fat, and trans fat.

**Sodium:** Check the sodium content on food labels, and choose the ones lowest in sodium. The majority of sodium we consume comes from processed foods. The Mediterranean diet is naturally low in sodium.

**Fiber:** Not only do you get this essential nutrient from fruits and vegetables but also in whole grains like breads, beans, rice, cereals, and pasta. Check the food label for the amount of fiber in the product, and choose ones that contain the most.

**Sugar:** The Mediterranean diet is naturally low in sugar. Check food labels for the amount of added sugar in the products you are purchasing.

Let's not forget the ingredient list, which can clue you in to other nutritional dilemmas. Ingredient lists are required on food labels for any food that contains more than one ingredient. Ingredient lists must be listed in descending order by weight. If you take a look at a cereal box, for example, and sugar is the first ingredient listed, that is a clue that the product contains mostly sugar.

Numbers aren't always what they seem, however. For instance, if a food has less than 0.5 grams of trans fat per serving, it can be listed as 0 grams on the Nutrition Facts label, but hydrogenated or partially hydrogenated oils will still be listed in the ingredient list. This will clue you in to whether a food contains trans fat, an unhealthy, artery-clogging fat. Although 0.5 grams of trans fat seems small, you could exceed recommended amounts if you eat multiple servings of that food.

## Percent Daily Value

Not sure if a serving of food has a little or a lot of a particular nutrient? That is where the percent Daily Value (%DV) comes in. You will find this information on the right side of the label for most of the nutrients.

This percentage, calculated for you on the label, is an average of how a single serving of a particular food meets the daily requirements for each nutrient, based on a 2,000-calorie diet. It is important to remember that %DV refers to what you need for the entire day, not in a single meal or snack. Depending on your individual calorie needs, you may need more or less than 2,000 calories per day. So for some nutrients, you may need more or less than what is listed as 100 percent of the DV. The %DV will provide you with a frame of reference to decide whether or not the food will provide an appropriate amount of a specific nutrient, and it can help you determine if a serving of food is high or low in a specific nutrient.

As a general guide to %DV:

- 5% or less DV is low. Aim for this amount for all nutrients that you want to limit in your diet.

- 10% to 19%DV is moderate. This indicates that the food is a good source of the nutrients you want to consume in greater amounts.

- 20% or more DV is high. This indicates that the food is an excellent source of nutrients you want to consume in greater amounts.

Trans fats, protein, and total sugars do not require %DV. Trans fats do not yet have sufficient data to establish a Daily Value. Protein only needs a %DV if the food claims to be high in protein or if it's to be used for children under 4 years old because protein is not indicated as a health concern. Total sugars have no %DV because no recommendations have been made for the total amount you should eat in a day.

There are plenty of good reasons to use the Nutrition Facts label. If you plan to follow a Mediterranean diet, the information it provides can be very helpful in choosing the right foods. Reading the label can take some practice, but once you master it, it can come in very handy. Be sure to scan the entire label and look at the whole food as opposed to only looking for one nutrient. For example, a food can be low in fat but not hold any other nutritional value, or it can be fat-free but loaded with sugar and/or sodium.

## Understanding Health and Nutrient Content Claims

Health and nutrient content claims also can appear on a food label. Both types of claims are strictly defined and regulated by the FDA and can help you easily find foods that meet your specific nutrition goals.

Nutrient content claims such as "low fat" or "high fiber" can make it easy to find foods that will help you reach your goals. When following the Mediterranean diet, you might look for claims that deal with fat, fiber, sodium, sugar, and cholesterol. These nutrient content claims usually show up on the front of the food's label or package for quick information. They pertain to a single serving and are an optional part of the label. An example might be the label term *free,* as in "fat free," "calorie free," or "sodium free." In these examples, *free* means the amount of fat, calories, or sodium in one serving of the food is so small that it probably won't have an effect on health. There are also regulated definitions for *low, reduced, high, good source, more, light, healthy,* and, on meat, *lean* and *extra lean.*

Just because a food is labeled "cholesterol free," however, doesn't necessarily mean it is healthy and will fit into the Mediterranean diet. Some foods contain hydrogenated or partially hydrogenated oils, which are trans fats. The same goes for foods labeled "sodium free," which could contain high amounts of sugar and, therefore, empty calories. Always check the Nutrition Facts label to get the whole story—even if a claim is included on the packaging.

Health claims link a food product or dietary supplement with a decreased risk for some chronic diseases and/or health related conditions. As with nutrient content claims, health claims are printed on the front of a food's label or packaging. These claims are optional and are reviewed and authorized by the FDA. Only certain health claims have been approved on foods, and these claims are supported by strong scientific evidence. Some of the health claims that might be of particular interest for the Mediterranean diet include the following:

- To make health claims about sodium and reducing the risk for high blood pressure, a food must meet requirements of a "low-sodium" food.

- To make health claims about dietary fat and risk of cancer, a food must meet requirements for a "low-fat" food. Fish and game meats may meet the requirements for "extra lean."

- To make health claims about reducing the risk for coronary heart disease, a food must meet the requirements of a "low-fat," "low-saturated-fat," and "low-cholesterol" food.

- To make health claims about a food that contains a fruit, vegetable, or grain product that offers a reduced risk of cancer, a food must meet the requirements for a "good source of fiber" and for a "low-fat" food.

- To make health claims about a food that contains a fruit, vegetable, or grain product that contains fiber, particularly soluble fiber, and lowers the risk of coronary heart disease, a food must meet the requirements for a "low-fat," "low-saturated-fat," and "low-cholesterol" food; have at least 0.6 grams of soluble fiber (without fortification) per serving; and list soluble fiber on the label.

- To make health claims about a food being low in fat and high in fruits and vegetables reducing the risk of cancer, a food must contain a fruit or vegetable, meet requirements for a "low-fat" food, and meet the requirements for a "good source" (without fortification) of at least one of the following: vitamin A, vitamin C, or dietary fiber.

Look for foods with these health claims, and you are bound to find a food that will fit well into your Mediterranean eating plan.

# The Mediterranean Foods Alliance

The Mediterranean Foods Alliance (MFA) was created in 2005 by the Oldways Preservation and Exchange Trust to help companies build their brands and businesses around the Mediterranean lifestyle. MFA found that even though people had heard about the amazing benefits of the Mediterranean diet and wanted to eat in the Mediterranean style, they were not always sure how to incorporate the diet into their everyday lives—or into their grocery store shopping carts. Members of the MFA help develop and publish Mediterranean diet educational resources that allow people to make healthy changes in their daily diets. The MFA also reaches out to the media to help increase the visibility of the Mediterranean diet across the United States.

The MFA is meant to be a resource for consumers, chefs, retailers, health professionals, and journalists—or anyone who wants to better understand and incorporate the Mediterranean diet.

Through membership in the MFA, companies support the work of educating consumers and health-care professionals about the benefits of the Mediterranean Diet. When a company becomes a member of the MFA, benefits are designed to provide the company and its product(s) greater visibility among health-conscious consumers and health-care professionals of all types. MFA helps them align their brand with the Mediterranean diet, and companies that become a member of MFA are offered, by Oldways, an optional small Mediterranean Diet Pyramid image to use on their product packaging.

## In This Chapter

To begin the gradual transition to a Mediterranean way of eating, you need to become familiar with foods you need to start adding and reducing. Stocking your kitchen and beginning to change the way you look at your food choices and meals are great ways to start. When food shopping, reviewing the Nutrition Facts label and any health and nutrition claims on food packages can help you make better food choices for a healthy diet.

# CHAPTER 6

# Olive Oil

Olive oil has been around for centuries, yet experts are still discovering new health benefits and ways to use it. Olive oil is the only oil that can be used as is, freshly pressed and minimally processed from the olive itself. Best of all, olive oil is free of cholesterol, sodium, trans fat, and sugar and is a rich and healthy source of monounsaturated fats and other essential nutrients, including antioxidants and phytonutrients.

# The History and Production of Olive Oil

Olive oil comes from olives, which are actually a fruit—hence the reason olive oil is put in the plant group of the Mediterranean Diet Pyramid.

There is a history of more than 6,000 years of olive tree cultivation in the Mediterranean region. At one time, the oil from olives was used not only for food but also for beauty treatments, fuel for oil lamps, medicinal purposes, and even soap-making. Currently, olive oil continues to grow in popularity and usage—it has become big business because its health benefits are well documented. Olive oil plays a part not only in Mediterranean cuisine but also in cuisines all over the world, including the Western culture of today.

Turning olives into oil is a delicate process. The oil is obtained by pressing and centrifuging the crushed olives. However, there are different techniques for the pressing, or extraction, process, and each individual grower has their own unique method. The way in which the olives are picked, shipped, handled, and pressed all play a role in the ultimate quality and grade of the oil.

You might find extraction methods described on olive oil labels. Cold extraction processes retain more nutrients as well as the color, flavor, and aroma of the olives. Heat extraction processes can take a toll on delicate olives and destroy much of the fragile nutrients with just about all the color, flavor, and aroma.

Most of the worldwide supply of olive oil is produced from olives grown in Greece, Spain, and Italy. Spain supplies about 45 percent of the world's olives. Spanish oil is usually golden yellow with a fruity, nutty flavor. Italian olive oil is often dark green with an herbal aroma. Italy is responsible for about 20 percent of the world's olives. Greek olive oil is generally highly flavored and aromatic. Greece grows about 13 percent of the world's olive supply.

Other areas, including California, Australia, and France, have begun producing olive oil as well. Olive oil from France and California tends to be milder in flavor and lighter in color. Australian olive oil, mostly exported to Asia and Europe, can vary a great deal in flavor, depending on where the olives were grown and whether the oil was produced from olives from a single region or a blend of olives from several regions. If you try a particular brand and don't like the flavor, try another until you find the one that suits your taste.

# Olive Oil and the Mediterranean Diet

Olive oil is essentially the backbone of the Mediterranean diet, at least partly due to the simple fact that olive trees are abundant in the Mediterranean region. With all its amazing health benefits, olive oil is the principal fat source in the Mediterranean diet and a daily staple in many Mediterranean homes, complementing the traditional flavors and dishes of the Mediterranean cuisine. It's not the only food that creates this diet's health benefits, but it is a major component.

# Olive Oil, Every Day

Olive oil is used abundantly in cooking, baking, marinating, and dressings throughout the Mediterranean region. It is one of the foods that contributes to the diet's high proportion of heart-healthy monounsaturated fats. To reap the health benefits of this healthy oil and to follow the guidelines of the Mediterranean diet, olive oil should be a part of your everyday diet.

Here are some tips for getting more olive oil in your daily diet:

- Use olive oil instead of dressing on your salads. Add a bit of red wine vinegar and lemon as well.

- Dip your 100 percent whole-grain bread in olive oil, and do away with the butter or margarine. Add a bit of oregano, black pepper, or Parmesan cheese for more flavor.

- Sprinkle freshly cooked vegetables, including baked potatoes and corn on the cob, with olive oil.

- Scramble your eggs or cook your omelets in olive oil instead of butter or margarine.

- Toss it into your favorite pasta with fresh veggies.

- Brush the bread for grilled sandwiches with olive oil instead of margarine or butter.

- Use olive oil to baste meat or seafood before and during grilling and roasting.

- Use olive oil in recipes in place of vegetable oils or other fats.

- Use olive oil, along with herbs and spices, to marinate meats, seafood, or vegetables before cooking.

- Use olive oil to prepare spreads or dips such as hummus.

- Stir-fry lean meat or seafood and your favorite vegetables in olive oil.

# Olive Oil's Health Benefits

Olive oil is a fat, but its high content of healthy, monounsaturated fats makes olive oil quite healthy. Studies have consistently shown that one of the key benefits to consuming olive oil is that it helps lower cholesterol. The monounsaturated fats help lower the LDL (or "bad") cholesterol and increase the HDL (or "good") cholesterol, and both of these are important factors for good heart health. The key to getting the health benefits from this oil is not just to *add* olive oil to your current diet but to use it as a *replacement* for unhealthy fats, as in the Mediterranean diet.

The Food and Drug Administration (FDA) provides qualified health claims for manufacturers to use that assert a relationship between consumption of oleic acid (a monounsaturated fat) in edible oils and a reduced risk of coronary health disease. One of the edible oils highest in oleic acid is olive oil.

Two current health claims include the following stipulations:

- "Supportive but not conclusive scientific evidence suggests that daily consumption of about 1½ tablespoons (20 grams) of oils containing high levels of oleic acid, when replaced for fats and oils higher in saturated fat, may reduce the risk of coronary heart disease."

- The claim also must make it clear that to achieve this benefit, these oils "should replace fats and oils higher in saturated fat and not increase the total number of calories you eat in a day."

With all the research being done on heart-healthy olive oil, researchers are finding even more health benefits. The rich supplies of polyphenols in olive oil, which are not found in many nut and seed oils, are natural antioxidants and have been shown to have anti-inflammatory and anticoagulant properties. This is central to evidence that olive oil can lower cholesterol, blood pressure, and the risk for heart disease as well as protect against certain cancers and even osteoporosis.

Olive oil is well tolerated by the stomach and may have a protective function against ulcers, gastritis, and gallstones. In addition, the omega-3 fatty acids in olive oil help keep blood cells from sticking together, increase blood flow, and help reduce inflammation, making these fats useful for preventing not only cardiovascular disease but also inflammatory conditions such as arthritis. Because of the antioxidants, phytonutrients, and healthy fats olive oil contains, it also may help slow down the process of aging and the many chronic conditions that follow.

# Olive Oil's Nutritional Properties

Olive oil is considered a monounsaturated fat. As with other oils, it is made up of more than one type of fat, but it is predominantly comprised of monounsaturated fatty acids (or oleic acids). In fact, no other naturally produced oil has such a large monounsaturated fat content. From a nutritional standpoint, the fat content in a typical olive oil averages about ...

- 75 percent oleic acid (an omega-9 monounsaturated fat),

- 10 percent linoleic acid (an omega-6 polyunsaturated fat),

- 1 percent linolenic acid (an omega-3 polyunsaturated fat), and

- 15 percent saturated fat.

The U.S. dietary reference intakes for essential fatty acids currently recommends consuming omega-6 and omega-3 fats in a ratio of 10 to 1. It is amazing how nature provides nearly just that ratio in olive oil.

Fat isn't the only component in olive oil. This oil is rich in essential vitamins and antioxidants such as thiamin; riboflavin; niacin; and vitamins A, C, E, and K. You can even find a bit of iron and other essential nutrients in it. It also is full of polyphenols and flavonoids, both of which are powerful phytonutrients and health promoters. In fact, choosing an olive oil with a green or yellow tint ensures you are getting plenty of those polyphenols, a powerful antioxidant.

Olive oil outweighs other fats when it comes to its content of health-promoting monounsaturated fats. Even fats that contain decent amounts of monounsaturated fats contain far too much saturated fat, as shown in the following table.

## A Comparison of Fats

| Type of Fat | Monounsaturated | Polyunsaturated | Saturated |
| --- | --- | --- | --- |
| Olive oil | 75 percent | 10 percent | 15 percent |
| Canola oil | 62 percent | 31 percent | 7 percent |
| Peanut oil | 48 percent | 33 percent | 19 percent |
| Palm oil | 39 percent | 9 percent | 52 percent |
| Butter | 30 percent | 5 percent | 65 percent |

(continues)

**A Comparison of Fats** (continued)

| Type of Fat | Monounsaturated | Polyunsaturated | Saturated |
|---|---|---|---|
| Corn oil | 25 percent | 62 percent | 13 percent |
| Soybean oil | 25 percent | 60 percent | 15 percent |
| Sunflower oil | 21 percent | 68 percent | 11 percent |
| Flaxseed oil | 18 percent | 73 percent | 9 percent |
| Coconut oil | 6 percent | 2 percent | 92 percent |

## Sorting Out Olive Oil Varieties

Choosing an olive oil can be confusing without the right information—there are different grades of olive oil, and some are more flavorful and provide more health benefits than others.

Olive oil is graded on taste, acidity level, and processing method. Certain types of olive oils are better for certain cooking methods and recipes. The many variables that go into producing olive oil such as the variety of olive, where the olive is grown, its ripeness when picked, the time of harvesting, the pressing technique, the packaging, and storage all can make remarkable differences in color, aroma, and flavor. Each type of olive oil carries its own classification, which is used to differentiate between all the varieties.

## Extra-Virgin Olive Oil

At the head of the class sit the extra-virgin olive oil (EVOO) varieties. These can include label classifications such as "premium extra-virgin" and "extra-virgin" oils. These are the highest-quality olive oils made from the first pressing of the olives with no heat or chemicals and very low levels of acidity (no more than 0.8 percent). Acidity levels correspond with the type of olives used as well as with storage and production methods. A low acidity level is a key factor in a great-tasting, high-quality olive oil. Extra-virgin olive oil has the lowest acidity level, but as it gets older, the acidity can rise a bit and change the flavor slightly. These oils are unrefined and contain higher levels of antioxidants, particularly vitamin E and polyphenols, because they are less processed. For your health's sake, extra-virgin olive oil is the best choice.

Extra-virgin olive oils come in a wide range of flavors. Flavor is determined by many factors, including the type and ripeness of olive used, growing conditions, harvesting methods, storage, and pressing methods. In general, the deeper the color, the more flavor the oil yields. The color of these high-quality oils should be a deep greenish-gold color.

Extra-virgin olive oil is great for dipping bread into; as a dressing or marinade; and for drizzling over vegetables, stews, or fish. The highest-quality extra-virgin olive oils have a buttery taste and can be used to replace other fats, such as butter or margarine, on breads. Because heat can change both flavor and nutritional content, to properly appreciate extra-virgin olive oil's excellent aroma and flavor, it is best used in uncooked dishes or as a finishing touch.

When shopping for a high-quality extra-virgin olive oil, look for bottles that are certified by the International Olive Oil Council (IOOC). IOOC-standard oils must meet certain criteria before being placed into a specific category. These olive oils cannot be combined with any other type of oil, and they must pass through a certified panel of tasters, meet analytical criteria, and prove genuineness and purity.

## Virgin Olive Oil

Next in line is virgin olive oil. These oils can include label classifications such as "fine virgin" and "semifine virgin." Virgin olive oil, like extra-virgin olive oil, is made from the first pressing of the olives. It is produced with no chemicals or high heat and is unrefined. The difference between the two oils and their grade is around 1 percentage point of acidity. However, in the world of olive oils, that's all it takes to distinguish between great oils and very good oils. Virgin olive oil is nice for salad dressings and marinades and also works well in uncooked dishes. The taste is not quite as pronounced as extra-virgin olive oil, but it still has a good flavor.

Fine virgin olive oil must have a good flavor by industry standards and an acidity level of no more than 1.5 percent. This oil is less expensive than extra-virgin olive oil, but it is very close in quality. Virgin olive oil also must have a good flavor, but the acidity can be no more than 2 percent. This oil is good for cooking, but it has enough flavor to be enjoyed uncooked.

Semifine virgin olive oil must have an acidity level no higher than 3.3 percent. It is best used for cooking because the flavor is not strong enough to be enjoyed in uncooked dishes.

## Pure or Refined Olive Oil

One more step down the ladder, you will find olive oil that can be labeled as "pure olive oil" or "refined olive oil."

Pure olive oil consists of a blend of both refined olive oil and virgin olive oil.

Refined olive oil is obtained by refining virgin olive oil, or chemically treating it using charcoal and other chemical and physical filters, to neutralize strong tastes as well as acid content. Oils that are further refined after the first pressing can no longer carry the title "virgin."

These oils carry a much milder flavor and are good for sautéing, where virgin oils are not due to their low smoke point. (An oil's smoke point is the temperature at which it smokes when heated. If an oil is heated past its smoke point, it is no longer good for use or good for you. Refined olive oils have a slightly higher smoke point than unrefined olive oils—about 410°F/210°C versus 400°F/200°C, respectively.) These oils also are ideal for basting and grilling and are a good choice for pasta dishes.

## Lite Olive Oil

The word *lite* refers to oils that have been refined. Lite olive oil is also called "light" or "mild" oil. These words don't mean the oil is lower in fat or calories but rather refer to its light or mild flavor. These oils are highly refined or processed to extract the last bit of possible oil from the olives.

Lite oils contain the same amount of healthy monounsaturated fats as all the other olive oils, but much of the color, aroma, and flavor is lost due to the refining process. Other nutritional content is lost, too, such as vitamins and antioxidants.

These oils are more suitable for cooking or baking and using in recipes where strong flavor is not desired. The refining process also gives these oils a higher smoke point, making them a better candidate for high-heat cooking methods.

# Storing Olive Oil

Now you know olive oil will be a staple in your pantry. But how long should it stay there? How should it be stored?

Oils can be fragile and need to be handled with care. The four enemies of olive oil are age, heat, air, and light. Restricting all these will greatly extend the oil's shelf life and keep it from turning rancid, which would destroy all its healthy antioxidant properties.

Because heat, air, and light do so much damage to olive oil, your best bet is to keep it in a dark, cool cupboard. Tinted glass or stainless-steel bottles make optimal containers. Avoid other metals such as iron or copper, which can create toxic compounds when they come in contact with olive oil. Also avoid most plastics because oil can leach out toxic compounds from the plastic.

The cap or lid on the container needs to be tight to keep out unwanted air.

Storage temperature is important. Room temperature—about 70°F (21°C)—will do just fine. Keep the oil out of cupboards that are near your oven or other heat sources. If your kitchen seems to be too warm most of the time, try refrigerating your oil. You can keep small amounts at room temperature for daily use and put the remainder in the refrigerator. Keep in mind that refrigerated olive oil will solidify and turn cloudy until it is returned to room temperature. Oil experts don't recommend storing premium extra-virgin olive oils in the refrigerator because condensation can develop and affect the flavor. Your best bet for these oils is room temperature. Other olive oils do fine with refrigeration.

Because of olive oil's high content of monounsaturated fat, when stored properly, it can be stored for longer than other oils. In fact, high-quality olive oils retain their quality and flavor for at least 1 year, while lower-quality olive oils last only a few months. Unopened, olive oil keeps for as long as 2 years.

Olive oil doesn't get better with age—in fact, as it ages, acidity rises, flavor diminishes, and nutritional content decreases. Extra-virgin olive oils keep a bit longer because they start with a lower acidity level. Not all bottles carry bottling or "use by" dates, but it's worth checking if the bottle does have one before you buy. Don't let your olive oil just sit in the cupboard—use it!

Bright light can destroy an oil. In some grocery stores, especially ones open 24 hours, bottles of olive oil can sit under bright lights all day long. When shopping, opt for bottles that are not stored on the top shelf or at the front of the shelf in the light. Instead, grab a bottle from the second row where direct light doesn't reach it. Also, look for brands that come in dark-colored bottles. Be sure the bottle is free of dust, too, which might signify it has been sitting on the shelf for quite some time.

# Cooking with Olive Oil

Cooking with olive oil is a great way to include its health benefits in your daily diet. Olive oil helps bring out the natural flavor of foods, herbs, and spices. The extra-virgin and virgin varieties are your best choices to use uncooked or cooked at a low to medium temperature. Refined olive oil and olive oil grades are better choices for high-heat cooking such as sautéing.

(In the recipes later in this book, we specify when we'd recommend using extra-virgin olive oil and otherwise call for "olive oil" so you can decide which variety you'd like to use—virgin, refined, or another grade.)

Remember, smoke point is important. An oil's smoke point is the temperature at which it smokes when heated, and at that point, any oil is basically ruined. Olive oil generally has a higher smoke point than most other oils, but the refined or lower-quality olive oils have the highest smoke points.

Whether you are using olive oil to sauté, stir-fry, or panfry, here are some tips:

- Heat the pan or skillet over medium heat, and when the pan is hot, add the olive oil and heat it to just below its smoke point before adding food. The food should sizzle when added to the oil. If it doesn't, the pan and the oil aren't hot enough.

- Pat-dry the food before placing it in the oil. This ensures a crispy exterior.

- Brush meat, seafood, and vegetables with a bit of olive oil when you're grilling or broiling. This enhances the flavor, seals in the juices, and produces a crispier exterior. Don't forget to brush the grill, too, to keep the food from sticking.

- Use the lower-quality olive oils for stir-frying or panfrying because they are better for high-heat cooking methods.

- Use olive oil for cooking with foods that contain a high acid content, such as vinegar, wine, lemon juice, or tomato, to help balance the acidity.

- Add 1 tablespoon olive oil to boiling water before adding pasta. This helps eliminate sticking and clumping.

- Remember that olive oil, although healthy, is a fat that contains a lot of calories, so use it in moderation.

# Baking with Olive Oil

Most people are used to baking with butter or margarine, but few of us think about olive oil when it comes to baking. Baking with olive oil gives your baked goods a healthier kick, and it can help produce lighter-tasting breads, cakes, and other baked goods. Substituting olive oil for butter drastically reduces the amount of saturated fat and cholesterol in your baked goods, too. You also will use less fat when baking with olive oil, and that means fewer calories. The best choices for baking are the lite, light, or mild varieties of olive oil because they can stand high heat and have a much milder flavor.

When you are baking or just cooking in general, replacing bad fats with good fats can be easy. When a recipe calls for a vegetable oil or another type of fat like butter or margarine, simply use olive oil instead.

As a general guide, substitute an equal amount of olive oil for the same amount of another cooking oil and three-quarters the amount of olive oil when substituting for butter or margarine.

The substitutions in the following table help you replace butter or margarine with olive oil in your favorite recipes.

## Butter/Olive Oil Substitutions

| Butter | Olive Oil |
| --- | --- |
| 1 teaspoon | ¾ teaspoon |
| 2 teaspoons | 1½ teaspoons |
| 1 tablespoon | 2¼ teaspoons |
| 2 tablespoons | 1½ tablespoons |
| ¼ cup | 3 tablespoons |
| ⅓ cup | ¼ cup |
| ½ cup | ¼ cup + 2 tablespoons |
| ⅔ cup | ½ cup |
| ¾ cup | ½ cup + 1 tablespoon |
| 1 cup | ¾ cup |

## In This Chapter

Olive oil is made from olives, which are actually classified as a fruit. Olive oil's primary fat component is monounsaturated fat, which is known for its health benefits, but it also contains essential vitamins and antioxidants. There are several classifications of olive oil, determined by the processing method, and some are considered higher quality than others. Olive oil is great for cooking and can even be used in baking.

# CHAPTER 7

# Whole Grains

We often refer to a large part of the grain food group as "comfort foods." Those tasty complex carbohydrates such as bread, rice, cereal, and pasta help make us feel satisfied and content.

Add the word *whole,* and these grain foods are much more than comfort foods; they are an essential part of a healthy diet. Health experts continually advise us, both young and old, to eat more whole grains.

If whole grains are so healthy, why do people eat so few of them? It could be that we don't know exactly what whole grains are and why we should eat them.

# What Are Whole Grains?

All grains are a good source of complex carbohydrates, vitamins, and minerals. However, whole grains kick it up a notch by also including more fiber and additional essential nutrients, including antioxidants. Whole grains are termed "whole" because they are made of the entire seed of the grain: the bran, germ, and endosperm. Whole grains can be eaten whole, cracked, split, or ground.

The Whole Grains Council offers the official definition: "Whole grains or foods made from them that contain all the essential parts and naturally-occurring nutrients of the entire grain seed in their original proportions. If the grain has been processed (e.g., cracked, crushed, rolled, extruded, and/or cooked), the food product should deliver the same rich balance of nutrients that are found in the original grain seed."

## Whole Grains Versus Refined Grains

Grains are broken down into two subgroups: whole grains and refined grains. Whole grains are much more efficient than refined grains for increasing your fiber intake, providing essential nutrients, and contributing to good health.

We already know that a whole-grain food is made from the entire grain kernel. The bran is the outer layer of the grain and supplies antioxidants, B vitamins, trace minerals, and fiber. The germ, nestled inside the endosperm, is tiny but packs a powerful punch, supplying B vitamins, vitamin E, trace minerals, antioxidants, essential fats, and fiber. The endosperm, or the inner part of the grain kernel, contains most of the protein and starchy carbohydrates. The endosperm supplies only small amounts of vitamins and minerals and no fiber.

Whereas whole grains contain all three parts of the kernel, refined grains contain only the endosperm. Whole grains contain all the fiber and most of the nutrients, and refined grains are basically whole grains that have been processed or milled and have had the bran and germ removed. Milling provides the grain with a finer texture and improves the shelf life; however, it also strips away dietary fiber, iron, and essential vitamins. When the bran and germ are stripped away, about 25 percent of a grain's protein and most of the key nutrients are lost.

Examples of whole grains include the following:

- Amaranth
- Barley
- Buckwheat
- Bulgur
- Corn
- Oats, including oatmeal
- Popcorn
- Quinoa (technically a seed but commonly thought of and cooked like a grain)
- Rice, wild and brown
- Rye, whole
- Sorghum
- Spelt
- Teff
- Whole-wheat bread, buns, tortillas, crackers, and rolls
- Whole-wheat flour
- Whole-wheat pasta

Examples of refined grains include the following:

- Baked goods (unless made with a whole-grain flour)
- Breads, buns, and rolls made from white or refined flour
- Crackers made from white or refined flour
- Flour tortillas made from white or refined flour
- White flour
- White pasta or noodles
- White rice

## Adding Back Nutrients

Because so many nutrients are stripped away during the milling process of refining grains, most of these grains are enriched, meaning that some of the nutrients that were lost during processing are added back to the food. These are nutrients that were naturally present in the food to begin with.

In enriched grains, particular amounts of B vitamins and iron are added back, but fiber is not. This justifies why it is best to choose whole-grain foods rather than foods made from refined grains.

Dietary guidelines recommend that all adults eat at least half their grains as whole grains, which is about three to five servings per day. The more the better though, so don't be shy about those whole grains!

# Whole Grains and the Mediterranean Diet

Whole grains form the foundation of the Mediterranean diet and are included in the largest food section of the Mediterranean Diet Pyramid (see Chapter 3), the plant group. The pyramid suggests basing every meal on these highly nutritious complex carbohydrates. The more whole grains you include in your daily diet, the closer you are following the Mediterranean diet and the more health benefits you will reap.

According to the Whole Grains Council, the average American eats less than one serving of whole grains per day, and 40 percent of Americans never eat whole grains. If following the Mediterranean diet is your goal, it's time to work on increasing your consumption of whole grains. Health experts agree that even small amounts of whole grains can put you on the road to better health.

# Whole Grains' Health Benefits

The medical evidence speaks for itself: it confirms that whole grains reduce the risk of heart disease, stroke, cancer, type 2 diabetes, and obesity. Replacing refined grains with whole grains can significantly improve total cholesterol, LDL ("bad") cholesterol, hemoglobin A1c (a measure of blood sugar), and C-reactive protein (a measure of inflammation). Whole grains also have been associated with a lower incidence of gastrointestinal issues such as constipation and diverticulosis.

Studies show that just three servings of whole grains a day can greatly reduce your risk for many chronic diseases. Other health benefits of whole grains include helping reduce inflammatory diseases, colon cancer, and hypertension (high blood pressure).

# Whole Grains' Nutritional Properties

Whole grains are an abundant source of healthy nutrients. They contain antioxidants (vitamin E and selenium), B vitamins (thiamin, riboflavin, niacin, and folate), and minerals (iron, magnesium, and selenium). In addition, they are packed with dietary fiber and phytonutrients that contain antioxidant properties. When all these nutritional components work together in a whole food, the result is powerful protection for health.

# Choosing Whole Grains

How do you ensure that the foods you are choosing are indeed whole grain? Whole grains currently take up about 10 to 15 percent of grocery shelves. It can sometimes be a challenge for consumers to find these healthier whole grains among the sea of refined grain foods.

The key is to carefully check food labels. Don't be fooled by the color of a product or certain wording. For example, just because a loaf of bread is brown in color does not necessarily mean it is made from whole-wheat flour and is, therefore, a whole grain. Many times, breads labeled "wheat" are actually colored with molasses or caramel coloring, or they are made with a mixture of both refined and whole-wheat flours, where proportions vary. You may come across descriptive words such as *multigrain, stone-ground, cracked wheat, 100 percent wheat* (meaning wheat is used, but not necessarily whole wheat), *bran,* or *seven grain,* just to name a few. These might sound nutritious, but unfortunately, they do not guarantee a whole-grain product—and often they are not whole grain.

To determine if a food product is actually whole grain and contains whole-grain ingredients, look for the word *whole* on the package, such as *whole wheat* or *whole grain,* and check to see if whole grains appear among the first items in the ingredient list. Not all whole grains have the word *whole,* so look for other whole-grain ingredients such as brown rice, bulgur, graham flour, oatmeal, and wild rice.

Use the Nutrition Facts label (see Chapter 5) to choose foods with a higher percent Daily Value (%DV) of fiber. The more fiber a food contains, the better chance there is a decent amount of whole grains in the product. If the product has 20 percent or more %DV for fiber, it's considered a high-fiber food.

You also can check for one of many grain authorized health claims by the FDA on the label including, "Diets low in saturated fat and cholesterol and rich in fruits, vegetables, and grain products that contain some types of dietary fiber, particularly soluble fiber, may reduce the risk of heart disease, a disease associated with many factors." Foods that display this specific claim must contain at least 0.6 grams of soluble fiber and declare that on the Nutrition Facts label as well as meet the nutrient content requirements for a food that is low in fat, saturated fat, and cholesterol.

The Whole Grains Council has developed three Whole Grain Stamps to help consumers easily choose whole-grain foods. You can find the stamps on hundreds of foods currently, with more to come. Each stamp displays how many grams of whole-grain ingredients are in a serving of that specific food. Here's what to look for:

- **100% Stamp:** All of the food's ingredients are whole grain. There is a minimum requirement of 16 grams (one full serving) of whole grains per labeled serving with this stamp.

- **50% Stamp:** At least half of the food's ingredients are whole grain. There is a minimum requirement of 8 grams (half a serving) of whole grains per labeled serving with this stamp.

- **Basic Stamp:** The food contains at least 8 grams (half a serving) of whole grains but may contain more refined grains than whole grains.

*(Used by permission. Oldways Whole Grains Council, www.wholegrains council.org.)*

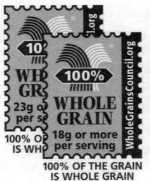
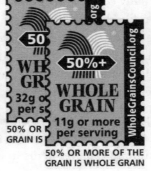
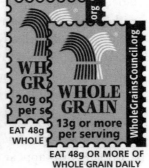

# Popular Grains of the Mediterranean

There are loads of whole grains out there to try, and many are traditional to the Mediterranean diet. Now is the time to tantalize your taste buds and begin sampling some of these tasty whole grains. You might already be familiar with some, such as rice, cereal, pasta, and breads, but there are many more that may be new to you. Let's take a look at the grains popular in the Mediterranean diet.

## Whole-Wheat Bulgur

Bulgur, a whole grain with a mild, nutty flavor, is a staple in the Mediterranean diet. It is cracked wheat that has been partially cooked to be quick-cooking. Bulgur is especially high in fiber, protein, and minerals but low in calories and fat. In fact, bulgur contains more fiber than oats, buckwheat, or corn.

This versatile grain comes in three grinds: fine, medium, and coarse. The finest grind is perfect for hot breakfast cereals and desserts. The medium grind is preferred for grain salads such as tabbouleh, stews, soups, and multigrain baked goods. Coarsely ground bulgur can be used for pilaf, stuffing, and casseroles.

Bulgur makes a great meat extender and, because of its high protein content, a nutritious meat substitute in plant-based meals. Bulgur is used much like rice in the Mediterranean diet and combines well with many foods.

## Hulled Barley

Barley is a cereal grain that is only lightly milled and retains much of its soluble and insoluble fiber. With hulled barley, only the outermost hull of the grain is removed, which makes for a chewier grain and a more nutritious whole-grain food. In fact, hulled barley is the only form of barley that is considered a whole grain. Varieties such as scotch barley and barley oats retain more of the bran than pearled barley, but none of these forms are considered a whole grain.

Hulled barley makes a healthy choice for use in grain salads, soups, risotto, and stews, or as a stuffing for vegetables. It has a wonderful chewy texture, making it an interesting addition to your meals, and can be a nice alternative to rice.

## Whole-Grain Couscous

Whole-grain couscous is a coarsely ground semolina pasta made from whole-grain durum flour. It is not always made from whole grains, so be sure it is labeled as either "whole wheat" or "whole grain." It's widely used in Middle Eastern countries but is becoming much more popular in American dishes.

Couscous has a light flavor and is very similar to rice in shape, color, and texture. In fact, it is almost a perfect mixture of both rice and pasta. Couscous very nicely absorbs the flavors of Mediterranean foods such as herbs, spices, vegetables, stews, lamb, seafood, or chicken.

## Polenta

Polenta is a common food in the Mediterranean region and is a must when discussing whole grains. Polenta is made from ground cornmeal; however, you want to avoid degerminated cornmeal because this has the germ removed and, therefore, is not a whole grain. Your best bet is to buy stone-ground, whole-grain cornmeal and use that to make polenta to ensure you have a whole-grain product.

The word *polenta* can refer to the dish or to the actual ground cornmeal itself. To make polenta, cornmeal is boiled in water to make a porridge-type dish—something that is better known in America as cornmeal mush. Traditionally, polenta can take some time to prepare; however, a form of quick-cooking polenta is gaining popularity. After polenta is cooked, it can be left in the refrigerator overnight to allow it to harden into a doughlike texture. At that point, it can be baked and cut into squares almost like cornbread.

Polenta can be served in numerous ways: baked, in stews, and as a bread substitute. Cooked polenta can be used much like pasta as a base for sauces, toppings, vegetables, seafood, and meats.

## Quinoa

Quinoa—which, as has been mentioned, is technically a seed but is commonly thought of and cooked like a grain—is popular with the people of the Mediterranean and becoming more well-known in American kitchens, too.

Quinoa is light and fluffy, with a slightly crunchy texture and nutty flavor when cooked. It is quite high in protein and antioxidants, with nearly twice the amount of protein as whole grains, and is considered a complete protein, making it a great choice as a meat substitute or for use in vegetarian diets. (A complete protein, or whole protein, provides the body with an adequate proportion of all nine essential amino acids needed for optimal health. Most complete proteins come from animal sources such as meats, seafood, and dairy products, with very few coming from plant sources.) It also is a high-fiber food, with a whopping 5 grams of fiber per cooked cup.

Quinoa is very versatile and can be eaten as a breakfast cereal; mixed with vegetables; or added to soups, stews, and salads. It also can be used to make flour for breads or used as a substitution for pasta, couscous, or rice.

# Flours to Discover

When reaching for a flour for baking, many of us probably tend toward white all-purpose flour. White all-purpose flour is made from wheat that has been refined, stripping away the layers that contain all the nutrients and, therefore, is not a whole grain. In other words, it is wheat flour, but not whole-wheat flour—and as we've discussed, the nutritional difference between refined and whole-grain flours is quite significant.

Refined flours are not the type of flour you would find in most homes around the Mediterranean. Many different whole-grain flours have a much higher nutritional content and create a more complex taste and heartier texture because they include the bran and germ of the grain. The good news is that these flours can work just fine in your favorite dishes and baked goods.

Whole-grain flours don't last as long as refined flour, so when buying them, be sure to check the sell-by date to ensure you are getting the freshest available. These flours should be stored in the refrigerator or freezer in an airtight container—be sure to set out the flour and allow it to get to room temperature before using. You can expect most of these flours to last about three months, so only buy what you will use in that time. Whole-grain flours can cook differently than white all-purpose flour, so you may have to alter recipes slightly to get the end product you are looking for.

Here are some tips to help you add whole-grain goodness to your cooking and baking:

- Use whole-grain flour in simple recipes that you have made before and in recipes that call for only a small amount of flour. It might be helpful at first to find recipes that actually call for whole-grain flour.

- Research online or in cookbooks which flours work best for different foods or baked goods (such as breads versus cakes). You can get started with the list of flours later in this chapter.

- Start slow by substituting at least half all-purpose flour with whole-grain flours such as spelt or whole-wheat flour.

- Because whole-wheat flours absorb more liquid than refined white flour, you may need to add additional liquid in small portions, a little at a time, to get the consistency you need.

- Sift flour before and after measuring to help improve texture.

- You may need to use more leavening agent (such as baking powder or baking soda) to help with the rising properties of whole-grain flour.

- Put a pan of water in the oven while baking to help retain moisture; whole-grain flour tends to be drier than refined flour.

- Because some whole-grain flours are gluten free, if you are baking bread leavened with yeast, half of the flour you use must be a gluten-containing flour.

With a little practice, you will be able to find the combinations of refined and whole-grain flours that suit your needs. By adding some whole-grain flour to white all-purpose flour, you can begin to add fiber and other essential nutrients to your favorite baked goods. The more you know about the different whole-grain flours, the easier it will be to work with them.

## Whole-Wheat Flour

Whole-wheat flour has a high gluten content and a coarse texture. It is sometimes referred to as "whole-wheat bread flour" and is ideal for bread baking due to its ability to rise. Whole-wheat flour is higher in fiber and protein than refined white flour. Because bread made with 100 percent whole-wheat flour can be somewhat coarse and heavy, and doesn't keep long, it's best to mix in 30 to 50 percent refined flour to lighten the texture. Your bread will taste better, and you will still be getting the benefit of using a whole grain.

## Spelt Flour

Spelt flour is close in flavor and texture to whole-wheat flour. It contains no wheat but does contain some gluten. However, the gluten in spelt is a bit fragile, so it's important not to overmix your dough or batter because the gluten gives baked goods their elasticity and structure. Spelt is a popular and easy substitute for wheat flour in most breads, baked goods, and other recipes. It is a bit nuttier and sweeter than whole-wheat flour, is high in protein, and has a strong nutritional profile.

## Barley Flour

Barley flour is a delicate, low-gluten flour that is made by grinding whole barley. This flour is moist and has a sweet, nutlike flavor. As with many other whole-grain flours, it can be used to replace part of the wheat flour (white or refined flour) in baked goods and recipes to provide a unique flavor and texture as well as a kick of nutrition. Try substituting ⅓ cup barley flour in place of your regular flour for a more tender product. Barley flour also can serve as a thickener in soups and sauces instead of using refined flour.

## Whole-Rye Flour

Rye flour is milled from whole rye berries and grains of rye grass. It provides moisture and density to baked goods and is low in gluten. Rye flour can be bought in a variety of colors: dark, medium, and light. The color depends on how much bran is removed during the milling process.

Dark rye flour, the least-refined form of rye flour, is high in nutrients—even higher than whole-wheat flour. Pumpernickel flour is a type of dark rye flour that is used to make pumpernickel bread. The medium-colored rye flour is most common and is still quite nutritious because most of the bran is left. Light rye flour is the most refined or has the most bran removed, making it the least nutritious.

Equal proportions of rye and wheat flour (white or refined flour) work well in yeasted and quick breads to help the rising process. Rye flour has a slightly sour taste, making it a great flour to use for rye bread and sourdough bread.

# Cooking Whole Grains

You can consume whole grains daily, even without cooking them, simply by eating whole-grain breads, cereals, and other prepared whole-grain foods. However, that isn't the only way to enjoy them. You also can include them in many of your favorite dishes and recipes by making easy substitutions. Because some of these whole grains may be a little different from what you're used to, here are some guidelines:

- Cooking most whole grains is very similar to cooking rice: put the dry grain in a pan of water or broth, bring to a boil, and simmer until the liquid is absorbed. Cooking times vary depending on the grain type, so read package directions.

- For grains that are tougher and take longer to cook, presoak them in the allotted amount of water for a few hours before cooking.

- Try batch cooking when you cook grains. They will keep for at least three or four days in the refrigerator, and they take just a few minutes to warm up. You can toss them into salads, stews, and soups.

- Look for quick-cooking grains, such as instant brown rice—but be sure you are buying a whole-grain product. Review the Nutrition Facts label to ensure you are getting the fiber you expect.

# Tips for Going Whole Grain

If you want to follow the Mediterranean diet, it's time to start adding healthy whole grains to your daily diet. Be adventurous and try some whole grains you've never tasted and maybe have never heard of. Forget the myths that whole grains don't taste good or that they are difficult to work into your daily diet. You'll be pleasantly surprised to discover how wrong those myths are!

Here are some tips to get you started:

- Try rolled oats, barley, buckwheat, or other whole grains as your breakfast cereal topped with fresh fruit.

- Substitute a mixture of unrefined whole-grain flour for refined flour in your baked goods and as thickeners.

- Step up your breakfast foods by making pancakes or muffins using a combination of whole-grain flours.

- Don't restrict yourself to the same whole grains every day. As with other food groups, variety is best to ensure you get the most nutritional benefits from all types of whole grains.

- Choose whole-grain breads and cereals. Making simple changes like choosing a whole-grain breakfast cereal instead of a refined, sugary cereal and whole-wheat bread in place of white bread can make big changes to your nutritional intake.

- Try whole-grain rice and other side dishes. This easy change can add so much flavor to your dishes. You might be surprised at how much better brown rice tastes than white rice, for example. Add something new to your pilaf or other side dishes, like couscous, barley, or bulgur.

- Try buying whole-grain pasta or a pasta that is a blend of whole-grain and white flours. Use them with your favorite sauces or in casseroles, soups, and cold salads.

- Check out new recipes from sources like the Whole Grains Council (wholegrainscouncil.com) to sharpen your whole-grain cooking skills.

- Short on time? Add cooked bulgur, brown or wild rice, whole-wheat couscous, or barley to your favorite canned or homemade soup for an instant serving of whole grains.

- Jazz up your bread stuffing with cooked bulgur, wild rice, or barley.

- Add ¾ cup uncooked oats to each 1 pound (450g) of ground turkey or ground chicken breast to make meatballs, stuffed peppers, burgers, or meatloaf. Whole grains add flavor and make a great meat extender.

- Stir in a handful of oats to your plain, nonfat yogurt along with some fruit.

- Do something simple like snacking on popcorn. What could be easier than air-popped popcorn? Just be sure it isn't covered in butter and salt.

- Use oat bran as a coating for fish or chicken.

The key is to begin finding ways to fit in whole grains anywhere you can. It doesn't take a lot of whole grains to get your daily recommended amounts, but shoot for as many as you can. Always check food labels and ingredients lists to ensure you are actually buying whole-grain products, and don't stop learning about and trying a variety of whole grains.

## In This Chapter

The foundation of the Mediterranean diet is built on plant foods, including whole grains. A whole grain, by definition, includes the whole seed: bran, germ, and endosperm. Whole grains are much more nutritious than refined grains and are packed with fiber. Foods need to include the word *whole,* in most cases, if they are truly a whole grain. Always read the Nutrition Facts label and ingredient list, and look for the Whole Grain Stamp. Don't be afraid to cook and bake with whole grains and whole-grain flours, and look for new ways to add them to your daily diet. They can be tasty and nutritious, and they add some wonderful new flavors.

# CHAPTER 8

# Fruit

Fruit is one of the most natural foods in the world—abundant in nutrition and variety, readily available, and packed with sweet goodness. Yet it also is one food many of us take for granted. Studies show that 90 percent of Americans don't eat enough fruit.

Eating a colorful variety of fruit can provide a wide range of valuable nutrients that are essential for good health, and there are proven links that eating more fruit can lead to lowered risk for some chronic conditions. No wonder fruit is a major component of the Mediterranean diet.

# Fruit and the Mediterranean Diet

The Mediterranean Diet Pyramid (see Chapter 3) recommends basing every meal on healthy plant foods, and that includes fruit. (You might be starting to notice a pattern: every time we discuss a plant-based food, we mention the foundation of the Mediterranean Diet Pyramid. Plant-based foods are what this diet is truly founded on.) The keys are to include fruit as often as possible and to consume a wide variety to ensure you reap all the nutritional benefits.

You might be surprised to learn that some of the fruits included within this Mediterranean Diet Pyramid group include olives, avocados, dates, and pomegranates. It also contains more familiar fruits such as strawberries, apples, grapes, and pears.

# Fruit's Health Benefits

No matter what kind, whether it's native to the Mediterranean region or more common on American grocery shelves, fruit is simply a healthy food. Eating more fruit as part of an overall healthy diet has been shown to reduce the risk of stroke, cardiovascular diseases, type 2 diabetes, and certain cancers, such as colon and stomach cancers, as well as lower blood pressure. A diet rich in fruit can lower the risk of digestive issues such as constipation and diarrhea by providing dietary fiber and regulating bowel movements. When you make the simple change of eating fruit in place of sweets, junk foods, or other foods with added sugar and fat, you may even lose weight or better maintain a healthy weight.

# Fruit's Nutritional Properties

Fruit is naturally low in fat, sodium, and calories and contains no cholesterol, saturated fat, or trans fats. Most fruit contains about 80 percent water, so fruit even contributes to your overall daily fluid intake. Most fruit is rich in potassium, which is helpful in maintaining a healthy blood pressure. Some of the most valuable nutrients found in fruit include dietary fiber and antioxidants such as vitamin C and vitamin A. Eating a variety of colorful fruits can provide plenty of plant compounds and phytonutrients, such as flavonoids, carotenoids, and phenols—all of which are beneficial to your health and can help lower your risk for various chronic health conditions. Consuming a variety of fruits incorporates a broader range of nutrient consumption in your diet.

Fruit gets its sweetness from fructose, the natural sugar found in fruit. Today we are taught to think of sugar as something to avoid or limit; however, there are many different types of sugar, from naturally occurring sugars, like the fructose in fruit and the lactose in dairy products, to added sugars, like those added to cookies, baked goods, soft drinks, and other processed foods. The difference is that foods like fruit that contain naturally occurring sugars are also loaded with essential nutrients for good health. On the other hand, added sugars, which are refined sugars, are usually found in foods that provide empty calories with little to no nutritional value.

In the body, the natural sugar in fruit acts much the same way added sugar does. Our bodies don't know the difference, so for people with diabetes, this could pose an issue. However, if you have diabetes, it's important to still strategically include fruit in your meal plan to help manage diabetes. Fruit is high in fiber, which can help delay the absorption of sugar into the bloodstream and maintain blood sugar levels. Speak with a registered dietitian nutritionist or certified diabetes care and education specialist about how to safely include fruit in your meal plan.

# Popular Fruits of the Mediterranean

You already know fruit is a vital part of the Mediterranean diet, but you might not be familiar with some of the most popular fruits in those regions. Let's take a look at a few of the more widely eaten Mediterranean fruits.

## Olives

Olives are the fruit of the olive tree. Olives, and olive oil, are staples of the Mediterranean diet (see Chapter 6). In fact, although olives are grown all over the world, the primary source continues to be the Mediterranean region.

Olives are far too bitter to be consumed in their natural state, right off the tree, and require some processing (fermentation or curing) before they are considered edible. The color of olives depends on their ripeness as well as the processing method used. You can find the unripe green olives or the fully ripened black variety.

Olives are small but plentiful in heart-healthy monounsaturated fats, vitamin E, iron, copper, and a variety of beneficial phytonutrients, and they even contain some fiber. You can use olives in salads, on pizza, in pasta dishes or main dishes, as a predinner appetizer (as they often do in the Mediterranean), or just by themselves as a snack. Varieties of olives consumed include Kalamata, Manzanilla, Sicilian, and Gaeta.

Keep in mind that olives can be high in sodium and are quite high in fat, unlike most other fruits, so they are best eaten in moderation.

## Avocados

Avocados are commonly thought of as a vegetable because they don't have the same sweet flavor most fruits have, but they are a fruit—and a staple in the Mediterranean region as well as in the United States. Avocados are native to Mexico and Central America, and in the United States, avocados are grown in California and also some in Florida and Hawaii. The avocado tree has a long harvest season, so avocados can be found in most grocery stores year-round.

Avocados pack a powerful nutritional punch, with their especially high levels of protein, fiber, niacin, thiamin, riboflavin, folate, vitamin E, zinc, potassium, magnesium, and numerous phytonutrients. Avocados are cholesterol and sodium free; they are high in fiber; and as a bonus, most of their calories come from heart-healthy monounsaturated fat. With all the healthy components of avocados, they may help lower blood pressure and reduce the risk of high blood pressure, stroke, and heart disease. In addition, avocados are known to be a substantial source of lutein (a type of phytonutrient called a carotenoid), which comes from the yellow pigment in the avocado. Lutein has been shown to help maintain eye health as we age. Because of their relatively higher fat content—about 5 grams of fat per serving—avocados tend to be high in calories, so moderation is the key for this nutrient-dense fruit.

Avocados ripen after they have been picked, so buy ones that are a bit under-ripe, or firm but not rock hard. Give each a quick squeeze; if it gives a little, it's good, but if it is too soft, it's overripe. You can store avocados at room temperature in a brown paper bag for about three or four days until they ripen and soften a bit. You can store ripe avocados in the refrigerator for about two or three more days.

Avocados can be used in salads, on sandwiches, on toast, in creams, in cold soups, and for well-known dishes like guacamole. Do not cook avocados, except maybe to warm them up a bit, because this makes them bitter. To prepare an avocado, cut a washed and ripened avocado lengthwise all the way around the pit. Rotate or twist the halves to separate. Slide the tip of a spoon underneath the pit, and gently lift it out. To remove the peel, hold the avocado cut side up, and, starting at the small end, remove the skin using a butter knife, spoon, or your fingers.

# Figs

Figs are the fruit of the ficus tree and are believed to have originated in western Asia, but they eventually found their way to the Mediterranean. The best-quality figs are grown and produced in the Mediterranean region, where it is dry and warm, although some are grown in California, too.

Figs are available fresh or dried. Dried figs are most common because fresh figs do not transport well and, once picked, do not last very long. Dried figs contain abundant amounts of calcium, iron, fiber, protein, and potassium as well as two phytonutrients (flavonoids and polyphenols). One quarter cup of dried figs provides a whopping 5 grams of fiber, which is 20 percent of the recommended daily value. They contain no fat, sodium, or cholesterol.

Figs make a great sweet and nutritious snack and, considering their unique flavor and texture, pair well with meat, poultry, fish, stews, and vegetables. Figs make a flavorful and nutritious contribution to cookies and other baked goods—in fact, figs contain a natural chemical, humectant, that absorbs water and extends the freshness and moistness of baked products. Fig purée is a great substitute for fat in many baked-good recipes.

You can store dried figs in unopened packages in the cupboard for up to six months. After the package is opened, the figs should be stored in a container with a tight-fitting lid in the refrigerator. Fresh figs won't last long at room temperature, so they should be stored in the refrigerator, where they will last for several days.

# Pomegranates

Hugely popular in the Mediterranean region, pomegranates are increasingly beloved around the world for their superfood qualities. Pomegranates, especially the juice, contain several phytonutrients, including tannins, polyphenols, and anthocyanins. In fact, pomegranate juice contains more antioxidants and phytonutrients than red wine or green tea. Research has pointed to these antioxidants and phytonutrients as being beneficial in helping protect the body from several chronic diseases, such as heart disease, rheumatoid arthritis, and certain cancers. New research also has found that certain phytonutrients in pomegranates may possibly reduce the risk of a type of breast cancer called hormone-dependent breast cancer. In addition, the nutrients in pomegranates can help slow the aging process and neutralize free radicals, which can damage body cells, tissues, and DNA and cause chronic health issues. Pomegranates are low in calories and a good source of fiber, vitamin C, calcium, potassium, and iron.

Pomegranates take a little bit more work than other fruits. After cutting and peeling back the leathery outer skin, you will find the sweet-tart seeds of the fruit, the arils. You can pick out the arils and store them in the refrigerator to enjoy in salads, yogurt, sauces, and almost anything else you want to add a powerful health punch to. A medium pomegranate yields about ½ to ¾ cup of seeds. During the winter months, when cold-weather produce starts to become boring, pomegranates—which only make an appearance as fresh fruit September through January—can really spice up your fruit life. Whether you eat the seeds or drink the juice, you are doing your body a healthy favor by choosing pomegranate.

If you take medication on a regular basis, talk to your doctor before trying these tasty fruits because pomegranate juice can interfere with the metabolism of certain medications.

## Dates

Dates are another popular fruit in the Mediterranean region. Available in stores year-round, dates can be soft, semi-dried, and dried. In the Mediterranean, desserts and snacks rely heavily on dried fruits such as dates because of their intensely sweet flavor.

Dates are virtually fat free as well as cholesterol and sodium free. They contain few calories yet are rich in fiber and boast a vast amount of nutrients essential for optimal health, including vitamin C, vitamin K, vitamin A, calcium, iron, potassium, manganese, magnesium, and copper. They are rich in the B-complex vitamins, containing $B_6$, niacin, pantothenic acid, and riboflavin. In addition, dates contain many of the health-promoting phytonutrients, such as tannins, beta-carotene, lutein, and zeaxanthin. The phytonutrients in dates help protect the body from free radicals and can help protect against certain cancers. In addition, dates have some anti-infective, anti-inflammatory, and anti-hemorrhagic properties. They are said to be an excellent treatment for intestinal problems and have a laxative effect.

Look for fresh dates in the produce section of the supermarket, or find dried dates near the raisins and prunes. Fresh dates should be stored in a well-sealed container. They can last up to two months at room temperature or up to eight months in the refrigerator. Store them in the freezer, and they will last for several years. Dried dates will last up to a year if refrigerated. Whether you are choosing fresh or dried dates, look for plump fruit with unbroken skin that appears smoothly wrinkled. If your dates have been stored for a while and look dried out, put them in a bowl of warm water for several minutes to rehydrate.

A small amount of chopped dates can bring a lot of flavor to many dishes, such as salads, dressings, sauces, gravies, toppings, syrups, and more. Dried or soft dates can be eaten plain for a sweet snack. They also can be stuffed with almonds, walnuts, or cream cheese.

# More Popular Fruits

Some of the more exotic fruits of the Mediterranean might be new and exciting to you, but don't overlook the everyday fruits native to your area. They, too, can be nutritional powerhouses with great value, availability, and flavor. In fact, many of these fruits are also eaten on a daily basis in the Mediterranean.

## Strawberries

Strawberries—which are just as popular in the Mediterranean as they are in the United States—have a lot more to offer than just their sweet, delicious flavor. They are low in calories and high in fiber, especially soluble fiber. They include essential nutrients such as folate, vitamin C, manganese, and potassium, just to name a few. And you may be surprised to learn that a serving of about eight medium strawberries contains more vitamin C than an orange!

The anthocyanins in strawberries are the phytonutrients that provide the berry's rich, red color and have been shown to serve as a potent antioxidant that helps protect cell structures in the body and prevent oxidative damage in the body's organ system. Strawberries are also quite high in a phytonutrient known as phenols, making them a heart-protective fruit, an anticancer fruit, and an anti-inflammatory fruit all in one.

To get their full nutritional benefit, it is best to enjoy strawberries when they are in season, from April to July. Purchasing them from local markets ensures you get even more of their nutritional value because they begin to lose nutrients soon after they are picked. Strawberries are highly perishable and should be purchased only a few days prior to use. It is best to store them in a colander or special fruit container in the refrigerator to allow air to circulate around them. Remove the caps from the strawberries only after you wash them and right before eating them.

Along with strawberries, don't forget other berries, such as blueberries, raspberries, and blackberries, all of which are high on the nutritional score sheet as well.

## Grapes

Grapes are common in both the Mediterranean diet and the typical Western diet. American varieties are available mostly in the months of September and October, while European varieties are available all year long.

Grapes are full of beneficial nutrients, such as manganese, potassium, vitamin C, thiamin, and vitamin $B_6$, but studies show that red grapes get their health benefits from a category of phytonutrients called polyphenols. The three types of polyphenols in grapes (found mostly in the skins and seeds of the fruit) with the biggest health benefits are flavonoids, phenolic acids, and resveratrol. Flavonoids are what give grapes, grape juice, and red wines their vibrant purple color. The darker the grapes, the higher the concentration of flavonoids. Flavonoids, phenolic acids, and resveratrol all help decrease the risk of heart disease and stroke. Red grapes also contain anthocyanins, tannins, carotenes, inositol, and other health-protective phytonutrients.

Grapes are simple fruits and require no more prep than a simple washing. They make a great snack or addition to salads. For a cool treat in the hot months, try eating frozen grapes. Because grapes are quite perishable, always store them in the refrigerator.

## Oranges

Oranges are part of the citrus fruit family and available October through February. Oranges contain high levels of vitamin C, potassium, vitamin A, and B-complex vitamins. Peel into one juicy orange, and you can fulfill your daily requirement for vitamin C.

Oranges are bursting with healthy doses of beneficial antioxidants and phytonutrients, such as beta-carotene, flavonoids, and lutein, which appear to help reduce inflammation, lower cholesterol and blood pressure, and reduce the risk for heart disease. They are high in soluble fiber and low in calories—but only if you stick to the whole fruit instead of juice. When oranges are juiced, much of the pulp and, therefore, the fiber is gone. Many store-bought juices contain added sugar, preservatives, and other artificial ingredients, so read labels closely, opt for 100 percent fruit juice, and drink in moderation.

Oranges can be stored at room temperature, but they keep better and longer—up to two weeks—in the refrigerator. Oranges make a satisfying sweet snack and are a great addition to a green salad. Try mixing chopped oranges with plain, low-fat vanilla yogurt and a sprinkle of almonds or walnuts for the perfect Mediterranean-style snack.

## Apples

Apples come in many varieties, and all are low in calories, contain no fat or sodium, and are packed with fiber. You can find just about any flavor of apple to fit your taste, from tart to sweet. "An apple a day keeps the doctor away" partly thanks to apples' long list of phytonutrients that function as antioxidants as well as flavonoids and phenolic acids that support heart health. Apples are also full of vitamin C. Several studies have associated eating apples with a reduced risk of some types of cancers, heart disease, asthma, and type 2 diabetes.

One of apples' strongest nutritional attributes is fiber. Just one small apple can provide about 3 to 5 grams of soluble fiber called pectin. However, keep in mind that the fiber, as well as many of the antioxidants and phytonutrients, is contained in the fruit's skin, so peeling the apple removes most of its health benefits. Whole apples are a much better nutritional choice than apple juice because the juice lacks fiber and other phytonutrients and may contain added sugars. Apples should be quite firm when you purchase them and stored in the refrigerator for better nutrient retention.

Apples are another simple fruit that take nothing but a wash to prepare. In addition to eating them raw, you can add them to salads, baked goods, or stuffing. Apples make a delicious duo with protein foods such as cheese, peanut butter, or chicken.

# Fruit for Dessert

Fruit is naturally sweet and filled with every imaginable nutrient needed for good health. In the Mediterranean, fresh fruit is the typical, and preferred, daily dessert. People of the Mediterranean regions rarely consume high-calorie, high-sugar, and fat-laden desserts. Fresh fruit can help satisfy that momentary craving for something sweet after a meal and is far better for your health.

Other than simply grabbing a fresh piece of fruit, there are many other ways to enjoy fruit as a dessert. Grilled fruit is just one example and is a delicious treat to end a summertime meal. Check out the wonderful fruit dessert recipes in Chapter 23 for more ideas.

# Fresh Isn't the Only Option

Fresh is only one option for enjoying fruit. Frozen, canned, and dried fruit are also available—and often just as nutritious.

The nutrients in some fresh fruit can begin to deteriorate as soon as it is picked. If you're not buying local, and the fruit has been sitting a long time in the store, much of the nutritional value may have been lost. However, most frozen and canned fruit (as well as vegetables) are processed within hours of harvest, so much of their flavor and nutritional value are preserved.

This doesn't mean frozen and canned are always best, but they are an option when your favorite fresh fruit is out of season or you don't have it in the house. Stocking your kitchen with all types of fruit ensures you always have some on hand.

The one problem with canned and frozen fruit is that they may include added sugar, so be sure to check food labels. Buy canned fruit that is canned in water or its own juice rather than syrup, and look for frozen fruit that is unsweetened.

The other option—and it is a good one—is dried fruit. A wide variety of fruits are available dried, including apples, apricots, bananas, cherries, cranberries, dates, figs, pineapples, plums (prunes), and raisins, to name a few. Compared to their fresh counterparts, dried fruits have a much longer shelf life and usually contain more fiber, iron, potassium, and selenium. However, with that comes a higher calorie and carbohydrate content in the form of natural sugar, so serving sizes are much smaller. Dried fruit tends to lose some vitamins, such as B vitamins and vitamin C, during the drying process. Some manufacturers add back these vitamins, so check for this information on the label. Sulfur is often added to dried fruit to preserve color. You will find "Contains Sulfites" on the label for those people who are sulfite-sensitive. Be aware, too, that some dried fruit may have added sugar. For example, sugar is often added to dried cranberries because they are so tart; few people would eat them if they didn't have added sugar. It may add a few more calories, but it doesn't take away from the nutritional content of dried fruit.

Dried fruit makes a great snack, or you can use it to top hot or cold cereals and yogurt. You also can add dried fruit to baked goods, stuffing, salads, trail mix, and couscous or other grains.

The bottom line is that canned, frozen, and dried fruit can complement, not replace, your daily intake of fruits—they are simply another option. Choose fresh when possible, but keep other forms on hand.

What about fruit juice? Fruit juice can be another option for fruit intake, but it is not normally recommended because most of the fiber and some of the other nutrients are removed during processing. If using fruit juices, use them only occasionally, and be sure the label states the juice is 100 percent juice with no added sugars. Of course, there will be naturally occurring sugars in the fruit juice. If you are using grape juice as an alternative to wine, drink it in moderation and ensure it is 100 percent juice with no added sugar.

# Tips for Eating More Fruit

Experts suggest consuming at least five servings of fruits and vegetables every day. By adding plenty of fruit to your daily diet, you will be tapping into a rich source of nutrients that will help protect your health. The good news is that it might not be as hard as you think to consume all the fruit you need. Here are some tips to help you get more fruit into your daily routine:

- Make fruit convenient by keeping some washed and ready to be eaten in the refrigerator. The easier it is to eat, the better chance it will be eaten.

- Use fresh or dried fruit for quick snacks, especially when you have a sweet tooth. Fruit travels well and makes the perfect on-the-go snack.

- Sneak fruit into meals. Add dried cranberries to green salads, peaches or pineapple to your baked ham or grilled chicken, blueberries to your favorite pancake recipe, or chopped dates to muffins. The possibilities are endless.

- Start your day by adding fruit to your hot or cold breakfast cereal, eating it plain, or mixing it into a smoothie. You can blend all kinds of frozen fruit, along with veggies such as spinach, into a smoothie.

- Add fresh or dried fruit to plain yogurt or low-fat cottage cheese.

- Add pineapple slices on top of your pizza.

- Serve tuna, chicken, or egg salad in an avocado half instead of on bread.

- Add fresh or dried fruit to your green salads for a well-balanced, satisfying lunch or dinner. With so many combinations of fruits and vegetables, you can make a completely different salad every day of the week.

- Do as they do in the Mediterranean region, and serve fruit-based desserts. Widen your horizon and wake up your taste buds by trying new-to-you fruits.

Don't let cost scare you away from enjoying fruit more often. Many people are under the impression that fruit is too expensive to enjoy daily. That is far from the truth when you compare how much money you spend on other foods, especially junk foods. Replace those foods with fruit, and you won't be spending any extra. And buy fruits that are in season at your local market for more economical options. But remember, only buy what you will eat within a few days so you don't waste fruit or money.

## In This Chapter

Fruit is one of the foundations of the Mediterranean Diet Pyramid. Eating plenty of fruit as part of an overall healthy diet can help lower your risk for stroke, heart disease, type 2 diabetes, and certain cancers. Fruits are full of vitamins, minerals, fiber, antioxidants, and phytonutrients, all of which are important for good health. Popular fruits of the Mediterranean include olives, avocados, figs, pomegranates, and dates. However, you don't need to get fancy as long as you are eating a variety of fruit each day. Dried, canned, and frozen fruits are additional options if fresh fruit isn't available, but try to use fresh as often as possible.

# CHAPTER 9

# Vegetables

Vegetables are a significant component of the Mediterranean diet, and they need to be part of your everyday life, too. Vegetables come in such a variety of colors, flavors, and textures, even the pickiest of eaters can find something to like. Vegetables offer valuable nutrients that are essential for good health, and years of research have proven that eating more vegetables can lead to lowering the risk for some chronic health conditions.

# Vegetables and the Mediterranean Diet

The foundation of the Mediterranean diet is made of plant-based foods, and that includes vegetables in a big way. The Mediterranean Diet Pyramid (see Chapter 3) recommends basing every meal on healthy plant foods, including vegetables. That means doing your best to eat them at every meal and even as snacks when possible. The key, as with fruits, is to eat a large variety and a rainbow of colors to get the mix of nutrients your body needs.

Mediterranean cuisine incorporates loads of vegetables. Some vegetables typical to the Mediterranean region might seem unusual to you, but it isn't only these vegetables that provide health benefits. Many of the vegetables popular in the Mediterranean regions may be ones you are already familiar with and use quite regularly, such as tomatoes, spinach, bell peppers, peas, and potatoes. Others may be new to you, such as eggplant, arugula, grape leaves, and artichokes. No vegetable is off limits. Any and all vegetables get you on the right track to a Mediterranean way of life.

The simplest preparation—sautéing your vegetables in olive oil with a few herbs and spices—guarantees they are never tasteless or boring. Take peas, for example. Sauté them in olive oil with scallions and fresh tomatoes, and you have the perfect Mediterranean vegetable dish. (See Chapter 22 for more side dish recipes.)

# Vegetables' Health Benefits

It's impossible to argue the fact that vegetables are good for you. The vitamins, minerals, antioxidants, phytonutrients, and fiber vegetables contribute to your daily diet undoubtedly lead to better health. Eating more vegetables as part of an overall healthy diet has been shown to reduce the risk of stroke; heart disease; hypertension; type 2 diabetes; and many types of cancers, including stomach, colon, and lung cancers. With their high content of insoluble fibers, vegetables also may lower the risk for diverticulosis, a condition of the large intestines. (See Chapter 16 for more information about fiber.)

When you add more vegetables to your lunch box or dinner plate, or work in veggies at snack time, you boost your intake of the essential nutrients your body needs to help protect itself from disease and maintain normal function. In addition, consuming more vegetables can fill you up, leaving less room for junk foods and other calorie-, sugar-, and fat-laden foods. This leads to weight loss and better maintenance of a healthy weight.

# Vegetables' Nutritional Properties

Vegetables are nutritional powerhouses. Most vegetables are naturally low in calories, carbohydrates, fat, and sodium. They contain no cholesterol, saturated fat, or trans fat. Vegetables provide vitamins, minerals, antioxidants, and phytonutrients such as flavonoids, carotenoids, and indoles. Vegetables also supply the all-important dietary fiber, both soluble and insoluble. Brightly colored vegetables, especially dark green, yellow, orange, and red, are particularly rich in phytonutrients and antioxidants. According to experts, the more brightly colored a vegetable is, the more health-protective benefits it provides.

Most veggies are major sources of potassium, folate, and two powerful antioxidants: vitamin A and vitamin C. In addition, they deliver other essential nutrients, including phosphorus, magnesium, calcium, selenium, iron, manganese, copper, zinc, and vitamin E. Not all vegetables are created equal, and nutritional content differs, so vary your choices daily—and remember that color counts as well.

# Popular Vegetables of the Mediterranean

Vegetables are an important part of the Mediterranean diet, and the variety of vegetables in the region is so abundant, you likely can find several that please your palate. Many of the vegetables eaten in this region are vegetables you probably enjoy already. Let's look at a few of the more common veggies of the Mediterranean.

## Artichokes

The artichoke is a strange-looking vegetable. It's a large thistle-type plant native to the Mediterranean regions, but it also can be grown in the United States, primarily in California.

Artichokes are chock-full of nutrition and contain no fat, cholesterol, or trans fat. They offer a unique array of nutrients; are a good source of protein; and also contain potassium, magnesium, folate, the antioxidant vitamin C, and dietary fiber. They are rich in fiber, containing a whopping 10 grams of fiber in a large (120-gram) artichoke and approximately 7 grams of fiber in ½ cup of cooked artichoke hearts. This makes them one of the vegetables highest in fiber content. If that's not enough to convince you to try this vegetable, know that artichokes also contain an array of some of the most powerful health-promoting phytonutrients with antioxidant properties, including flavonoids (such as quercetin and rutin), anthocyanins, gallic acid, polyphenols, caffeic acid, and silymarin.

When choosing artichokes, look for ones that are dark green, heavy, firm, and have tight leaves. If the leaves appear to be opening, are loose, or are turning brown, the vegetable is probably past its prime. Artichokes are normally available year-round, but the peak season is from March to May. Artichokes should be stored, unwashed, in the refrigerator in a plastic bag. Your best bet is to eat artichokes within five days of purchase. You can cook artichokes in many different ways, including microwaving, steaming, grilling, boiling, braising, sautéing, and pressure cooking. You can cool the cooked artichokes completely, cover them, and store them in the refrigerator for up to a week.

Cooked artichokes can be eaten either hot or cold. The leaves are edible and the best place to start: simply pluck a leaf (use your fingers if you want!); place it between your front teeth; and pull to get the soft, tender flesh that sits at the bottom of the leaf. Discard the rest of the leaf.

When all the leaves are gone, what's left is the most popular part of the plant: the heart. Scoop out the fuzzy choke that guards the heart, and eat the remaining tender heart of the artichoke as is or use in your favorite dips, stir-fries, omelets, and more.

# Eggplant

Eggplants are very popular in Mediterranean, Asian, and Middle Eastern cuisine and are growing in popularity in the United States.

Numerous varieties of eggplants are available, ranging in color from dark purple (which is probably the most familiar), to red, green, white, and yellow, depending on the variety. Technically, eggplants are a fruit, but they are generally thought of and prepared as a vegetable. Eggplants look similar to squashes, with a tubular or pear shape, and are generally quite large. The flesh has a mild flavor but soaks up the flavor of other foods, herbs, and spices it's cooked with.

Eggplants are low in calories and fat; rich in fiber; and a good source of potassium, iron, protein, folate, manganese, vitamin K, thiamin, niacin, vitamin $B_6$, pantothenic acid, magnesium, phosphorus, copper, and vitamins A and C (two powerful antioxidants). In addition to featuring a multitude of vitamins, minerals, and antioxidants, eggplants contain health-protective phytonutrients such as phenolic compounds and flavonoids. With only 20 to 30 calories per 1 cup cubed, eggplants are very nutrient dense—loads of nutrition and very few calories.

Eggplants are very versatile and great when stuffed with a variety of ingredients or broiled, baked, grilled, or sautéed. In the Mediterranean, they are often used as appetizers, substituted for pasta in lasagna dishes, and used in place of meat in parmigiana. You can use them in a sandwich or add them to soups and stews.

Eggplants are available all year long, but their peak season is August through September. Look for eggplants that are shiny with a smooth skin containing no bruises or blemishes. An eggplant should be heavy for its size and have a solid sound when tapped. Smaller eggplants generally are sweeter, more tender, and have a thinner skin and fewer seeds. To be sure the eggplant is ripe, press the side with your finger; if it doesn't make an indentation, it's not ripe. If it does make an indentation but doesn't bounce back, it's overripe and most likely will be bitter. Choose one that is ripe but not too ripe because you can't store eggplants for very long. It is best to use them within a few days of purchase or harvest from your garden. Store them in a cool, dry place for a few days; if you must store them longer, keep them in the refrigerator in a plastic bag. They can be very delicate and can bruise easily, so be careful when handling them.

Eggplants, along with other vegetables such as potatoes, tomatoes, sweet peppers, and chile peppers, are classified as nightshade vegetables. Alkaloids, a specific substance found in these types of vegetables, can compromise joint function in people that are highly sensitive, although effects of food on joint function varies greatly among individuals. Cooking can lower the level of alkaloids by about 40 to 50 percent. However, people with joint problems (such as arthritis) or who are highly sensitive to alkaloids may benefit from avoiding this category of vegetables. Speak with your doctor before making any decisions.

## Zucchini

Zucchini may not seem like an exotic vegetable, but it is one of the more common vegetables of the Mediterranean. It is popular in the United States as well.

Zucchini is rich in fiber and a great source of antioxidants, vitamin A, and vitamin C. Zucchini also contains folate, potassium, magnesium, copper, riboflavin, manganese, phosphorus, thiamin, and vitamin $B_6$. It boasts health-promoting phytonutrients called carotenoids, specifically beta-carotene and lutein. With its high water content, zucchini is quite low in calories: only about 10 calories in ½ cup raw zucchini and 14 calories in the same amount cooked.

Zucchini is the most popular variety of summer squash and is available year-round. However, those ripened during the summer months are known to be more flavorful, with the peak season being May to August. Zucchini has a shape and color similar to a large cucumber, and its edible flowers are popular in French and Italian cooking.

Zucchini is quite versatile and can be used as a basis for all types of dishes, including pasta sauces, soups, stews, and main dishes. You can even grate it and sprinkle it on salads and sandwiches, run it through a spiralizer for zucchini "noodles," or add it to homemade breads and muffins. Zucchini has a high water content, so steaming or cooking it as quickly as possible with very little water is recommended. If you overcook zucchini, you basically end up with mush.

Take care when handling zucchini because they can bruise easily, and choose smaller ones because larger zucchini can be less flavorful and more bitter. Look for a moist stem and a shiny skin free of cuts and bruises. Like most other vegetables, zucchini is perishable, so only buy what you need. They are best stored in the refrigerator in a plastic bag, preferably in the crisper drawer, for about five days. Do not wash the zucchini until you are ready to use it. It is best to wash it well before eating and leave on the skin because the skin contains the majority of the nutrients.

# More Popular Vegetables

All vegetables count when you are following the Mediterranean diet; it makes no difference whether they started out in the Mediterranean regions or in your own backyard. The key is to include them daily and to eat a variety. Some of these vegetables are likely very familiar to you, and you might be surprised to find out just how common they are in the Mediterranean, too.

## Tomatoes

Botanically speaking, the tomato is considered a fruit; however, because most of us think of and prepare them as vegetables, and because they are more nutritionally like that of a vegetable, that is how they are more commonly classified. Tomatoes are just as popular in the United States (and many other countries) as they are in the regions of the Mediterranean. In fact, in the United States, tomatoes are second only to potatoes in quantity consumed.

Tomatoes are an excellent source of a variety of nutrients, including vitamins C, A, and K. They also are a good source of potassium, molybdenum, manganese, fiber, chromium, and thiamin. In addition, they deliver vitamin $B_6$, folate, copper, niacin, riboflavin, magnesium, iron, pantothenic acid, phosphorus, vitamin E, and even a bit of protein. One of the highlights of tomatoes' nutritional content is the powerful antioxidant lycopene, which gives tomatoes their red color.

There are literally thousands of varieties of tomatoes that vary in shape, color, and size. The most common shapes are round (such as beefsteak or globe); oval (such as roma or plum); and smaller, round, bite-size tomatoes (such as cherry and grape). Yellow tomatoes tend to be less acidic than their red counterparts.

Although tomatoes are available in your grocery store all year long, the peak season—when the best-tasting tomatoes show up—is from July through September. (Nothing marks the summer months better than a red, juicy, vine-ripened tomato!) Tomatoes are extremely versatile and can be used in an infinite variety of ways, including on pizza; in sandwiches; as ketchup; or in soups, casseroles, salads, dips, salsa—and the list goes on.

Choose tomatoes that are round, full, and heavy for their size. The skin should be tight, not shriveled, and free of bruises and blemishes. Store your tomatoes in a cool, dark place— preferably with the stem side down—and use them within a few days of purchase. Don't store uncut tomatoes in the refrigerator if you don't have to. A too-cold temperature changes the texture of the tomato's flesh and diminishes the flavor. Once the tomato is cut, leftover portions should be covered and refrigerated.

## Mushrooms

Mushrooms are a type of fungus. They are not plants, but they are often classified as a vegetable because of their similar nutritional value and culinary uses. Mushrooms are considered a vegetable on the USDA's MyPlate as well as on the Mediterranean Diet Pyramid. Mushrooms come in endless varieties, with the most common being portobello, white, shiitake, and enoki.

Mushrooms are loaded with a large variety of nutrients associated with good health. They are rich in selenium, a mineral that acts as an antioxidant and is critical for strengthening the immune system, and the disease-fighting antioxidant known as ergothioneine. Mushrooms are the only "vegetable" that contain vitamin D. In addition, they provide copper, potassium, and B vitamins (including riboflavin, niacin, and pantothenic acid).

People enjoy mushrooms not only for their taste but also for their versatility. They can be used as an ingredient for dishes such as pizza, pasta, soups, stews, salads, sandwiches, burgers, wraps, casseroles, stir-fries, meat dishes, vegetable dishes, and more. You can add mushrooms to just about any dish for a nutritional boost. You even can use portobellos in place of meat by grilling them and serving them on a bun.

Choose mushrooms that are firm and have a fresh, smooth appearance. The surface should not look dried out. You can keep mushrooms up to a week in the refrigerator. Store them in their original container for optimum freshness, and, once opened, store them in a paper bag to prolong their shelf life. Do not freeze fresh mushrooms. Cooked mushrooms can be frozen and will last up to a month in the freezer. Be sure to clean mushrooms well, but only right before using them.

## Carrots

This popular root vegetable boasts a sweet, crunchy taste that makes them a favorite of adults and children alike. Versatile and full of nutrition, carrots were originally cultivated in central Asia and the Middle Eastern countries.

Carrots are an excellent source of phytonutrients, especially beta-carotene, which possesses antioxidant properties, comes from the carotenoid group, and gives carrots their deep orange color. In fact, they contain more beta-carotene than any other vegetable. Ever hear that carrots can help you see better? Well, here's why: beta-carotene helps protect vision, especially night vision. In addition, this phytonutrient can be converted into vitamin A in the liver. Carrots are high in fiber and supply manganese; niacin; potassium; and vitamins A, $B_6$, K, and C.

Carrots can be eaten raw or cooked. Always wash carrots by gently scrubbing them right before eating. They should be peeled, especially if they're not organically grown. Carrots can be used in many ways: added to salads, soups, stews, casseroles, breads, and muffins. You can use them as a side dish (on their own or mixed with other veggies) or as a quick and healthy snack.

Choose carrots that are firm, smooth, relatively straight, and bright in color. Carrots are a hardy vegetable and will keep longer than others if stored properly. The trick with carrots is to try to minimize the amount of moisture they lose. Store them in the coolest part of the refrigerator in a plastic bag or airtight container. You should be able to keep them for about two weeks. If you purchase carrots with the greens attached, cut off the greens before storing.

Prepackaged baby carrots can be a great way to have carrots readily available for snacking or to use in your favorite recipes. Baby carrots are not babies, but rather mature carrots that have been whittled and peeled down to a smaller, more convenient size.

# Going for the Super Greens

Chances are your salads are comprised of iceberg lettuce—a salad green that is much less nutritious than its more colorful counterparts—and a few fresh veggies. Maybe a little cheese and some croutons—and can't forget the ranch dressing.

There is a better way! To make your salads healthier and give them a Mediterranean flair, start by choosing dark green leafy vegetables for the base of your salad. Top them with any vegetable or fruit you like, beans or nuts, and a wonderful extra-virgin olive oil–based salad dressing. Now that's a salad!

Most of us don't consume the 1½ to 2 cups dark green leafy vegetables recommended by the USDA's Guidelines for Americans, yet the Mediterranean diet highly emphasizes these superfoods. Dark green leafy vegetables are "super" because they are loaded with essential nutrients including but not limited to calcium; iron; folate; potassium; antioxidants (including vitamins A and C); and vitamins D, E, and K. Furthermore, they are very low in fat and calories and are great sources of fiber. Research suggests that the phytonutrients found in dark leafy green vegetables may help prevent certain types of cancer as well as promote heart health.

Greens can be used in a variety of ways, including in salads; sautéed in olive oil as a side dish; blended into smoothies; or added to soups, side dishes, stir-fries, sandwiches, and more. They also can be used as a wrap with your favorite fillings.

Choose greens that are fresh with a deep green color. Look for tender, brightly colored leaves with few wilted or yellowed spots. Always wash greens thoroughly before using, and store them in the refrigerator, unwashed in a plastic bag, for up to three days.

A vast variety of greens can boost your diet to Mediterranean greatness and spice up any salad or dish, including the following:

Arugula has a spicy, peppery taste. It is rich in vitamins A and C and calcium, and it's extremely low in calories. It can be cooked or eaten raw; however, with its strong flavor, when eating it raw, mix it with some milder greens. Arugula is popular in salads, stir-fries, soups, and pasta sauces.

Kale has a slightly bitter flavor and belongs to the group of vegetables that includes collards, cabbage, and brussels sprouts. Kale is rich in vitamins A, $B_6$, C, and K and is a good source of fiber, copper, manganese, calcium, and potassium. Kale is tasty when added to soups, stir-fries, pasta, and sauces. You can even try it as a pizza topping or dried into chips!

Spinach is a popular green with a sweet yet bitter flavor. It is one of the most nutritious greens, providing an excellent source of manganese; folate; magnesium; iron; riboflavin; calcium; potassium; and vitamins A, $B_6$, C, and K. Spinach contains at least 13 different types of health-promoting flavonoid compounds (phytonutrients). It can be eaten raw in salads, cooked as a side dish, or added to your favorite recipes like lasagna or pasta. As with other greens, it is quite low in calories.

Romaine lettuce is a popular salad green with a crisp texture. Although it is extremely low in calories and has a high water content, it is actually quite nutritious. Romaine is an excellent source of folate, manganese, chromium, and vitamins A and C. It is a good source of fiber, thiamin, riboflavin, potassium, iron, molybdenum, and phosphorus.

Swiss chard is very similar to spinach in taste; it also has a bit of a bitter flavor. It's rich in vitamins A, $B_6$, C, E, and K as well as potassium, magnesium, manganese, iron, and fiber. Additionally, it is a good source of copper, calcium, thiamin, riboflavin, folate, zinc, niacin, and protein. It is very tasty, whether eaten raw in salads or cooked. It can be tossed into pasta or used as a wrap for your favorite fillings, in omelets, or in place of spinach in dishes like lasagna.

Mustard greens taste much like arugula with a spicy, peppery flavor. This green is jam-packed with nutrients and phytonutrients, including folate; calcium; manganese; and vitamins A, C, K, and E. Mustard greens are delicious in salads, sautéed, added to pasta, or served with beans and rice.

Dandelion greens are a quick-cooking green with a bitter but tangy flavor. These greens are a great source of calcium, iron, potassium, and vitamins A and K. They are best when eaten in a salad or on a sandwich, sautéed with other vegetables, or steamed.

# Tips for Vegging Out

It's not hard to add more vegetables to your diet, and it will be worth your effort in the long run. Experts suggest consuming at least five servings of a combination of fruits and vegetables every day. The most effective combination is two servings of fruit and three servings of vegetables, especially green leafy vegetables, daily.

On the Mediterranean diet, you will be limiting certain foods that you might be used to eating. To avoid feeling like you're missing those foods, try to eat a variety of vegetables instead to please your palate. Here are some tips to work in more vegetables into your daily diet:

- Always keep fresh veggies in the refrigerator. Having them cleaned and ready to eat makes them easier to grab as a healthy snack.

- Keep an assortment of bagged vegetables in the freezer so you can easily add them to soups, side dishes, or casseroles when you don't have fresh on hand.

- Get creative with your cooking and add vegetables—or extra vegetables—to sauces, soups, side dishes, casseroles, salads, and pasta. You can never have too many vegetables!

- Use vegetable purées as pasta toppers or as a base for soups and sauces. You can even use a spicy vegetable purée to spread on breads, crackers, or tortillas or as a dip with raw veggies.

- Spice up your morning omelet or scrambled eggs with mushrooms, onions, red peppers, grated zucchini, spinach, or chopped broccoli. Veggies aren't just for dinner anymore!

- Forget the bread! Wrap your favorite sandwich filler in a romaine lettuce leaf, or scoop out a cucumber to fill.

- Try a vegetable sandwich for lunch wrapped in your favorite tortilla or wrap.

- Fill half of your dinner plate with vegetables.

- Serve soup, stew, chili, pasta, tacos, or rice in a scooped-out whole tomato or pepper. Be sure to eat the bowl!

- Add chopped spinach, kale, or other greens to soups, stews, casseroles, or smoothies. You can even add shredded carrots or zucchini.

- Make a point to serve a salad full of dark green leafy vegetables with every dinner.

- Set a goal of trying a new vegetable every week, whether it's a side dish or part of a new recipe. You may just find a new favorite!

Should you always choose organic, locally grown produce? Recommendations for the Mediterranean diet do emphasize locally grown foods, and in a perfect world, we would all enjoy fresh, local, organic produce. But in the real world, it's not always available, or it may be a bit more than your budget allows, so do the best you can. Shop local markets if possible, or at least look for locally grown produce in your neighborhood grocery store. If your choice is organic, all the better. If neither is possible and the best you can do is produce from your supermarket, that will work. The important thing is that you are including more vegetables (and fruit) in your daily diet.

## In This Chapter

Vegetables are one of the foundation foods of the Mediterranean Diet Pyramid. Eating more vegetables as part of a healthy diet has been shown to reduce the risk of stroke, heart disease, hypertension, many types of cancers, type 2 diabetes, and possibly diverticulosis. Vegetables are loaded with disease-fighting and health-promoting vitamins, minerals, antioxidants, phytonutrients, and fiber. Popular vegetables of the Mediterranean include artichokes, eggplant, zucchini, and dark green leafy vegetables. However, any variety of vegetables will do if you are consuming enough. Eating more vegetables every day does not need to be difficult, but it does take a little planning and preparation.

# CHAPTER 10

# Seafood

People of the Mediterranean region have long known about seafood's tremendous nutritional health benefits, and fish and other seafood are a staple protein in the Mediterranean diet.

Perhaps you don't think you like fish. Just as with vegetables, there may be some kinds you have yet to try that you actually might really like! Fish and shellfish come in a vast assortment, and they have different tastes and textures to please even the pickiest of palates. The key is to try them.

# Seafood and the Mediterranean Diet

The Mediterranean diet is a plant-based eating style; however, it is not without its healthy protein sources. It is not surprising, being that the Mediterranean regions are surrounded by water, that one of the recommended and popular protein sources is seafood. Fish and shellfish are readily available to people of the Mediterranean. The seafood group includes everything from salmon to sardines to squid—and many more.

One of the key ideas of the Mediterranean diet is eating more fish and less meat. Seafood is one step up from the plant group on the Mediterranean Diet Pyramid (see Chapter 3), which recommends eating small to moderate amounts of fish and shellfish at least two times per week.

# Seafood's Health Benefits

We know that the health benefits of the Mediterranean diet do not come from just one group of foods but from a combination of healthy foods. Seafood is one piece of that puzzle. Fish and shellfish are chock-full of omega-3 fatty acids, better known as "healthy" fat. These healthy and essential fatty acids protect our heart, decreasing the risk for heart disease. They cannot be produced by our bodies; therefore, we must get them from the foods we eat.

Research has shown that the omega-3 fatty acids in seafood may decrease the risk of sudden death due to arrhythmias (abnormal heartbeats). These fats also help decrease triglyceride levels. In addition, eating seafood that contains omega-3 fatty acids has been associated with reducing the decline of cognitive function associated with aging as well as lowering the risk of Alzheimer's disease and stroke. Other health benefits include strengthening the immune system; providing anti-inflammatory properties; relieving joint pain; improving skin and hair condition; improving circulation; reducing blood pressure; and helping in the development of a baby's brain, nerves, and eyesight during pregnancy. Eating seafood may even help reduce the symptoms of depression, anxiety, and attention deficit hyperactivity disorder (ADHD). The bottom line is that seafood is good and good for you—so eat more fish and shellfish!

# The Experts Agree

Still not convinced that seafood needs to be a part of your weekly diet? Experts seem to recommend fish and shellfish across the board. Not only does the Mediterranean diet encourage the consumption of fish, but so do other reputable organizations and sources.

The American Heart Association (AHA) recommends including at least two servings (about 3 ounces/85g cooked) of fish per week. The AHA recommends eating more fatty fish like salmon, mackerel, herring, lake trout, sardines, and albacore tuna (fresh or canned).

The 2020–2025 Dietary Guidelines for Americans recommend including 8 ounces (225g) of fish per week (based on a 2,000-calorie diet) for adults.

The American Diabetes Association recommends including fish at least two times per week. The National Cholesterol Education Program recommends that people choose fish more often.

The National Academies (Institute of Medicine) state that seafood is part of a healthy diet and can be substituted for other protein sources that are higher in saturated fat.

# Seafood's Nutritional Properties

Seafood is low in calories and low in unhealthy saturated fat—with most being low in cholesterol as well. This makes it a great source of high-quality protein and a much better source of protein than other animal sources. On average, depending on the type, fish contains about 22 grams of protein per 3.5-ounce (100g) cooked serving, or about 6 grams per 1 ounce (30g).

Seafood contains long-chain polyunsaturated omega-3 fatty acids, specifically eicosapentaenoic acid (EPA) and docosahexaenoic acid (DHA), which are nutrients found almost exclusively in seafood. The content of omega-3 fatty acid in seafood varies depending on the type of fish or shellfish, with fattier fish being higher. The fattiest seafood tends to be cold-water varieties, such as salmon, lake trout, mackerel, eel, sardines, herring, fresh albacore tuna, fresh bluefin tuna, orange roughy, and anchovies. Leaner seafood includes Pacific halibut, catfish, tilapia, cod, swordfish, flounder, haddock, pollock, shrimp, crabs, crayfish, squid, octopus, oysters, sea bass, and clams.

There is not yet an official intake guideline or recommended daily allowance (RDA) for EPA and DHA. However, consuming two, 4-ounce (115g) servings of fatty fish per week provides you with the amount of these essential fatty acids you need for good health.

We know that most seafood is loaded with omega-3 fatty acids, but it doesn't end there. Fish is filled with a variety of essential vitamins and minerals. It's a good source of B vitamins, and fattier fish provide vitamins A and D. Many fish are also a natural source of calcium, phosphorus, iron, potassium, zinc, magnesium, and copper.

Shrimp and a select variety of other seafood often get a bad rap for being too high in cholesterol. However, although the amount of cholesterol you eat is definitely important, there are other factors to consider. These types of seafood may contain moderate amounts of cholesterol, but they also are low in saturated, or unhealthy, fat. If you are consuming other foods on the Mediterranean diet that are low in cholesterol, saturated fat, and trans fat (the latter two of which can raise blood cholesterol levels), eating shrimp or other seafood higher in cholesterol is acceptable in moderation. How you cook the shrimp or seafood also counts, so deep-fried or swimming in butter is out. Other seafood higher in cholesterol includes squid, octopus, crayfish, clams, crab, oysters, scallops, and lobster. If you have high cholesterol and are concerned about your seafood selections, speak with your doctor or a registered dietitian nutritionist.

# Selecting Seafood

The more confident you are when shopping for seafood, the more likely you will be to purchase and consume it. To get started, you should know that the category of seafood includes finfish such as salmon, tilapia, and flounder as well as shellfish such as shrimp, clams, and oysters. Follow a few of these helpful tips when shopping for seafood to ensure you purchase high-quality, safe seafood that will fit your personal needs and preferences:

- Always buy fresh or frozen seafood from a reputable source.
- Check that the seafood at the fish counter is properly iced, well refrigerated, and kept in a clean display case.
- Choose the fish that is best for your recipe. Lean fish is best for baking, poaching, and microwaving, while fattier fish tends to do better when grilling and roasting because it won't dry out as quickly.
- Peak-quality finfish should be firm to the touch and have stiff fins and scales that are tight to the skin. The skin should be moist and shiny and not dry and dull.

- If fish has a strong fishy or sour smell, it's not fresh. Fresh fish should have a mild, fresh, and ocean-like odor.

- If you're buying a whole fish, look at the eyes. If the fish is fresh, the eyes are bright, clear, and protruding (as opposed to dull, hazy, and sunken in). Peak-quality shellfish is generally sold live. Unless they are frozen, canned, or cooked, lobsters, crabs, and crayfish should be living when sold. Clams, mussels, and oysters must be sold live if they are still in their shells. If their shells are removed, they should have a mild, fresh smell.

- If fish or shellfish is frozen, it should be free from freezer burn with no drying or discoloration, mild in odor, and free from ice crystals. Look for any signs of thawing and refreezing, such as freezer burn.

- Choose cooked shrimp with pink to reddish shells. For other crustaceans, the shells should be bright red.

- Stay away from cooked seafood that is displayed alongside raw seafood to avoid cross-contamination.

- Don't purchase seafood that is more than one or two days old, and avoid it if it has been in a display case for extended periods, even if on ice. If you don't know, don't be afraid to ask when the fish came in. The fresher it is, the better it will taste.

- If fresh fish is not available, buying fish or shellfish that has been frozen at sea is your next best option. You are better off buying salmon or other fish that has been frozen and then recently thawed than buying fresh fish that has been sitting, unfrozen, for several days.

- The easiest preparation option is to purchase fillets or steaks, both of which are ready to cook.

# Popular Seafood Choices of the Mediterranean

Seafood is prominent in many Mediterranean dishes and recipes. Some of the more popular choices may be varieties you already prepare and enjoy. Much of the common seafood included on the Mediterranean diet include fattier fish, which are higher in omega-3 fatty acids. However, there are also leaner choices, and it's best to consume a variety.

According to the Mediterranean Diet Pyramid, some common varieties include abalone, cockles, clams, crab, eel, flounder, lobster, mackerel, mussels, octopus, oysters, salmon, sardines, sea bass, shrimp, squid, tilapia, tuna, whelk, and yellowtail. Keep in mind that any type of fish or seafood will do when it comes to following the Mediterranean diet, but choose fattier fish more often—at least once per week.

# Salmon

Just as it is in the United States, salmon is one of the more common finfish in the Mediterranean regions. Salmon is a fish that even people who don't care for fish tend to enjoy. These fish are classified as either Pacific or Atlantic, depending on where they're caught. There is one type of Atlantic salmon and five types of Pacific salmon: Chinook (or king), sockeye, coho, pink, and chum. They range in color from pink to red to orange, and some are fattier than others, depending on the variety, where they are caught, and whether they are wild or farm-raised.

Salmon is low in mercury content and has a high nutritional content. It's an excellent source of protein and is low in calories and saturated fat. Salmon is a great source of omega-3 fatty acids and has the perfect health-supportive ratio of omega-3 to omega-6 fatty acids. (Omega-6 fatty acids are another group of essential fatty acids necessary for health. However, we don't have as much of a problem getting them in our diets as we do with omega-3 fatty acids. See Chapter 15.) Salmon is a good source of vitamin D; in fact, a 4-ounce (115g) serving of wild salmon provides all the vitamin D you need for the day—there aren't too many foods that can make that claim. That same serving of fish contains vitamins $B_6$ and $B_{12}$, niacin, selenium, phosphorus, and magnesium.

You can buy salmon frozen, fresh, canned, or smoked. Frozen salmon can taste great because it is usually flash-frozen soon after being caught. Look for fish that is wrapped well and free of ice crystals, visible blood, and discoloration on the skin and flesh. Fresh salmon can be purchased whole or in the form of steaks or fillets. Don't buy fresh salmon if it has a strong fishy smell. Canned salmon is almost always wild and contains a significant amount of calcium because there are small but edible bones of the fish included. Smoked salmon is a method used to preserve the fish, but it can be high in sodium as well as price.

Due to salmon's fat content, it holds up well to many different cooking methods without drying out. It is thick enough to grill and fatty enough to bake, poach, broil, or panfry. When baking or grilling, cook it just until it flakes to keep it from drying out.

Salmon is a versatile fish and pairs well with a wide variety of flavors. It is not a delicate fish, so it does well with sauces, rubs, herbs, and marinades. Following are a few ideas:

- Put a salmon fillet on a piece of foil. Top it with capers, crushed garlic, and a bit of lemon juice. Drizzle a small amount of olive oil and white wine over the top. Fold the foil so the edges seal into a packet, and bake it at 350°F (175°C) for about 15 to 20 minutes or until flaky.

- Poach salmon in a large skillet with 1 inch (2.5cm) of vegetable broth and a little fresh dill. Serve it with a dollop of nonfat plain Greek yogurt.

- Marinate salmon steak in olive oil, honey, and lime juice overnight, and cook on the grill until flaky. Or try it in an air fryer for a quick and easy dish.

- Marinate salmon in olive oil and diced garlic, and bake until flaky.

- Substitute canned salmon for canned tuna in any recipe.

There is a growing controversy about which is best: wild or farmed salmon. Farmed salmon is regulated by the U.S. Department of Agriculture and the Food and Drug Administration. It is typically Atlantic salmon and comes from fish farms that breed fish for human consumption. Wild salmon is regulated by the Environmental Protection Agency, which has stricter guidelines. It is typically one of the five types of Pacific salmon. Farmed salmon is usually fattier with more calories, offering more omega-3 fatty acids. However they also, on average, contain more environmental contaminants, such as polychlorinated biphenyls (PCBs) and mercury, because these contaminants are stored in fat.

The bottom line is that, whenever possible, you should choose wild over farmed salmon. This goes for other fish and shellfish as well. If only farmed salmon is available, the health benefits of the fish may outweigh the risk of the possible contaminants. To help reduce your exposure, trim the skin and visible fat off the fish, and prepare it by grilling or broiling to help reduce a significant portion of the fat.

## Tuna

Tuna is found in the Mediterranean Sea as well as in the Pacific, Atlantic, and Indian oceans. Fresh tuna is frequently enjoyed by coastal populations, while canned tuna is the number-one-consumed fish for Americans. Tuna is one of the fattier types of fish and is a good source of omega-3 fatty acids. Tuna comes in several varieties, including yellowfin, bluefin, and albacore (also called "white"). Albacore is one of the top fish sources of omega-3 fatty acids.

In addition to being a good source of omega-3 fatty acids, tuna is an excellent source of niacin, selenium, and high-quality protein. It's also a very good source of thiamin, vitamin $B_6$, potassium, phosphorus, and magnesium.

As with all fresh fish, choose fresh tuna that has no strong fishy odor. Tuna needs to be kept cold and is very perishable. Canned tuna is available in chunks or solid and can be packed in oil, broth, or water. Because most canned versions packed in oil use an oil high in omega-6 fatty acids, and most Americans already consume too many of these fats, it is best to choose tuna packed in water or broth. Some varieties are canned in broth as a flavor enhancer but can be higher in sodium. Rinsing canned tuna can drastically reduce sodium, and "no salt" and "reduced sodium" versions are available for those watching their sodium intake.

Tuna is a meaty fish and is sold fresh or frozen as steaks or fillets. Tuna is also sold as pieces as in the canned versions. If you haven't tried fresh tuna, you don't know what you're missing. The fresh version is much higher in omega-3 fatty acids and other nutrients, tastes delicious, and can be prepared in a variety of ways. Because the Mediterranean diet is all about eating fewer processed foods, fresh tuna is clearly the way to go when possible.

Here are a few ideas:

- Try tuna steaks on the grill. Marinate first with olive oil, lemon juice, and garlic.

- Replace canned tuna with freshly cooked tuna in your tuna salad recipes or in other salads.

- Cut tuna steaks or fillets into chunks, and skewer along with mushrooms, onions, tomatoes, peppers, or other vegetables. Marinate and then cook on the grill.

- Oven-roast tuna with paprika, chopped tomato, garlic, onion, and sweet bell peppers.

- Season tuna with a little salt and pepper or your favorite herbs and spices, grill, and serve over fresh, ripe figs.

## Sardines

Sardines are tiny fish that can be found on coasts all over the world, including near many Mediterranean regions. In fact, sardines were named after an island of the Mediterranean called Sardinia, where they were once quite abundant. More than 20 different species of small fish are sold as sardines around the world. Canned sardines in most supermarkets are usually small sprat or herring fish but, when canned, are considered and labeled as sardines. Pilchard is known as the "true" sardine.

Sardines are among the healthiest choices when it comes to fish and are delicious and inexpensive. Sardines might be tiny, but they provide a powerful punch of omega-3 fatty acids (2 grams per 3-ounce/85g serving) and are caught in the wild. They are low in contaminants like mercury because they are so small and so low on the food chain. They feed on organisms such as algae and, therefore, do not ingest the heavy metals, like mercury, that other fish do.

They are an excellent source of iron, vitamin $B_{12}$, and tryptophan. They also provide protein, calcium, phosphorus, selenium, niacin, and vitamin D. In fact, the canned variety, which usually includes soft, edible bones, has about 35 percent of the recommended daily value for calcium. If bones are removed, so is much of the calcium.

Sardines can be purchased fresh or canned; however, fresh sardines will not keep long (only a day or two) and they don't freeze well, so use them quickly. Choose whole sardines that have a clean smell, are firm to the touch, and have bright eyes. Sardines packed in olive oil are the preferred canned form (as opposed to those canned in soybean oil or other oils), but they also come packed in water as well as sauces such as tomato or mustard. Always check the can for an expiration date to ensure freshness.

You can cook and serve sardines in a variety of tasty ways. Here are a few ideas:

- Serve canned sardines broiled on whole-wheat toast for a simple, classic appetizer.

- Combine skinless, boneless sardines with half of a diced avocado. Drizzle with Worcestershire sauce, black pepper, and a dash of olive oil for the perfect healthy snack.

- Wrap fresh sardines in grape or fig leaves, and grill with olive oil and lemon.

- Sprinkle sardines with lemon juice, extra-virgin olive oil, and a touch of garlic or your favorite herb or spice.

- Try combining sardines with chopped onion, olives, chopped tomatoes, or fennel.

# Cooking Seafood

The best way to enjoy fish is baked, grilled, broiled, poached, stir-fried, sautéed, air-fried—basically, any way that isn't deep-fried. Avoid heavily battered fried fish as well as highly processed fish products like fish sticks. Choose low-fat, low-sodium seasonings such as herbs, spices, lemon juice, or other flavorings when cooking and serving seafood. Extra-virgin olive oil always makes a good base for marinades. Fish is generally a quick-cooking food; if thawed, it only needs to cook about 10 minutes for every 1 inch (2.5cm) of thickness. To check if fish is done, use a knife to cut into the thickest part and pull it aside. If it begins to flake, it is probably done. Another clue is that when the fish becomes opaque, it is ready to eat. When you remove the fish from the heat, let it stand for a few minutes to finish the cooking process.

If you are not a fish lover, get creative with recipes to keep it interesting and tasting great. Check out the recipes in Part 4 for some delicious ideas.

# A Few Issues

There always seem to be a few issues, no matter what the food, and seafood is no exception. One common issue when it comes to fish and shellfish is whether taking a fish oil supplement can replace actually eating seafood. Another concern is whether there is too much mercury, or other contaminants, in fish to deem it safe.

## Using Fish Oil Supplements

Maybe you are not a fish lover, but you do love the idea of all the essential nutrients, especially those omega-3 fatty acids, that fish provide. There has been an ongoing controversy about fish oil supplements and whether they are as beneficial as eating fish. Fish oil supplements usually come in the form of capsules, and most contain both DHA and EPA, two forms of omega-3 fatty acids found in fish, especially fatty fish.

The American Heart Association (AHA) says that increasing your consumption of omega-3 fatty acids through foods is preferable; however, people with coronary artery disease or high triglycerides may not be able to consume enough omega-3 fats by diet alone. For these people, the AHA suggests speaking with their doctors about the use of fish oil supplements.

The position of the American Dietetic Association (ADA) on nutritional supplements is that they can help some individuals meet their individual nutrient needs if their diet is inadequate due to extenuating circumstances. They recommend a food-based approach for the intake of fatty acids such as omega-3s, but for individuals who do not eat fish, other options can be pursued, such as foods fortified with these fatty acids or possibly supplements.

The bottom line? Currently there is no one answer that fits all. Most experts recommend getting your omega-3 fatty acids from foods, which includes more than just seafood. However, most seem to agree that supplements, in the correct dosage, can be used to "supplement" the diet but not completely take the place of foods that contain omega-3s.

If choosing a fish oil supplement, take a good look at the label. A supplement may list 1 gram (or 1,000 milligrams) of fish oil, but that doesn't mean it's all coming from omega-3 fatty acids. The amount of EPA and DHA are the most important components because these are the true indicators of the amount of heart-healthy omega-3 fatty acids in the supplement. For example, if the label states that the 1,000-milligram fish oil supplement contains 250 milligrams of EPA and 250 milligrams of DHA, then it has a total of 500 milligrams of omega-3 fatty acids, not 1,000 milligrams. In addition, check the label for a 3:2 ratio of either

3 parts EPA to 2 parts DHA or vice versa. Research suggests that either ratio is optimal for producing heart-healthy benefits.

Fish oil has Generally Recognized as Safe (GRAS) status in the United States. However, currently there is no standard RDA for EPA and DHA in the form of supplements. The FDA has concluded that fish oil supplements providing no more than 5 grams per day of EPA and DHA combined are safe when used as recommended. More than 5,000 milligrams (or 5 grams) from fish oil supplements is not recommended unless instructed by a health professional. Ongoing research points out that it is reasonable for most people to get up to 1,000 milligrams or 1 gram of combined EPA and DHA daily.

Consult with your health-care provider before taking a fish oil supplement (or any supplement), especially if you have a medical condition, are taking prescription medications, or have food allergies. Always let your doctor know if you are taking fish oil supplements because they can inhibit blood clotting, which may cause excessive bleeding for some people. And if you decide that fish oil supplements are the way to go, be forewarned: taking more than the recommended dose can increase your risk of bleeding and bruising, which isn't likely to happen from foods.

When it comes to fish oil supplements, use only reputable brands that are pharmaceutical grade, which means the supplement has met freshness and purity standards and often contains a higher potency of EPA and DHA in a single capsule. Because the FDA does not regulate supplements, it's best to look for one that has met purity and freshness standards through third-party testing (such as ConsumerLab.com), which you can find by looking at the label for a certification seal, visiting the company's website, or calling its toll-free number. Contaminants such as mercury and PCBs can accumulate in fish oil just as they do in fish, so look for supplements made from purified fish oil.

## Mercury Levels

Although seafood is abundantly healthy, balancing its benefits with its concerns about mercury and contaminant levels may leave you a bit confused. Don't give up on fish though, because it is still an excellent choice. You should be knowledgeable about this issue, but it should not keep you from making seafood a part of your diet.

Nearly all fish and shellfish contain traces of mercury; however, for most of us, the risk of mercury in fish is not much of a health concern. The concern is mostly for pregnant women because some fish contain high levels of mercury that could harm an unborn baby or a young child's developing nervous system. For this reason, the FDA and the Environmental Protection Agency advise women who are or may become pregnant, nursing mothers, and young children to avoid some types of fish that are higher in mercury and to eat fish and shellfish that contain lesser amounts of mercury instead. The FDA advises those who are pregnant or breastfeeding to consume between 8 and 12 ounces (225 and 340g) per week of a variety of seafood from choices that are lower in mercury.

The advisory states for this population ...

- Do not eat shark, swordfish, king mackerel, marlin, orange roughy, tilefish (Gulf of Mexico), and tuna (bigeye) because they contain the highest levels of mercury.

- Eat up to 12 ounces (340g; two average meals) a week of a variety of fish and shellfish that are lower in mercury, such as shrimp, canned light tuna, salmon, pollock, sardines, and catfish. Albacore (white) tuna, fresh or canned, has more mercury than canned light tuna; you may eat up to 4 ounces (115g) of albacore tuna per week.

- Check local advisories about the safety of fish if caught in local lakes, rivers, and coastal areas. If you cannot find information on local fish, eat up to 6 ounces (170g) per week of fish caught from local waters, and do not consume any other fish that week.

Even with these advisories in mind, the AHA's recommendations are to eat two servings of fish per week. At 4 ounces (115g) per serving, that is well below the FDA's and the Environmental Protection Agency's safe limit of 12 ounces (340g) per week. Eating a variety of fish and following the recommendations ensures that you can still enjoy fish, feel safe, and reap all its health benefits.

For more information and to stay on top of all new advisories and recommendations, go to fda.gov/food/consumers/advice-about-eating-fish.

# Tips for Eating More Seafood

Fish might not have been part of your diet before, but now that you know about its health benefits and how easy it can be to prepare, you may have changed your mind. Because following the Mediterranean diet is your ultimate goal, adding these foods is a must. Here are a few ideas to help get you started:

- Ease seafood into your diet by replacing one meat-based meal per week with one that contains fish or seafood. Work your way up to at least two meals per week.

- Add canned tuna or salmon to your salads to boost protein and nutrition.

- Prepare your seafood with olive oil, garlic, herbs, and spices to add flavor. Try breading fish with whole-wheat flour and a few breadcrumbs and sautéing it in olive oil.

• Don't forget: it isn't just fish that offers nutritional benefits. Also try other seafood such as shrimp, crab, lobster, oysters, and mussels.

• Be sure you are buying fresh fish for the best flavor.

• Halibut, fresh tuna, salmon, and swordfish steaks marinated and cooked on the grill make a delicious and healthy alternative to red meat.

• Experiment with fish-based soups such as clam chowder or lobster bisque.

• Learn how to cook fish properly. Overcooking fish makes it tough and dry, which hinders the flavor. Remember that fish is cooked when its flesh turns opaque and flakes easily when poked with a fork.

• If you enjoy leaner fish such as tilapia or catfish, consider adding another serving of a fattier fish to your weekly menu to boost your intake of omega-3 fatty acids.

## In This Chapter

Fish and shellfish are a main protein source in the Mediterranean diet. Heart-protective omega-3 fatty acids are one of the most important nutrients that seafood provides. Fattier, cold-water fish contains higher amounts of omega-3 fatty acids. If you are considering supplementing your diet with a fish oil supplement, consult your health-care provider first. By following the recommendations of the American Heart Association and the Environmental Protection Agency, you can eat fish safely, focusing on all the nutrition and health benefits they provide without worrying about ingesting too many contaminants.

# CHAPTER 11

# Nuts, Seeds, and Legumes

Nuts, seeds, and legumes are all essential additions to a healthy diet and should not be overlooked. These foods are a category of plants that have pods (or fruits) and include beans, peas, lentils, and peanuts, among others. Nuts are anything with an edible kernel and hard shell. Nuts and legumes are technically seeds, but the seeds we discuss in this chapter are the smaller edible plant seeds that are meant for eating rather than for yielding more plants. This group of foods might be small in size, but they're big on nutrition—and a big part of the Mediterranean diet.

# Nuts, Seeds, and Legumes and the Mediterranean Diet

Nuts, seeds, and legumes are all included in the plant group, which is the foundation of the Mediterranean Diet Pyramid (see Chapter 3). The pyramid recommends eating an abundance of, and basing most meals on, plant-based foods. That includes legumes, nuts, and seeds.

Nuts and seeds are commonly eaten as a snack, nuts are a popular ingredient in many desserts, and the Mediterranean diet is filled with fabulous dishes using many different varieties of legumes. A wide variety of these three foods are used in the Mediterranean regions, including almonds, hazelnuts, walnuts, pine nuts, sesame seeds, sunflower seeds, lentils, chickpeas, fava beans, cannellini beans, and split peas.

# Nuts' and Seeds' Health Benefits

At one time, nuts were given a bad rap for their high fat and calorie content, but now they are known worldwide as a healthy food. Seeds also provide a fairly high dose of fat. But both nuts and seeds contain the heart-healthy type of fat, giving them a health-friendly reputation. Research has found that people who eat nuts on a regular basis have a lower risk for heart disease and sudden cardiac death. Studies also have found that nuts can lower LDL or "bad" cholesterol levels in the blood. The benefits of nuts and seeds are still under the microscope, but more research and results are emerging all the time.

Nuts and seeds may be high in calories due to their fat content, but because of their nutritional makeup, they can help reduce hunger by making you feel full and satisfied. Moderation is the key, but nuts and seeds, along with a healthy diet and exercise, may actually help you lose weight or maintain a healthy weight. The fiber in nuts and seeds helps prevent constipation and hemorrhoids. The powerful antioxidants they provide can help slow the aging process and lower the risk of many age-related health conditions.

In a very large study concerning the health benefits of nuts, researchers analyzed data from more than 210,000 health professionals during a span of 32 years. They discovered that, compared to those who never or almost never ate nuts, participants who ate 1 ounce (30g) of nuts five or more times per week had a 14 percent lower risk of cardiovascular disease and a 20 percent lower risk of coronary heart disease during the study period.

In addition to a variety of nuts, you should include seeds, which may offer the same health benefits.

The best approach to using nuts and seeds to your advantage and reaping all their health benefits is to eat them in moderation and as a replacement for, not an addition to, foods in your diet that are high in saturated fats and/or trans fats. Nuts and seeds contain quite a bit of fat, and even though most of the fat is a healthy fat, it can still add up to a lot of calories. The Dietary Guidelines for Americans recommend consuming 1 ounce (30g) per day to reduce the risk of chronic disease. Sticking to a smaller portion ensures you get all the health benefits without getting too many the calories.

As with most other foods we have discussed, not all nuts and seeds are created equal, and many differ in their nutritional makeup. At the top of the list for heart health are walnuts, almonds, hazelnuts, and pecans. Your best bet is to eat a variety of nuts and seeds.

# Legumes' Health Benefits

Legumes are a family of plants whose seeds develop inside pods and include beans, peas, lentils, peanuts, and soynuts. With their soluble fiber content, legumes can help lower LDL or "bad" cholesterol levels, thus lowering the risk for heart disease. Soluble bean fiber has a low glycemic index, so it's valuable to people with diabetes because it helps slow the absorption of sugar into the bloodstream, helping control blood sugar levels. Beans' rich source of antioxidants has been linked to lowering the risk for several types of cancer, including colon cancer.

A bonus for dieters: legumes are low in calories, and foods that have a low glycemic index and are high in fiber, like beans, can help keep hunger at bay by filling you up. Including beans in your diet on a regular basis also can aid in digestion and normalize bowel function, which can help prevent constipation and hemorrhoids.

Basic legumes supply a load of heart-protective, disease-fighting benefits for very little cost, and, in the form of peanuts or soynuts, are as simple to consume as popping a handful into your mouth.

# Nuts' and Seeds' Nutritional Properties

The Mediterranean diet is filled with healthy fats, but more than olives and olive oil provide these good fats. You could say nuts and seeds are high-fat foods; however, the fats they contain are ones you definitely want to include in your diet.

Nuts and seeds provide plenty of both monounsaturated and polyunsaturated fats, contain very little saturated fat, and have no trans fat. Some, such as walnuts, Brazil nuts, flaxseeds, and pumpkin seeds, contain omega-3 fatty acids, but they contain a different source from that found in fish. They contain the plant-based source of omega-3 fatty acids known as alpha-linolenic acid (ALA), which the body can convert, in small amounts, to EPA and DHA, the fatty acids found mostly in fish.

Nuts and seeds also contain vitamin E, a powerful antioxidant known for enhancing the immune system, protecting the nervous system, and lowering the risk for heart disease. They also are a great source of vitamin A, phosphorus, potassium, folate, magnesium, copper, selenium, protein, and fiber. Seeds are among the best plant sources of both iron and zinc.

Some nuts and seeds, such as cashews, pecans, and walnuts, contain plant sterols, a compound found in vegetable oils that can help lower cholesterol levels. These plant sterols are now being added to many food products, such as margarines, but in some nuts and seeds, they are a natural occurrence. Nuts and seeds also contain a variety of health-promoting phytonutrients, including flavonoids.

# Legumes' Nutritional Properties

Legumes are among the most versatile and nutritious foods available. Most are low in fat and contain no cholesterol or trans fats. Some, such as soybeans, navy beans, and kidney beans, contain the plant-based source of the heart-healthy ALA omega-3 fatty acids. Legumes are rich sources of folate, copper, potassium, and magnesium, and most are also a good source of iron and B vitamins. Legumes are a bountiful source of both soluble and insoluble fiber, too; just 1 cup of legumes can provide as much as 15 grams of fiber—that's half of the daily requirement for adults. Legumes also are a great source of protein, offering a whopping 15 grams of protein in a 1-cup serving, and soybeans offer even more! Just about all plant-based foods offer various health-promoting phytonutrients, but the legume family is at the top of the list as one of the most phytodense food sources. These include flavonoids, isoflavones, and more. Legumes, especially black, red, and brown beans, are among the richest sources of antioxidants. In addition, like nuts and seeds, legumes offer plant sterols.

Beans also are known for their gas-causing effects. However, if they are soaked in water for at least a few hours before they are cooked, they will cause less flatulence and, as a bonus, be easier and faster to cook. Using canned beans also can reduce gas because the canning process eliminates some of the gas-producing sugars.

# Storing and Preparing Nuts, Seeds, and Legumes

Nuts are sold either shelled or unshelled, and either fresh or, more commonly, dried. Unshelled nuts can be kept for up to a year and unhulled seeds keep for several months if stored in a cool, dark, dry place. Shelled nuts and seeds will not keep as long and are more prone to rancidity. They should be kept in an airtight container in the refrigerator and used by their expiration date. Most nuts and seeds can be eaten raw, but toasting them helps intensify their flavor. (To toast, place nuts or seeds in a single layer in a small skillet and set over medium heat. Cook, stirring occasionally, for 5 to 7 minutes or until lightly browned—keep an eye on them because they can burn quickly. Or toast in a preheated 400°F/200°C oven for 5 to 7 minutes.)

The best part of legumes, besides their star nutritional profile, is that they are available year-round, inexpensive, and versatile. The bland taste of beans makes them the perfect sponge to soak up the flavor of other ingredients in a dish. Most can be found dried or canned and have long shelf lives. They are the perfect addition to your pantry to whip up a Mediterranean-style dish in no time. However, a little planning may be needed because many dried beans are best soaked before cooking. You can always cook a big batch of beans and freeze them for later use.

# Popular Nuts and Seeds of the Mediterranean

Nuts and seeds play an important role in the traditional diet of the Mediterranean and throughout the world. A large variety of nuts and seeds are common to the Mediterranean, and many may be in your pantry already, including almonds, cashews, hazelnuts, pine nuts, pistachios, walnuts, and sesame seeds, just to name a few.

Although nuts are a healthy food source, it's important to realize that peanuts and tree nuts are among the top foods linked to allergic reactions. Tree nuts include almonds, cashews, walnuts, pecans, pistachios, Brazil nuts, hazelnuts, and chestnuts. People with allergies to peanuts and tree nuts must be diligent about reading food labels, asking questions, and being on the lookout for hidden ingredients so they can avoid nuts at all costs.

# Walnuts

Walnuts have one of the highest contents of omega-3 fatty acids of all nuts and seeds, making them a very heart-healthy food. They are a good source of monounsaturated fats, manganese, and copper. Eating walnuts has many potential benefits, including heart health, lowering cholesterol, improving cognitive function, anti-inflammatory benefits, bone health, and even lowering the risk for gallstones. Walnuts are a heart-healthy food, certified through the American Heart Association's Heart-Check program. The Heart-Check mark is a quick and reliable way for consumers to identify foods that meet the nutritional standards set by the American Heart Association.

Walnuts, along with pecans and chestnuts, have some of the highest antioxidant contents of all tree nuts. Walnuts specifically contain an antioxidant called ellagic acid that helps support the immune system and may help protect against several types of cancer. Walnuts also contain high levels of the essential amino acid l-arginine, which helps keep the inner walls of the blood vessels smooth, reduces the risk for hypertension, and helps lower blood pressure.

Walnuts are a delicious way to add a boost of nutrition, flavor, and crunch to any dish, including baked goods, soups, stews, sauces, cooked vegetables, stuffing, and salads. In addition, they make a convenient and highly nutritious snack.

# Pine Nuts

Pine nuts are a major part of the cuisine throughout the Middle East and Mediterranean regions. This particular nut is especially high in protein, with just 1 ounce (30g) of pine nuts yielding about 4 grams of protein. This makes them a great protein choice for those on a vegetarian diet. Like walnuts, they are a good source of the amino acid l-arginine, which helps protect the heart. Pine nuts are high in monounsaturated fats and low in saturated fat, and they have the highest concentration of a specific monounsaturated fat called oleic acid that helps lower triglyceride levels in the body. They also are a good source of fiber and iron and an excellent source of magnesium. In addition, they contain copper; zinc; thiamin; riboflavin; potassium; manganese; selenium; folate; niacin; and vitamins A, $B_6$, E, and K. Pine nuts supply plenty of health-promoting antioxidants and phytonutrients as well.

Pine nuts have a sweet, buttery flavor and delicate texture. They are especially good in salads and can be used in desserts. They are best known for their use in pesto, a sauce traditionally made from pine nuts, fresh basil, garlic, grated cheese, and extra-virgin olive oil. (See page 223 for our Pesto recipe!) Pine nuts make a perfect on-the-go snack and can be eaten raw or lightly toasted in the oven with a bit of olive oil, which not only enhances their flavor but also adds even more heart-healthy monounsaturated fats. Shelled pine nuts tend to go rancid quickly and should be stored in the refrigerator to prolong their shelf life and maintain their nutritional content.

## Sesame Seeds

Sesame seeds are popular in many Middle Eastern dishes. They add a nutty taste and are available in a variety of colors, including brown, red, black, yellow, and ivory.

These seeds are a very good source of copper, manganese, magnesium, calcium, iron, phosphorus, thiamin, and zinc. Sesame seeds are a good source of fiber and healthy monounsaturated fats, and they contain a phytoestrogen known as lignan that is an antioxidant and may have anti-cancer effects. In addition, they contain a substance called phytosterols, which may help block cholesterol production. Sesame seeds also may lower cholesterol levels and blood pressure, fight cancer, provide relief from rheumatoid arthritis, support bone health and vascular and respiratory health, and boost the body's antioxidant capacity. With the combination of nutrients that sesame seeds contain and the possible health benefits, you have plenty of reasons to add them to your diet.

Sesame seeds with their shells should be stored in an airtight container in a cool, dark, dry place. After the seeds are hulled, like many other nuts and seeds, they are more prone to rancidity and should be stored in the refrigerator or freezer.

The nutty flavor of sesame seeds can add a special touch to even the most basic dish. They are perfect in salads, dressings, vegetables, rice dishes, stir-fries, and baked goods such as breads and muffins. Sesame seeds are the main ingredient in tahini (sesame seed paste) and in the Middle Eastern treat halvah. Tahini can be spread on breads and drizzled with honey for a sweet treat. Tahini is also used in hummus.

# Popular Legumes of the Mediterranean

Because the Mediterranean diet is mostly a plant-based eating style, legumes play a significant role. They are filling, full of protein and other essential nutrients, inexpensive, and versatile, and they make the perfect replacement for red meats and other high-fat meats. Legumes encompass a wide variety of beans, lentils, peanuts, and peas. Legumes such as cannellini beans, chickpeas, fava beans, kidney beans, green beans, lentils, split peas, and peanuts are common to the Mediterranean.

# Lentils

Lentils are a staple in Middle Eastern cuisine and in dishes throughout the world. Compared to other dried legumes, lentils are quick and easy to prepare. They also tend to absorb the flavors from the foods and seasonings they are cooked and served with. Lentils are sold either whole or split and come in red, brown, and green varieties. The most commonly sold lentil in grocery stores is the brown variety, but green and red lentils usually can be found at specialty food stores. Canned lentils can be just as nutritionally loaded as those you cook yourself; however, choose ones without added sodium.

Lentils may be small, but they are packed with plenty of nutrition. Lentils are rich in protein without all the fat and cholesterol of animal sources, making them a common meat substitute in vegetarian dishes. Lentils are excellent sources of folate and molybdenum and are a good source of soluble and insoluble fiber, manganese, iron, phosphorus, copper, thiamin, and potassium. Lentils also provide various phytonutrients that have an antioxidant effect and can help protect from diseases such as cancer. If you were to look at a chart of fiber in foods, you would discover that legumes, like lentils, lead the pack. The soluble fiber in lentils can lower cholesterol and the risk for heart disease as well as help control blood sugar in people with diabetes. Lentils' insoluble fiber may help prevent constipation and digestive disorders.

Store lentils in an airtight container in a cool, dry, dark place for up to 12 months. Lentils need no presoaking as other legumes do and cook quickly. Cooked lentils can be stored in the refrigerator in a covered container for about three days. Use them in salads, pastas, rice dishes, cooked vegetables, soups, and stews.

# Peanuts

Peanuts are popular in American culture, but they are also a very common legume in the Mediterranean regions. Don't let the word *nut* in the name fool you; technically, peanuts are a legume, although they have a nutrient profile closer to that of a nut.

Like nuts and unlike most legumes, peanuts are high in the polyunsaturated fats and heart-healthy monounsaturated fats emphasized in the Mediterranean diet. The type of monounsaturated fat found in peanuts is oleic acid, which is also found in olive oil. Peanuts contain no cholesterol or trans fats, both of which raise cholesterol levels and risk for heart disease and stroke. Peanuts are a terrific source of protein, providing about 7 grams in just 1 ounce (30g) of raw peanuts. Peanuts also are a good source of fiber and other essential nutrients, including vitamin E, niacin, folate, copper, riboflavin, phosphorus, magnesium, and manganese. Just 1 ounce (30g) of peanuts provides 16 percent of your daily needs for vitamin E, which has been shown to act as an antioxidant reducing the risk of heart disease.

Peanuts are rich in health-promoting phytonutrients, including resveratrol, which falls in the polyphenol group. This phytonutrient is also found in grape skins, red wine, and grape juice and is thought to be one of the compounds responsible for many of the health benefits associated with the Mediterranean diet. Peanuts' nutritional components can help reduce risk of heart disease, stroke, cancer, gallstones, Alzheimer's disease, and cognitive decline.

Peanuts come raw or roasted (roasting is said to optimize their antioxidant content), shelled or unshelled. It's important to store shelled peanuts, especially raw ones, in a tightly sealed container in the refrigerator or freezer because heat, humidity, and light can all cause rancidity. They will keep this way for up to three months in the refrigerator and six months in the freezer. Unshelled peanuts should be kept in a cool, dark place; keeping them in the refrigerator will extend their shelf life to about nine months.

Peanuts, especially raw ones, need to be stored correctly because in the wrong environment, they can grow a highly dangerous fungus called aflatoxin, which is a known carcinogen. Throw away peanuts that are discolored, shriveled, or moldy.

Peanut butter is another peanut choice, but it lacks the fiber of whole peanuts and may have salt, sugar, and trans fats added during processing. Flavored and roasted peanuts can be high in sodium.

Peanuts are versatile and can be used in a number of ways. They are great sprinkled on tossed salads, added to sautéed chicken and vegetables, sprinkled on yogurt, mixed with raisins and other dried fruit, or eaten plain as a snack.

## Cannellini Beans

The variety of beans is endless, but the cannellini bean, also known as the white kidney bean or fazolia bean, is a favorite in the Mediterranean region. It is known for its smooth texture and nutty flavor and is commonly found in minestrone soup or bean salads. Cannellini beans hold up well during cooking and readily absorb flavors of foods, herbs, and spices they are cooked with.

Cannellini beans are low in calories and fat and are an excellent source of fiber, helping lower cholesterol, promote heart health, and control blood sugar. Just 1 cup cooked yields about 11 grams of fiber and 15 grams of protein. They are an excellent source of iron, magnesium, and folate.

Cannellini beans can be bought canned or dried. Dried beans should be stored in an airtight container and have a very long shelf life. Cannellini beans should be rinsed and then soaked overnight before boiling, slow-cooking, or pressure-cooking. One cup of dried cannellini beans yields approximately three cups of cooked beans. In recipes that call for cannellini beans, you can substitute great northern or navy beans. The cooked beans can be added to soups, stews, and chilis or served on their own with your favorite seasonings. They even can be puréed to a paste and seasoned to serve on crackers or sandwiches.

# Nuts for Desserts

The people of the Mediterranean are not big on sweets (although they may indulge a little from time to time), so nuts are a main dessert ingredients. Traditional Mediterranean cuisine relies heavily on unprocessed foods, like nuts and fruit, making their desserts dramatically different from the cookies, cakes, pies, and other high-fat and high-sugar desserts so popular in Western culture. You won't miss them though. The crunchy, nutty, fruity desserts of the Mediterranean diet will delight and satisfy your palate—and, better yet, fulfill your dietary requirements without leaving you wanting more when your meal is over. Check out the delicious dessert recipes in Chapter 23.

# Tips for Eating More Nuts, Seeds, and Legumes

The Mediterranean diet encourages eating more nuts, seeds, and legumes as part of your daily diet, but these may be foods you haven't thought much about until now. The following tips help you add these healthy foods on a daily basis:

- Add legumes to soups, stews, chilis, and casseroles. Even if your recipe doesn't call for them, try adding some for flavor and a nutritional boost.

- Try puréed beans as the basis for dips (like hummus, which is puréed chickpeas), or season for spreads on flatbread. (See page 228 for our tasty Hummus recipe.)

- Add cooked dried beans such as chickpeas, kidney beans, or black beans to salads. You can also toss in nuts or seeds for a little extra crunch.

- Use canned beans instead of dried beans. They can be just as nutritious and are often more convenient. Drain and rinse the canned beans before using to lower the sodium content.

- Eat a handful of nuts or seeds as a quick snack.

- Sprinkle chopped nuts on top of your favorite yogurt.

- Use crushed nuts as a coating for chicken or fish instead of breadcrumbs.

- Add nuts in pasta or vegetable dishes for flavor and crunch.

- Top your morning oatmeal or cold cereal with a few walnuts, almonds, or your favorite nut.

- Top your favorite cheese with chopped nuts as an appetizer.

- Add ground nuts to homemade bread or muffins.

As you add more legumes to your diet, be sure to drink enough water to help your digestive system handle the increase in fiber. Remember, too, that nuts and seeds are high in calories, so eat them in moderation.

## In This Chapter

Nuts, seeds, and legumes are an essential component of the plant-based group on the Mediterranean Diet Pyramid. Nuts, seeds, and legumes all contribute to heart health and offer many other health benefits as well. Many nuts, seeds, and legumes provide the plant-based omega-3 fatty acids (ALA). Legumes are high in protein, fiber, phytonutrients, and other essential nutrients for good health and are a good substitute for meat. Nuts are a main ingredient in many Mediterranean desserts. Adding more nuts, seeds, and legumes to your daily diet is easier than you might think!

# CHAPTER 12

# Other Proteins

The Mediterranean diet is full of healthy protein sources, the majority of which are seafood, grains, legumes, nuts, and seeds. A smaller portion of protein is available in other sources, including meat, poultry, eggs, cheese, yogurt, and milk. These other sources include some very unhealthy food choices. The key is learning how to choose foods from each group that are healthier and fit the Mediterranean diet.

# Meat and Poultry

Meat and poultry do not play a huge role in the Mediterranean diet, but they do play a part. Meat and poultry are acceptable protein choices on the diet, but depending on cut, grade, and preparation, they can add a lot of saturated fat and cholesterol to your diet, so the right choice means everything.

One step up from seafood on the Mediterranean Diet Pyramid is the poultry, eggs, cheese, and yogurt group; one step up from that is the red meat group, at the very top of the pyramid along with sweets. The higher up on the pyramid you go, the less consumed those foods are on the Mediterranean diet. (See Chapter 3 for more on the pyramid.)

Poultry is recommended in moderate portions, every two days or weekly. It is suggested you bake or broil your poultry because deep-fried foods don't fit into the Mediterranean diet. Red meat, at the top of the pyramid, is recommended less often—preferably no more than a few times per month. Specifically, consumption should be limited to a maximum of 12 to 16 ounces (340 to 450g) per month, with leaner versions being the preferred choice. (Not sure what "lean" means? Here are the approved definitions from the U.S. Department of Agriculture [USDA]: lean is less than 10 grams of total fat, less than 4.5 grams saturated fat, and less than 95 mg of cholesterol; extra lean is less than 5 grams of total fat, less than 2 grams of saturated fat, and less than 95 mg of cholesterol.)

Red meat contains a lot of saturated fat and cholesterol, both of which are bad for your heart and do not fit in a heart-healthy diet such as the Mediterranean diet. However, plenty of healthy protein choices are heart healthy and make perfect substitutions. If you must have a burger, for example, try making it out of ground turkey or chicken breast instead of ground beef to eliminate a lot of saturated fat and cholesterol.

When it comes to moderation and portion size, you have to think smaller than a 12-ounce (340g) steak; a reasonable portion of meat on the Mediterranean diet is about 3 ounces (85g). That is about the size of the palm of your hand or a deck of playing cards. Try including smaller portions of meat with meals, and for this diet, think of meat as more of a side dish, with vegetables and whole grains taking up most of your plate.

## Meat, Poultry, and the Mediterranean Diet

The Mediterranean diet may not revolve around meat, but it does have a place for it. People of the Mediterranean do eat small amounts of meat and even smaller amounts of red meat.

Chicken, turkey, duck, guinea fowl, pork, lean beef, lamb, veal, and even mutton and goat show up in the traditional diet more often than red meat.

Duck can be considered a lean poultry if you stick to the breast meat, remove all skin, and drain any fat. Guinea fowl makes a great alternative to chicken and can be cooked in any way that a small chicken would be cooked, such as roasting. This meat has a subtle gamy flavor and is high in protein and low in cholesterol. Lamb is nutrient-dense and lean with very little fat or marbling (fat within the meat that cannot be trimmed away); however, it contains some monounsaturated and polyunsaturated fats, which are very beneficial.

When it comes to meat, the key is to replace more meats and other animal-based proteins with plant-based sources, such as beans, nuts, seeds, and grains, and also seafood.

This doesn't mean that the Mediterranean diet is a vegetarian diet, and it doesn't mean you need to replace all the meat in your diet with plant sources and fish. As long as you choose lean red meat and poultry, you can enjoy meat in moderation, along with other sources of protein, and continue to follow the concepts and reap the benefits of the Mediterranean diet.

## Meat and Poultry's Nutritional Properties

Meat may have its good and bad points, but on the good side, it does provide essential nutrients that are vital for health and maintenance of our bodies. One bad point is that choosing the wrong foods and/or eating too much of them might contribute too much saturated fat and cholesterol to your diet, both of which have negative health implications. One good point is that meat and poultry provide a long list of nutrients, including B vitamins (niacin, thiamin, riboflavin, and $B_6$), vitamin E, zinc, and magnesium. Poultry contains a generous portion of some B vitamins that might not be as plentiful in red meat, but it does not contain as much iron as red meat.

Meat also provides a large proportion of our daily protein requirements. Animal protein is known as a complete protein, meaning it contains an ample amount of all the essential amino acids (the building blocks of protein) our body needs to function properly on a daily basis. There are 20 different amino acids; 9 of them are essential because our bodies cannot make them, so we must get them from foods we eat. Incomplete proteins (grains, legumes, nuts, seeds, and vegetables) are missing a few essential amino acids or do not have enough of these amino acids to make them complete proteins.

You can still get all the essential amino acids you need without eating animal protein by consuming a wide variety of plant foods. If you don't eat meat, you can still get complete proteins in eggs, milk, cheese, seafood, soy, quinoa, and a few select grains.

Red meat is a large contributor of iron in our diets. Other meats do contain iron, but red meat contains the most. Iron is used in the body to carry oxygen to organs, tissue, and blood. People who do not get enough iron, especially teenage girls and women in their childbearing years, may suffer from iron-deficiency anemia. Anemia can cause weakness, fatigue, a weakened immune system, and a general feeling of illness. Eating foods high in heme iron, such as meat, poultry, and fish, or eating foods with nonheme iron, such as fruits, vegetables, grains, and nuts, along with foods rich in vitamin C, can help the absorption of the iron and lower the risk of iron-deficiency anemia.

Heme iron is the form of iron found in animal foods and is much more absorbable in the body than the nonheme iron found in most plant foods. Eating an abundance of iron-rich plant foods can ensure that you meet your daily requirement. Eating meat and/or foods rich in vitamin C can enhance the absorption of nonheme iron from plant foods.

## The Best Cuts and Grades

To include meat in your Mediterranean diet, you must make smart choices. To do that, you need to know a little more about meat.

In the United States, certain meats, including beef, veal, and lamb, are graded by the USDA according to their marbled fat content, texture, appearance, and age of the animal. Pork is not graded, but it is inspected by the USDA Food Safety and Inspection Service (along with all meat, poultry, and eggs). Check the label to find the grade, which will help you determine the fat content. Nutritionally speaking, the nutrient content, including vitamins and minerals, is the same regardless of the meat's grade.

There are three grades of meat: prime, choice, and select. Prime has the most marbled fat and, unfortunately, because of that, is usually the most tender and juicy; choice has a moderate fat content; and select has the least amount of marbled fat. (For veal and lamb, the grade good is used instead of select.)

Poultry such as chicken and turkey offer high-quality protein and can be a lean animal-protein option. Other poultry may include duck, pheasant, and quail, which are leaner choices, especially without the skin. Poultry is not always a guaranteed lower-fat alternative to red meat; dark meat with the skin left on can carry lots of fat. For your leanest choice, you need to remove the skin (pure fat) and choose the white meat portions, such as the breast, which contains the lowest amount of fat. Trimming excess fat from poultry also helps reduce your fat intake.

# Shopping and Cooking Tips

Although meat contributes some very important nutrients to the diet, it unfortunately has a few downsides, including saturated fats and cholesterol, which can have some serious negative health implications. Diets high in saturated fats and cholesterol can raise LDL or "bad" cholesterol in the blood, increasing your risk for cardiovascular disease and stroke. The good news is that by choosing leaner cuts of meat, which are lower in fat, saturated fat, and calories; limiting the amount you eat; and using the correct cooking techniques, you can enjoy moderate amounts of meat as part of your regular diet.

Consider these tips when shopping for or cooking meat and poultry to ensure the leanest options:

- When buying meat such as beef, pork, lamb, and veal, look for lean and well-trimmed cuts with ⅛-inch fat trim or less. Lean cuts of beef include top sirloin, top and bottom round roasts, flank steak, or tenderloin. Lean cuts of pork include tenderloin, top loin roast, loin rib chops, or center loin chops. Lean cuts of lamb include leg, loin chop, arm chop, or foreshanks. Lean cuts of veal include rib or loin chop, roast, cutlet, or blade or arm steak.

- Look for the words *round* or *loin* when shopping for beef and *loin* or *leg* when buying pork or lamb.

- Choose select and choice cut meats, or look for labels that state "lean" or "extra lean."

- Both chicken and turkey can be bought ground, but be sure you are buying ground breast meat. If it doesn't say breast, then it is ground with dark meat and skin and can be just as high in fat as regular ground beef. Other lean cuts of poultry include skinless chicken breast, skinless turkey breast, or skinless Cornish game hen.

- Choose ground beef that is 90 percent lean or higher. Ground round is the leanest, followed by ground sirloin, chuck, and then regular ground beef.

- Be sure you buy fresh meat. Beef is usually a bright red color. Note the date on the package, and only buy meat that will still be fresh when you are ready to use it, unless you plan to freeze it immediately for later use.

- Use moist methods of cooking to keep leaner meats from drying out, such as braising, stewing, boiling, sautéing, or stir-frying, and drain off any fat.

- If using a dry method of cooking, such as baking or grilling, try marinades to tenderize the meat and keep it moist while cooking. Choose healthier marinades such as mixtures of herbs, spices, wine, lemon juice, or olive oil.

- Cooking meats melts away the marbled fat that you are not able to trim away. When cooking meat or poultry in the oven, put it on a rack in a pan so the fat drips away from the meat.

- After browning ground meat, drain the fat and rinse the ground meat with hot water. Blot with a paper towel to remove even more fat (as well as the water).

- Don't batter meat or poultry or slather them with creamy sauces, which adds fat and calories.

It is essential to be careful when handling raw meat. Cook it thoroughly, especially pork and poultry, to the recommended internal temperatures, and never thaw at room temperature. Wash your hands thoroughly both before and after handling raw meats. Use designated cutting boards for raw meats, and wash them, as well as any utensils used to cut the raw meat, thoroughly after each use.

# Eggs

Eggs are another high-quality protein source used in the Mediterranean diet. Eggs are grouped with poultry, cheese, and yogurt on the Mediterranean Diet Pyramid, where poultry and eggs are recommended to be consumed in moderate portions every two days or weekly. The pyramid specifically recommends consuming only up to seven eggs per week, including those used in cooking and baking. With their high protein content, eggs are included in the meat, fish, poultry, nuts, and beans group of the USDA's MyPlate.

## Eggs and the Mediterranean Diet

When we think of eggs, we think mostly of chicken eggs. In the Mediterranean, eggs often come from quail and duck as well. Quail eggs are much smaller than chicken eggs and are among the most delicious. Duck and quail eggs are hard to come by in the United States, but they may be found in specialty food stores.

Eggs have a stronger presence in the traditional Mediterranean diet than meat does. They are used for omelets, sauces, soups, dessert recipes, and for cooking and baking in general. They also are often boiled to be eaten as a breakfast food, with chopped tomatoes and other veggies, or as stuffing in tomatoes.

## Eggs' Nutritional Properties

Eggs are an inexpensive, convenient, and easy-to-prepare source of protein. A large egg provides about 6 grams of high-quality complete protein—in fact, eggs contain one of the highest-quality proteins.

Eggs are very nutrient-dense and low in calories, supplying only about 70 calories for one large egg. They also are a good source of folate; riboflavin; phosphorus; iron; and vitamins A, D, and B$_{12}$. Eggs are an excellent source of choline, a vitamin-like substance essential for the normal functioning of all our body's cells. Eggs provide phytonutrients, including lutein and zeaxanthin, both of which are included in the carotenoids group. These phytonutrients have been shown to be associated with eye health, skin health, cancer prevention, and slowing the effects of aging.

Many of these beneficial nutrients are found in the egg's yolk. The yolk also includes heart-healthy monounsaturated and polyunsaturated fats; about half of the egg's total amount of high-quality protein is found there as well. Unfortunately, the cholesterol and most of the fat is contained in the yolk, too.

Because eggs are high in cholesterol—about 200 milligrams per egg yolk—the American Heart Association (AHA) recommends consuming no more than one whole egg per day. However, the cholesterol in eggs shouldn't scare you away from eating them. In fact, the Food and Drug Administration (FDA) has recently proposed new guidelines that categorize eggs as a "healthy" food. If you comply with the recommendations of the Mediterranean diet of no more than seven egg yolks per week (or four if you have high cholesterol), and you follow the remainder of the diet (which is quite low in cholesterol), eggs can fit in just fine—and you won't be missing out on all the beneficial nutrients they provide. To reduce some of the fat and cholesterol in eggs, use whole eggs with extra egg whites when preparing eggs.

The Dietary Guidelines for Americans as well as the AHA have changed their recommendation of limiting cholesterol intake to 300 milligrams per day. Instead, it is recommended that you eat as little dietary cholesterol as possible, as well as saturated fat and trans fat (both of which can increase blood cholesterol levels) while consuming a healthy eating pattern.

# Dairy

Dairy foods such as cheese, yogurt, and milk are good sources of calcium and vitamin D, but they can be high in saturated fats because they are animal-based foods. Although consumed daily, dairy is not a big part of the traditional Mediterranean diet compared to the typical American diet.

# Dairy and the Mediterranean Diet

Dairy products are consumed in low to moderate amounts in the Mediterranean diet. People of the Mediterranean consume some calcium from dairy but also from plant-based sources such as dark green leafy vegetables, figs, seeds, almonds, tofu, and various beans.

Cheese and yogurt are grouped with poultry and eggs on the Mediterranean Diet Pyramid. The pyramid specifies daily consumption of cheese and yogurt (low-fat/fat-free, Greek versions are preferable) in low to moderate portions. More specifically, two servings (or more depending on your individual needs) are recommended per day, with one serving equaling 1 cup of low-fat or fat-free milk, 1 cup of low-fat or fat-free yogurt, or 1 ounce (30g) of low-fat cheese.

# Dairy's Nutritional Properties

Dairy products are one of the biggest sources of calcium, but that isn't all they provide. Dairy foods are a good source of potassium; phosphorus; protein; riboflavin; niacin; and vitamins A, D, and $B_{12}$. Beyond containing calcium, which helps strengthen bones and decrease your risk for osteoporosis, nutrient-rich dairy products can help improve overall nutrient intake and reduce the risk for chronic health problems such as hypertension. In addition, getting enough dairy may play a role in helping maintain a healthy weight.

It's not only the amount of protein in dairy but also the source of the protein that is important because not all proteins are created equal. The proteins in milk, casein and whey, are high quality—meaning they are complete proteins. Adequate intake of high-quality protein, especially whey protein, combined with resistance exercise has been shown to increase muscle mass and promote fat loss.

## Cheese

When we talk about cheese on the Mediterranean diet, it is not the processed, individually wrapped slices but rather flavorful and natural cheeses. Cheese in the Mediterranean commonly comes from sheep's and goat's milk, which are usually lower in cholesterol than cheeses made from cow's milk. Because cheese is made from milk, it is a great source of milk's natural nutrients, including calcium and protein.

Cheeses common to the Mediterranean include Brie, chèvre, Corvo, feta, fontina, goat, Manchego, mozzarella, Parmesan, Parmigiano-Reggiano, ricotta, and pecorino, just to name a few. The cheese you choose should not be processed cheese, and it should be naturally low in fat or a lower-fat version, if possible, to cut back on saturated fat. Some of the cheeses common to the Mediterranean may not be low in fat, but because many are so flavorful, you actually don't need to eat too much of it.

Not sure how to find a lower-fat cheese? When it comes to cheese labeling, low-fat cheese has 3 grams of fat or less per serving, reduced-fat cheese has 25 percent less fat than the same full-fat cheese, and fat-free cheese has less than 0.5 grams of fat per serving.

## Yogurt

Yogurt is a nutritious food that, in addition to protein, calcium, and its other essential nutrients, contains "friendly" or "good" live bacterial cultures that contribute to good gut health. These live active cultures may boost the immune system and aid in digestion. Be sure the label states "live and active cultures."

Yogurt is quite popular in the Mediterranean region, but basic, plain yogurt or Greek yogurt, not the fruited yogurt with added sugar you might find at your local grocery store. Greek yogurt is thicker and creamier than the yogurt Americans are used to eating. In Greece, this yogurt is usually made from sheep's or cow's milk, but most of the Greek yogurt in the United States is made from cow's milk. Making Greek yogurt requires a few extra steps, with one of the important being a filtering or straining process, which gives the yogurt a thicker consistency. Greek yogurt tends to be a bit higher in protein and lower in sugar. However, just as with regular yogurt, stay away from the full-fat versions, which can be high in saturated fats. And watch the added sugar.

In the Mediterranean, yogurt is used for more than just breakfast or a quick snack. People often sweeten yogurt naturally with fresh fruit or honey. Plain yogurt or Greek yogurt is used in dips, sauces, and dressings and served with meat and vegetables. A popular Greek dip called tzatziki is made with yogurt and used as a dip, spread, or condiment. (See our Chicken Tzatziki Pita recipe, page 265, to make your own tzatziki.)

## Milk

Milk certainly plays a role in a healthy diet, but is not a traditional part of the Mediterranean diet. In the Mediterranean, milk is used more frequently in preparing foods than for drinking, and most dairy foods are consumed in the form of cheese or yogurt.

If you are new to the Mediterranean way of eating and are struggling to cut down on your milk intake, you can swap your milk for unsweetened almond or soy milk since nuts and legumes are a staple of the diet. Lots of nondairy milk products are available; just be aware of added sugars, and opt for the unsweetened versions.

## In This Chapter

Meat and poultry are consumed on the Mediterranean diet as a protein source but in moderation and not on a daily basis. The leanest cuts of meat and poultry should be used when including them in the Mediterranean diet. Poultry is favored over red meat, which is placed at the very top of the Mediterranean Diet Pyramid. Consumed in moderation, eggs contribute high-quality protein as well as a host of other essential nutrients and can be part of this healthy diet. Natural, flavorful (not processed) cheese is a common dairy choice, with most cheese coming from sheep's or goat's milk. Both low-fat Greek and plain yogurts are common dairy choices. Milk is not the beverage of choice but is used quite often in preparing meals.

# CHAPTER 13

# Herbs and Spices

The Mediterranean diet is all about flavor, and that flavor is achieved not only from the foods consumed on this rich and varied diet, but also from the wide range of herbs and spices used to season those foods. A pinch of this and a dash of that adds flavor to your favorite dishes, gives them a Mediterranean flair, and adds a host of health benefits.

# Getting to Know Herbs and Spices

Although the terms *herb* and *spice* are often used interchangeably, the two are not the same. By definition, herbs are the fragrant leaves of plants or low-growing shrubs. Examples include thyme, basil, dill, oregano, and rosemary. Herbs can be used fresh or dried, with dried forms being either whole, crushed, or ground.

Spices, on the other hand, come from the bark, root, buds, seeds, stems, berries, or fruit of plants or trees. They normally come in only a dried version—except for garlic and ginger, which come in other varieties such as cloves or roots. Other examples of spices include paprika, allspice, and coriander.

Seasoning blends are usually a mixture of both herbs and spices. Some seasonings can contain quite a bit of sodium, such as garlic salt, celery salt, onion salt, or seasoned salt. Use these sparingly, and be sure to read the label.

Fresh herbs can be wonderful in cooking; however, sometimes they can be hard to find or expensive unless you grow your own, which isn't a bad idea. For longer staying power, treat fresh herbs like fresh flowers. Chop off the bottom edges of the stems, just like you would with fresh flowers, and place them in a glass filled with water to just cover the stems. You can leave them out on the counter or place them in the refrigerator door if your kitchen is warm. They'll last up to a week.

Dried herbs are a great alternative to fresh. Dried herbs and spices can spoil within a year, so buy only what you will use within a few months; check the date on the container. Store the herbs in a tightly covered container in a cool, dark, dry place, and do not refrigerate.

Because dried herbs are much stronger than fresh versions, different amounts should be used when cooking. As a general rule of thumb, 1 teaspoon of a dried herb equals 1 tablespoon of a fresh herb.

A few simple herbs and spices can help bring out the flavor of foods, but adding too much can overwhelm your dish. If you are not sure about flavor or strength, start with just ¼ teaspoon of dried herbs or spices per 1 pound (450g) of meat. You can always add more—but after you add it, you can't take it away.

# Herbs and Spices and the Mediterranean Diet

Herbs and spices have been a culinary tradition in the Mediterranean region for thousands of years and are used liberally in Mediterranean cooking. In fact, they are so essential to the Mediterranean diet, they are included in the plant-based group on the Mediterranean Diet Pyramid.

# Herbs and Spices' Nutritional Properties

Herbs and spices add plenty in the way of flavor and aroma to foods—not to mention helping retain flavor in foods—while reducing the need for salt, fat, and sugar.

Evidence-based research has proven that herbs and spices also may possess health-promoting characteristics. These flavorful recipe additions are rich in a broad range of antioxidants and phytonutrients.

# Popular Herbs and Spices of the Mediterranean

Many herbs and spices are common to the Mediterranean, but keep in mind that whether they are common to the Mediterranean or not, they can be a healthy part of your diet. Stick with your favorites, or experiment with something new. Either way, herbs and spices can add plenty of flavor, originality, and appeal to your foods and meals—and a boost of nutrition as well.

Popular herbs and spices of the Mediterranean include anise, basil, bay leaf, cardamom, cilantro, chiles, clove, cumin, dill, fennel, fenugreek, garlic, ginger, lavender, marjoram, mint, oregano, paprika, parsley, pepper, red pepper flakes, rosemary, saffron, sage, savory, sumac, tarragon, turmeric, thyme, and za'atar.

The following sections take a look at some of the most common herbs and spices used in Mediterranean cooking. You may already use some of these, but you may find a few new ones to try.

# Garlic

Garlic is a versatile seasoning and a customary addition in Mediterranean cuisine in sauces, soups, stews, cooked vegetables, salad dressings, casseroles, and grain dishes. It is also used on bread and for marinades or rubs. Garlic can come fresh as cloves, dried, minced, or powdered.

Numerous studies have found that regular consumption of garlic can potentially help decrease cholesterol and triglyceride levels, lowering the risk of heart disease. Studies also show that it may even help lower blood pressure and prevent certain types of cancer.

Garlic gets its potential health benefits from sulfur compounds called allicin and diallyl disulphide. Allicin is what gives garlic its pungent odor. This compound is a powerful antibacterial and antiviral agent that has been shown to protect against common infections like colds, flu, and some stomach viruses. Diallyl disulphide is also responsible for that strong garlic odor. This compound offers an antimicrobial effect as well as protection against colon cancer and cardiovascular disease.

Other helpful nutrients are vitamin C and selenium, both of which are antioxidants, and manganese and vitamin $B_6$.

# Mint

Mint is known to have originated in the Mediterranean regions, with spearmint and peppermint being the most widely used varieties. It is highly fragrant and best used fresh, although dried is also available.

Mint is full of essential vitamins, antioxidants, and minerals, including vitamin A (beta-carotene), vitamin C, thiamin, folate, riboflavin, manganese, magnesium, copper, potassium, iron, calcium, zinc, and phosphorus. With its rich nutritional content, it offers many health benefits. Mint has been used for centuries to aid in digestion and help relieve indigestion. In addition, it may help protect against certain cancers, inhibit the growth of bacteria and fungus, combat bad breath, relieve congestion, and ease breathing.

Both peppermint and spearmint are quite widely used in Mediterranean cuisine and add a fresh flavor to a variety of sweet and savory dishes. Mint, especially spearmint, is added to eggs, hot and cold teas, sauces, dressings (especially yogurt dressings), salads, cooked vegetables, soups, stews, stuffings, and fruits. Mint can be used in marinades for lamb or fish and added to rice, couscous, or bean dishes. A popular salad dish, tabbouleh, contains mint. Because of peppermint's strong aroma and flavor, it is popular mostly in dessert dishes.

## Thyme

Thyme is native to and widely used in Mediterranean cuisine. It has a highly aromatic scent, so it should be used sparingly, either fresh or dried.

Thyme not only adds a burst of flavor to foods, but also is filled with nutrients, including phytonutrients and flavonoids. These nutrients act as powerful antioxidants, which means they protect against free radicals and help protect our cells from chronic disease such as heart disease and cancer. This herb also contains iron; manganese; calcium; some dietary fiber; and vitamins A, C, and K. Thyme may positively benefit respiratory problems and aid in digestion. It also has antibacterial and antifungal properties.

Thyme is popularly used with tomato-based dishes and in soups, sauces, stuffings, and marinades. It makes a great addition to egg, bean, and vegetable dishes, and pairs well with poultry, seafood, and meats.

# Flavoring with Herbs and Spices

The possibilities are endless when it comes to using herbs and spices. Experiment by adding them slowly and using a variety of mixtures—and boost your antioxidant intake at the same time. Here are some ideas for spicing up snacks and meals with Mediterranean flavor:

- Add rosemary to roasted potatoes for a great side dish for meats or fish.
- Add crushed red pepper, paprika, or fresh garlic to hummus.
- Roll a log of goat cheese in cracked black pepper, chili powder, oregano, basil, thyme, or dill. Serve as an appetizer with olives, dried fruit, nuts, or grapes.
- Top fresh tomatoes with balsamic vinegar and extra-virgin olive oil. Add freshly chopped garlic and a dash of fresh or dried basil or oregano. Toss and serve along fish or meat or on top of salad greens.
- Add finely chopped fresh mint to your favorite mix of fresh fruit.
- Add oregano to whole-wheat pasta, and drizzle with olive oil. Add your favorite veggies.
- Top your favorite rolls with extra-virgin olive oil, rosemary, and sea salt.

• Add a pinch of thyme to your eggs before cooking.

• Add a sprinkle of thyme to lamb or pork chops before grilling.

• Sauté steamed spinach, garlic, and fresh lemon juice for a tasty side dish.

## In This Chapter

Herbs and spices are used widely in Mediterranean cuisine and are part of the Mediterranean Diet Pyramid. Garlic, mint, and thyme are just a few of the common herbs and spices used in Mediterranean cuisine.

# CHAPTER 14

# Wine

Wine has been enjoyed throughout history. On the Mediterranean diet, wine is a key component to the diet's healthy benefits. Wine has been consumed by people living in the Mediterranean region for centuries, and their good health points to the potential benefits of drinking moderate amounts of red wine.

If you're not a wine drinker, you'll be happy to know that drinking red or purple grape juice offers many of the same healthy benefits.

# Why Is Wine Heart Healthy?

The benefits of red wine have been studied quite a bit. Researchers have discovered that even though the French eat a diet high in saturated fats—with butter, croissants, creamy sauces, cheese, and other fatty delights—statistically, they have a significantly lower incidence of deaths from heart disease. Researchers have concluded that the mitigating factor in all this is the French people's regular consumption of wine.

It isn't just wine in general but red wine specifically that studies are now suggesting protects against heart disease. Studies propose that red wine may have blood-thinning and anticlotting properties that help lower the risk of heart attack and stroke in middle-age people. It may also help prevent additional heart attacks after someone has already suffered one. Other studies have indicated that red wine can help raise HDL ("good") cholesterol in the bloodstream, which acts as a protector for the heart and can help prevent artery damage by lowering blood levels of LDL ("bad") cholesterol. It may even help prevent LDL from forming.

A growing body of scientific research shows that wine is good for your heart and offers health protection in other ways. The phytonutrients found in red wine offer a significant boost of antioxidant protection, which has the potential to help prevent not only heart disease but also various forms of cancer, such as colon cancer, by inhibiting tumor development. Other studies have found that these phytonutrients may be helpful in the treatment of neurological diseases such as Parkinson's and Alzheimer's diseases and age-related memory loss.

Wine is not the cure-all, though. The health benefits of drinking moderate amounts of wine are enhanced when you eat a heart-healthy diet, exercise regularly, and eliminate harmful lifestyle habits such as smoking. Research continues on the health links to red wine, but so far things are looking positive.

# Wine and the Mediterranean Diet

Wine is a popular beverage throughout the Mediterranean and is a staple of the diet. Countless studies have shown that people from the Mediterranean region who regularly consume red wine in moderation have lower risks of heart disease. The guidelines of the Mediterranean Diet Pyramid suggest moderate consumption of wine, normally with meals, amounting to about one or two glasses per day for men and one glass per day for women. (One glass equals 5 fluid ounces/150ml.)

The pyramid also states that, from a contemporary public health perspective, wine should be considered optional and avoided when consumption puts an individual or others at risk. Wine is enjoyed with meals in the Mediterranean; recreational drinking is typically not part of the Mediterranean lifestyle.

If you have problems limiting your alcohol intake to the amounts recommended for good health, are pregnant, have a personal or family history of alcohol abuse, have heart or liver disease, have any other medical or health condition that warrants not drinking alcohol, or are on certain prescription medications, refrain from drinking wine or any other type of alcohol. If you have concerns, speak with your health-care provider.

# Wine's Nutritional Properties

It's no wonder that wine provides some health benefits—it comes from the grape, a fruit that is loaded with vitamins, minerals, antioxidants, and phytonutrients. Wine, especially red wine, contains loads of health-promoting phytonutrients. Two of the most powerful in red wine are subclasses of polyphenols, including flavonoids and resveratrol. Experts believe that polyphenols may help prevent chronic diseases such as cancer, heart disease, and inflammation.

Flavonoids are among the most potent and abundant in our food supply; more than 4,000 types have been identified. The flavonoids are further divided into subclasses depending on their differences in chemical structure. Catechin is an important flavonoid that is related to the flavanols subgroup. It's abundant in red wine and is found to reduce the risk of heart disease by exhibiting significant antioxidant power that may help prevent blood clots and the formation of plaque in the arteries. It also seems to play a role in healthy lung function. Catechins also can be found in green, black, and white tea; cocoa powder; dark chocolate; grapes; and plums.

Resveratrol falls under the nonflavonoid subclass of polyphenols. It is believed that resveratrol is one of the compounds responsible for the health benefits associated with the Mediterranean diet. It seems to be the key ingredient in red wine that helps prevent damage to blood vessels, reduce inflammation, increase HDL cholesterol, reduce LDL cholesterol, and prevent blood clots. In addition, resveratrol has been demonstrated to be a potent antioxidant and have anticancer effects. If you are not a wine drinker, you can find resveratrol in red and purple grape skin and juice, peanuts, blueberries, and cranberries.

Other foods rich in polyphenols include onions, apples, green tea, broccoli, red peppers, strawberries, some nuts, and even olive oil (especially extra-virgin olive oil).

Phytonutrients called saponins also have been found to be more concentrated in red wine. This compound is believed to prevent the absorption of cholesterol into the bloodstream and act as an anti-inflammatory, having implications in not only heart disease but cancer as well. Saponins also can be found in olive oil and soybeans. Proanthocyanidins, another phytonutrient, can be found in red wine as well as in grapes, grape juice, tea, cocoa, many different berries, and cranberries and cranberry juice. This phytonutrient may also help reduce the risk of heart disease and cancer as well as protect against urinary tract infections.

Tannins are also associated with wine and found in the skins, seeds, and stems of grapes. Because the skins supply color to the wine, red wines typically contain more tannins than white wines. Tannins act as a natural preservative for wine and give wine structure and texture. Tannins offer heart-healthy benefits and may also inhibit platelet clotting. Tannins also can be found in tea, coffee beans, certain fruits, chocolate, and some nuts. Red wine can be a trigger for migraine headaches in some people who are susceptible or sensitive to it, and some experts believe tannins are responsible. French red wines (especially Bordeaux), Italian reds (especially Barolo and Barbaresco), and wines made from cabernet sauvignon grapes are high in tannins. Wines lower in tannins include Burgundy and dolcetto, and wines made from pinot noir, Barbera, and Sangiovese grapes.

# Which Wines Are Best for Heart Health?

Many of the heart-healthy phytonutrients found in wine, including resveratrol and other polyphenols, are present in the skin and seeds of the grape. Because the skin is used in fermentation of red wine, the amount of health-promoting phytonutrients is much higher in red wines than in white or rosé wines, where the grape skins are removed earlier in the process.

In rosé wines, the skin is left on just a bit longer than with white wines. This gives them that rosy color and allows them to offer a bit more in the way of health benefits than white wine, but not nearly as much as red wine. The longer the grape skin is used in the fermentation process, the more phytonutrients the wine contains.

Although red wine is a good source of phytonutrients, not all red wines contain the same quantity. The amount of these phytonutrients (such as resveratrol) is not measured frequently in most wines, and it can change from year to year, depending on growing conditions of the grapes. Additionally, the phytonutrient levels in wine can deteriorate over time, so drinking younger wines may be more beneficial.

Several studies say cabernet sauvignon and pinot noir seem to be the highest in phytonutrients. If you are not a red wine drinker, switching from white wine might take some getting used to. In this case, you might go for a lighter red such as merlot. Choose red wines that are darker and have a more intense color and flavor because this generally indicates higher levels of phytonutrients. When possible, favor wines straight from the Mediterranean regions, particularly from southern France, Greece, Sardinia, Sicily, and other places in the southern part of Italy.

## Reds

Red wines are classified as light-bodied, medium-bodied, or full-bodied. The *bodied* part of the classification depicts the texture of the wine, and the light, medium, or full describes the weight that you might feel on your tongue when you drink the wine.

Light-bodied wines have fewer tannins and, therefore, have a milder flavor and mouthfeel. These wines tend to go better with bold-flavored foods and are typically lower in alcohol content. Examples of light-bodied wines include Beaujolais nouveau, pinot noir, and red Burgundy.

Medium-bodied wines contain more tannins so are in the middle of the road when it comes to robust flavor, texture, and mouthfeel. Examples of medium-bodied wines include merlot, Shiraz, and Chianti.

Full-bodied wines boast the highest tannin and alcohol content and give you stronger flavor with a heavier mouthfeel. Examples of full-bodied wines include Bordeaux, cabernet sauvignon, and zinfandel.

Most red wines taste best when served at about 65°F (18°C), which is a bit cooler than room temperature. They are best stored in a cellar or basement; if not, they should be chilled shortly before serving.

## Whites

Although white wine doesn't boast the health-promoting phytonutrient content that red wine does, most alcohol in moderation does have some benefits.

White wines are usually a yellow or golden color and are made from the juice and skin of an assortment of green-, gold-, or yellow-colored grape varietals. They also can be made from the juice, but not the skin, of certain red grapes. However, because the red color of the skin is where most of the phytonutrients come from, the difference in health benefits between white and red wines is quite substantial. Although your best bet is red wine, moderate alcohol consumption, even of white wine, may provide some health benefits, such as reducing the risk for heart disease or stroke.

Most white wines are much lighter and have less body than red wines, largely because they lack the tannins of red wines. Some popular white wines include Riesling, sauvignon blanc, pinot grigio, gewürztraminer, and chardonnay.

As a rule of thumb, white wines usually go best with lighter meals and foods that have a milder flavor.

# Pairing Red Wine with Food

The people of the Mediterranean enjoy red wine on a regular basis, but it is almost always consumed with meals. There are plenty of red wines to choose from, and you can find one to go with just about anything you are eating. The key is to consider what the main ingredients of your entrée will be. Choose a wine that will not distract from or compete with the food you are eating. Wine should add to your meal. There isn't much science behind selection of wine; it is mostly personal preference.

One quick rule of thumb is to balance flavor intensity. Do this by pairing light-bodied wines with lighter foods and medium- to full-bodied wines with richer, heartier, more flavorful dishes.

Cheese is a wonderful pairing with wine. Hard cheeses are usually stronger in flavor and tend to go better with red wines. Softer cheeses, usually milder in flavor, pair better with white wines.

Don't be afraid to experiment and bend the "rules" to account for your own preferences. All that matters is that the combination tastes good to you. If you are throwing a dinner party, it is best to stick with common pairings so you know for sure you have a combination that works for the majority of your guests.

Not quite sure where to start? Here are a few suggestions for some of the more popular red wines:

- Cabernet sauvignon is best with beef or steak, duck, roasts, spicy poultry, lamb, lentils, or strongly flavored cheeses such as cheddar or blue cheese.

- Merlot is best with veal, lamb, stews, salmon, tuna, beef, strong or aged cheeses, pasta with red sauce, heavy seafoods, barbecued chicken, or pork.

- Zinfandel is best with duck, beef, tomato sauce, or barbecue sauce.

- Pinot noir is best with veal, chicken, turkey, lean cuts of beef, lamb, salmon, or tuna.

- Syrah/Shiraz is best with lamb, meat stews, pasta with tomato sauce, barbecue sauce, and spicy dishes.

- Chianti is best with Italian dishes, tomato-based sauces, poultry, and steak.

# Everything in Moderation

It is important to reiterate that the guidelines of the Mediterranean Diet Pyramid suggest moderate consumption of wine, normally with meals, amounting to one or two glasses per day for men and one glass per day for women. (One glass equals 5 fluid ounces/150ml.) The Dietary Guidelines for Americans advises that those who choose to drink alcoholic beverages should do so sensibly and in moderation. Experts agree that alcohol should be consumed only in moderation.

Drinking too much alcohol can be addictive for some and is associated with other less-favorable health issues. Drinking more alcohol than the moderate amount recommended for probable health benefits can increase the risk for high blood pressure, high triglycerides, liver damage, obesity, certain types of cancer, and other problems.

If you have a weakened heart or other major health issues associated with your heart, you should avoid alcohol. If you take aspirin daily, you should avoid or limit your alcohol consumption based on your health-care provider's advice.

The benefits discussed in this chapter are associated with consistent, moderate consumption of red wine. Serious health implications are associated with both heavy drinking and sporadic binge drinking. If you are not sure if drinking red wine is right for you, speak with your health-care provider.

# What If You Don't Drink?

Red wine's probable health benefits look promising; however, they are certainly no reason to start drinking if you don't already do so. The American Heart Association (AHA) cautions people *not* to start drinking if they do not already drink alcohol. If you do drink alcohol, do so in moderation. The AHA recommends an average of one or two drinks per day for men and one drink for women, with 5 fluid ounces (150ml) of wine equaling one drink.

If you don't drink alcohol, there are other ways to get many of the same health benefits red wine offers. Several studies have suggested that drinking red or purple grape juice may have some of the same beneficial health effects as drinking red wine. In fact, studies on Concord grapes, which are used to make many brands of grape juice, have been underway for many years and have shown that these grapes are loaded with a vast variety of flavonoids and resveratrol, as found in red wine. Grape juice also can contain a lot of calories so, just like red wine, drink it in moderation. Always read the food label to ensure you are buying 100 percent juice and not a grape drink with added sugar.

Many foods in the purple/blue fruit group have many of the same phytonutrients as red wine, including blueberries, blackberries, strawberries, cranberries, purple or red whole grapes, plums (fresh or dried), and eggplant. Most fruits and vegetables offer benefits for heart protection and health, so include a variety of fruits and vegetables to maximize heart health, and stay physically active.

## In This Chapter

Research shows that red wine has heart-healthy benefits, anticancer effects, and neurological benefits. Red wine is loaded with health-promoting phytonutrients, including flavonoids and resveratrol. The guidelines of the Mediterranean Diet Pyramid suggest moderate consumption of wine with meals amounting to about one or two glasses per day for men and one glass per day for women. (One glass equals 5 fluid ounces/150ml.) If you don't drink, don't start. Try drinking 100 percent red or purple grape juice as an alternative.

# PART 3

# TREASURES OF THE MEDITERRANEAN DIET

The Mediterranean diet is, without a doubt, one of the healthiest. But what makes this diet so good for you? Part of it is the Mediterranean lifestyle as a whole, but the biggest part is the food.

This way of eating is so healthy for your heart and overall well-being. Part 3 takes a closer look at the foods popular in the Mediterranean diet and what makes them so good for you. You learn about fat, fiber, and other essential nutrients that make this not just a diet, but a change to your way of eating that you will want to adopt as your permanent way of life.

# CHAPTER 15

# Fat

For decades, warnings have swirled around the reality of how much fat we eat. We have been taught that low fat is the best approach to both losing weight and lowering our risk for heart disease. Although we know fat is an essential nutrient, the Mediterranean diet has proven to us that it is not just the amount of fat we eat, but more importantly, the *types* of fat we consume.

Fat can be a confusing topic, with good fats, bad fats, healthy fats, and unhealthy fats. This chapter helps you make sense of it all and better understand how to make fat work to your benefit in your diet.

# Fats Matter

Some people can't get enough fat and overeat in this food category; others fear fat and take it to the extreme by eating little to no fat. The keys are balance and sticking to a diet made of mostly healthy fats. Because fats *do* matter in our diet. They are an essential nutrient, and we could not survive without them. Here are a few jobs they have in the body:

- Fat, along with carbohydrates and protein, provides the body with a source of energy to power physical activity and basic functions that keep our body going.

- Fat supports cell growth and aids in the production of important hormones.

- Fat enables the fat-soluble vitamins A, D, E, and K and the phytonutrient carotenoids to be transported and absorbed through the bloodstream. Without fat in our diet, we would be deficient in these nutrients.

- Fat supplies essential fatty acids that our bodies cannot make and that we must get from the foods we eat.

- Fat helps promote healthy skin and hair.

- Fat supports and protects our vital organs and bones from injury and provides insulation as a fat layer under the skin, keeping us warm in cold weather.

- Fat adds flavor and aroma to foods and satiety to our diets.

# How the Mediterranean Diet Delivers Healthy Fats

People of the Mediterranean region certainly eat their fair share of fat, but it comes in the form of healthy fats and is balanced with other healthy foods, moderate portions, and regular physical activity. A low-fat diet may not always be the way to go because such diets can be lacking enough of these healthy fats. Thanks to the Mediterranean diet, the word *fat* doesn't seem quite so scary anymore. Even though the Mediterranean diet adds up to about 35 to 40 percent of total daily calories from fat sources, those fat sources contain mostly healthy fats.

Olive oil is the primary fat source in Mediterranean foods and cooking. As you learned in Chapter 6, olive oil is full of monounsaturated fats that, when used in place of unhealthy fats, have been proven to be heart healthy. Other healthy fats of the Mediterranean diet include polyunsaturated fats and omega-3 fatty acids, which are found in fish, seafood, nuts, seeds, olives, and heart-healthy oils. Olive oil, the most commonly used fat in the Mediterranean diet, contains zero trans fat and is lower in saturated fat than many other commonly used fats, such as butter or shortening.

The 2020–2025 Dietary Guidelines for Americans no longer specify an upper limit for how much fat you should consume daily. However, the dietary reference intake (DRI) for fat set by the National Academy of Sciences is 20 to 35 percent of total daily calories for adults. The American Heart Association recommends limiting saturated fat intake to less than 5 or 6 percent of total daily calories, with the rest coming from polyunsaturated and monounsaturated fats such as nuts, seeds, fish, and vegetable oils.

The Mediterranean diet is moderately higher in fat than other recommendations, but it is not the amount of fat that is the issue as much as it is the type of fat consumed. The Mediterranean diet is much higher in monounsaturated fats than the typical Western diet, with well over half of the fat calories coming directly from monounsaturated fats. The average American's fat intake is about 30 to 40 percent, with about 20 percent coming from unhealthy trans fats and saturated fats.

The idea is not to simply add healthy fat sources to the foods you already eat but to replace the bad fats in your diet with good fats.

# What Are Fats?

Fats belong to a group called lipids, a general term that refers to all fats, cholesterol, and fatlike substances. In scientific terms, fats are chains of carbon, hydrogen, and oxygen.

Some fats are solid at room temperature, while others are liquid. Whether they are solid or liquid, the fat we consume from food, termed triglycerides, is broken down in the body to fatty acids and glycerol. You may have had your blood triglyceride levels checked by your doctor if you have had a lipid profile or cholesterol test. Besides being found as fat in food, triglycerides also circulate in the bloodstream and are deposited in the body's fat cells. A high triglyceride level can be a risk factor for heart disease.

There are three types of fatty acids: monounsaturated, polyunsaturated, and saturated. Most fat-containing foods and oils contain a mixture of these fatty acids and are classified according to the dominant fat. Depending on the proportion of fatty acid content, they will either be liquid (such as olive oil) if they have more unsaturated fats or solid (such as butter) if they have more saturated fats.

Fats can be divided into two basic categories: good and bad. But whether good or bad, all fats are created equal when it comes to calories. Healthy or unhealthy, all fats are higher in calories (9 calories per gram) than the other two macronutrients, carbohydrates and protein (both 4 calories per gram). The biggest difference between fats is that the good fats are healthy fats and have health-promoting effects, and the bad fats have the opposite effect.

# The Good Fats

The good fats include monounsaturated fats, polyunsaturated fats, and omega-3 fatty acids. This is the category of fats most prevalent in the Mediterranean diet.

## Monounsaturated Fats

Foods found in the Mediterranean diet are most abundant in monounsaturated fats. Monounsaturated fats are deemed *mono* because they are missing one hydrogen pair on their chemical chain. There are many different types of monounsaturated fats, but oleic acid is the most common, comprising about 90 percent of fats found in the typical diet. These fats are typically liquid at room temperature but solidify when chilled.

These healthy fats are a good source of vitamin E, a powerful antioxidant that has been associated with reducing the risk of heart disease. Research shows that monounsaturated fats, when used to replace saturated or trans fats, can help lower total cholesterol and LDL ("bad") blood cholesterol, reducing the risk for heart disease and stroke. Research also has shown that these fats can reduce inflammation and possibly protect from some forms of cancer, as well as help increase insulin sensitivity, which aids the body in better utilizing glucose or blood sugar.

In addition, because fat takes longer to digest than protein and carbohydrates, these fats can increase satiety after a meal or snack. Consuming too many unhealthy fats can pose health problems, but fortunately, unsaturated fats (such as monounsaturated fats) do not pose health risks and even have a number of benefits. By adding them to your diet, you will feel fuller and more satisfied, which can help you stick to a healthier diet regimen by making it easier to control portion sizes and eat only at scheduled times.

Foods highest in monounsaturated fatty acids include olives and olive oil; canola, peanut, sunflower, and sesame oils; avocados; hazelnuts, macadamia nuts, almonds, brazil nuts, cashews, and pecans; sesame seeds and pumpkin seeds; and peanut butter.

## Polyunsaturated Fats

Polyunsaturated fats are another healthy fat found in the Mediterranean diet. These fats are deemed *poly* because, unlike monounsaturated fats, they have more than one missing hydrogen pair on their chemical chain. These fats are typically liquid both at room temperature and when chilled.

When polyunsaturated fats are consumed in moderation and used to replace saturated fats or trans fats in the diet, they can help reduce total cholesterol, lower LDL (bad) blood cholesterol levels, and lower blood triglyceride levels, thus lowering the risk for heart disease and stroke. These types of unsaturated fats include omega-6 and omega-3 fatty acids, which are essential to our health, but because the body cannot produce them, we must get them from the foods we eat. Polyunsaturated fats have many of the same health benefits as monounsaturated fats.

Foods highest in polyunsaturated fatty acids include soybean, corn, and safflower oils; walnuts, pine nuts, and butternuts; sunflower seeds, flaxseeds, and sesame seeds; and fatty fish and shellfish.

## Omega-3 Fatty Acids

Omega-3 fatty acids are a group of polyunsaturated fatty acids that provide numerous health benefits. The Mediterranean diet is loaded with omega-3 fatty acids, which is one of the reasons the people of this region tend to be healthier.

These fats play a crucial role in brain function and normal growth and body development. Research shows that omega-3 fatty acids help reduce inflammation and may have the power to reduce the risk of heart disease, cancer, and arthritis. They may help lower total cholesterol, increase HDL ("good") cholesterol, lower triglycerides, lower blood pressure, alleviate some symptoms of depression and other psychological disorders, improve skin disorders, and aid in eye health. These fats may also help prevent age-related mental decline and lower the risk for Alzheimer's disease. The list continues to grow as more research is done.

Omega-3 fatty acids are found mostly in fatty fish such as salmon, mackerel, halibut, tuna, and herring. In fish, they are found in the forms of eicosapentaeonic acid (EPA) and docoshexaeonic acid (DHA), both discussed in Chapter 10. These two types of omega-3 fatty acids provide the greatest potential health benefits. Omega-3 fatty acids also can be found in a variety of plant foods, including walnuts, soybeans, flaxseeds, pumpkin seeds, and numerous nut oils.

Just two servings a week of foods high in omega-3 fatty acids can give you what you need to reap their health benefits. As with the other healthy fats, they should replace the unhealthier fats, not be in addition to them. But don't go overboard—too much omega-3, in the form of supplements, can have health implications for some people.

## Omega-6 Fatty Acids

Omega-6 fatty acids are a group of polyunsaturated fats that you may not have heard as much about. They, too, are considered an essential fatty acid because they are necessary for our health; however, our body cannot make them, so we must get them from the foods we eat.

Just like omega-3 fatty acids, omega-6 fatty acids play a crucial role in brain function and normal growth and development. When used to replace unhealthy fats, these fatty acids have been shown to be beneficial in reducing blood cholesterol levels, therefore lowering the risk for heart disease and stroke.

The most common omega-6 fatty acids are linoleic acid (LA) and arachidonic acid (AA). The one we consume the most of, LA, is found mostly in nuts, seeds, and many vegetable oils, such as soybean, corn, safflower, and sunflower. Because many of these types of refined oils are used in processed foods, they also can be found in many snack foods, cookies, crackers, sweets, and even fast foods. The omega-6 fatty acids we consume the least of can be found in meat, poultry, eggs, and some fish.

There has been much controversy and confusion concerning omega-6 fatty acids. The problem revolves around how much of this fatty acid we should consume because it is believed that AA has pro-inflammatory properties, which can be linked to heart disease. Some believe these pro-inflammatory properties can be remedied with the proper intake or ratio of omega-3 fatty acids to omega-6 fatty acids.

Experts do agree that omega-6 fatty acids and omega-3 fatty acids should be consumed in varying degrees and that there should be some type of ratio or balance between them. The typical American diet is usually off-balance, providing excessive amounts of omega-6 fatty acids and low levels of omega-3 fatty acids. The Mediterranean diet provides a healthier balance between the two fatty acids, making it more heart healthy. The Mediterranean diet is more favorably balanced because it doesn't include as much of the meats, sweets, refined oils, and processed foods that are high in omega-6 fatty acids. Instead, the diet includes more foods higher in omega-3 fatty acids and contributes a better balance of the good foods that contain omega-6 fatty acids.

The key is a proper balance of these omega fatty acids. The solution is not only decreasing the amount of omega-6 fatty acids you consume but also increasing the omega-3 fatty acids. In general, you can cut back on omega-6 fatty acids and increase omega-3 fatty acids by reducing your consumption of processed foods and fast foods; replacing polyunsaturated refined vegetable oils with extra-virgin olive oil; and eating less meat and more fish, nuts, and seeds. However, the bottom line is that we do get more LA than AA in most of our diets. Omega-6 fatty acids are essential, are associated with a lower risk for heart disease and stroke, and can be a part of a healthy diet when balanced correctly.

# The Bad Fats

In the war on fats, the bad guys are saturated fats and trans fats. Fortunately, both of these types of fat are very limited on the Mediterranean diet.

## Saturated Fats

Saturated fats are one of the bad fats. The chemical structure of these fats is fully saturated with hydrogen atoms. This makes saturated fat solid at room temperature, unlike unsaturated fats that are liquid at room temperature.

Saturated fats are the main cause of high blood cholesterol levels, even more so than dietary cholesterol. And because many of the foods that are high in saturated fat are also high in cholesterol, it's a double whammy. Saturated fats trigger the liver to make more LDL (bad) cholesterol. This all adds up to a higher risk for heart disease, stroke, and some types of cancer.

Saturated fats are found naturally in most animal-based foods such as meat, poultry, butter, and whole or reduced-fat milk and milk products. In addition, many baked goods and fried foods contain high levels of saturated fat. Even though most vegetable oils contain more unsaturated fat, a few contain more saturated fat. Foods that contain coconut or coconut oil, or palm and palm kernel oils are high in saturated fats, but they do not contain cholesterol.

You can reduce your intake of saturated fats by using unsaturated fat sources (such as olive oil instead of butter or hydrogenated margarines), limiting or avoiding high-fat sauces, choosing leaner cuts of meat, avoiding processed meats, and consuming fat-free or low-fat dairy products. You also should check food label ingredient lists for both the amount of saturated fat in the product and ingredients to avoid, such as hydrogenated vegetable oil, shortening, coconut oil, palm kernel oil, or cocoa butter.

Just a small reduction in saturated fat in your diet can go a long way. A report by the National Cholesterol Education Program recognized that a 1 percent decrease in dietary saturated fat led to a 2 percent decrease in LDL (bad) cholesterol, which led to a 2 percent decrease in heart disease risk.

## Trans Fats

The worst fat you can eat is trans fat. These types of fats are created when a liquid vegetable oil is made more solid by the addition of hydrogen through a process called hydrogenation. These more solid fats gained popularity with manufacturers because they increase the shelf life and flavor of many baked and processed foods.

Trans fats have received more attention lately because researchers have found out just how dangerous they are to our health. Trans fats raise LDL (bad) cholesterol and lower HDL (good) cholesterol. In fact, some experts believe they can raise LDL cholesterol even more than saturated fats can. Consuming these fats increases your risk for heart disease and stroke and is also associated with a higher risk for developing type 2 diabetes.

Although a small amount of trans fats is found naturally in animal foods and dairy products, most are added to foods through hydrogenation. Trans fats are found in a large variety of foods, including fried foods, commercial baked goods, stick margarines, shortening, fast foods, snack foods, and any food that contains hydrogenated vegetable oils.

In January 2006, the FDA required that all manufacturers begin adding trans fat to their Nutrition Facts label on packaged foods to make it easier for consumers to see how much trans fat is in the foods they are choosing. However, products can be labeled as "0 grams of trans fats" if they contain 0 to less than 0.5 grams of trans fat per serving. You can spot trans fat in a product by reading the ingredient list and looking for the ingredients referred to as "partially hydrogenated oils."

Trans fats have absolutely no health benefits, and most experts agree that the less trans fat you eat, the better. Public health authorities recommend limiting the amount of trans fat you consume to no more than1 percent of your total daily calories. If you eat 2,000 calories per day, that means getting no more than 20 of those calories from trans fats—which is 2 grams or fewer per day.

You can decrease the amount of trans fats you eat by including more fruits, vegetables, whole grains, and fat-free or low-fat dairy products. Also include leaner cuts of meat, poultry without the skin, fish, seafood, legumes, nuts, and seeds. Limit your intake of commercial baked goods, crackers, cookies, snack foods, and other processed foods. Use olive oil instead of butter or margarine. Check food labels for trans fat, and look on ingredient lists for hydrogenated or partially hydrogenated vegetable oils. Most importantly, follow the Mediterranean diet, and trans fat will be a distant thought.

## Dietary Cholesterol

Cholesterol in foods is not really a fat, but a fatlike substance found only in animal foods such as meat, eggs, cheese, milk, and poultry. We do get cholesterol from the foods we eat, but our liver produces all we need—so no dietary cholesterol is required. Cholesterol does play an important role in the body, but it is when we have excess that problems occur.

Our body needs cholesterol for some very important functions, including making hormones, bile acids, and vitamin D. In addition, cholesterol is part of every body cell. Any unused excess cholesterol, whether from food or produced by our body, gets stored as plaque in the arteries, increasing the risk for heart disease and stroke. Limiting dietary cholesterol and the fats that raise blood cholesterol—saturated fats and trans fats—is part of the heart-healthy equation.

For people who already have high cholesterol, therapeutic diet guidelines can include as much as 10 percent of total calories from polyunsaturated fats and up to 20 percent from monounsaturated fats because these fats can actually help lower blood cholesterol levels and the risk of heart disease. This explains a lot when it comes to the Mediterranean diet, which is higher in both of these unsaturated fats and, therefore, a heart-healthy diet.

# Replacing Unhealthy Fats with Healthy Ones

Although most of us realize that too much of the wrong types of fat can be dangerous to our health, we live in an overweight society that continues to get bigger and more unhealthy. We may know what we should and shouldn't eat, but making it part of our everyday lifestyle is a struggle.

The most crucial strategy to remember is that you should not only add healthy fats to your diet but also replace the unhealthy fats with the healthy fats. Replacing unhealthy fats with healthier fats doesn't need to be a huge change, and from a health standpoint, it is worth the modification. Even small changes can add up to big benefits.

There are many ways to reduce the bad fat and increase the good fat. Following the Mediterranean diet will ensure you are on the right track. Here are a few other strategies to help you get started:

- Create your own salad dressings instead of using commercial dressings, which often can be overly processed and full of saturated fats. Mix olive oil with your favorite herbs and spices for a quick and healthy dressing.

- Throw out the butter and margarine, and use olive oil or canola oil instead on bread, vegetables, and pasta or in recipes.

- Replace some of the fat in baked goods with applesauce or other puréed fruit. Use canola oil or light or extra-light olive oil for baking cakes or muffins.

- Choose fat-free (skim) milk or plant-based milks (like almond milk) instead of whole or low-fat milk. Fat-free dairy milk has all the same nutrients as whole milk minus the saturated fat.

- Choose leaner cuts of meat, and eat moderate portions. Choose fish and vegetarian dishes more often.

- Read food labels, and avoid foods with partially hydrogenated oils or ones that contain trans fats on the Nutrition Facts label.

- When eating out, don't be afraid to ask the server what type of oil is used. If you are not sure, do not order anything cooked in fat.

- Try using low-fat yogurt to replace sour cream in recipes or baking.

- Snack on a handful of nuts instead of a bag of chips or other bagged items.

- Use avocado on a sandwich instead of mayonnaise.

- Replace one egg with two egg whites in recipes to cut back on fat and cholesterol.

## In This Chapter

Fats are necessary for our health and have important functions in the body. The Mediterranean diet is high in healthy monounsaturated fats found in olive oil, nuts, and seeds. The Mediterranean diet is also high in omega-3 fatty acids, a healthy polyunsaturated fat found in fish, seafood, nuts, and seeds. Most diets are too high in omega-6 fatty acids and too low in omega-3 fatty acids; the Mediterranean diet boasts a healthy balance. Saturated fats and trans fats are unhealthy fats and should be limited as much as possible; the Mediterranean diet contains very little of these unhealthy fats. The key to a healthy diet is not only adding healthy fats to your diet but also replacing the unhealthy ones already there.

# CHAPTER 16

# Fiber

Do you need to lower your cholesterol? Seek relief from persistent constipation? Want to lower your risk for certain cancers? Or need to get your blood glucose in check? If you answered yes to any of these questions, your solution just might be a high-fiber diet like the Mediterranean diet.

The cuisine of the Mediterranean is known for its fiber-rich content, and fiber helps in all of the above situations. Following the Mediterranean diet all but guarantees you get the fiber your body needs daily for optimal health in a tasty and nutritious way.

# What Is Fiber?

Fiber is the substance found in plant cell walls that gives plants their shape and structure. You may have heard of fiber being referred to as "roughage" or "bulk." Our bodies cannot digest or absorb fiber, so it basically comes in and goes out while performing some amazing things during its travels.

Dietary fiber, or the fiber found in foods, is referred to as a complex carbohydrate, but because it doesn't provide nutritional content or calories, it's not considered a nutrient. However, it is still listed on the Nutrition Facts label to help you identify foods rich in fiber. Although fiber falls under the carbohydrate category on the label, it does not provide the same number of calories as other carbohydrates nor is it processed in the body the same way other sources of carbohydrates are.

# Types of Fiber

Fiber is divided into two categories: soluble and insoluble. These fibers differ in their abilities to dissolve in water as well as their health effects on the body. However, one is not better than the other. In fact, they are both important to your health; the key is to eat a variety of fiber-rich foods every day to get enough of both types. Many foods contain both types of fiber, although some may contain more of one type of fiber than the other.

## Soluble Fiber

Soluble fibers dissolve in water. These fibers include pectins, gums, and mucilages, to name a few. Soluble fibers help lower LDL ("bad") cholesterol levels, which in turn can help reduce your risk for heart disease. The people of the Mediterranean region have a very low incidence and risk of heart disease. This amazing fiber also can help slow down the rate at which glucose (blood sugar) is absorbed by the body. This may help control blood sugar levels in people with diabetes and other blood sugar problems.

Generous quantities of soluble fiber can be found in legumes such as pinto beans, lima beans, navy beans, and soybeans; barley; fruits such as apricots, apples, pears, red currants, and grapes; vegetables such as artichokes, beets, carrots, cauliflower, and broccoli; and seeds such as flaxseeds, sesame seeds, and sunflower seeds.

## Insoluble Fiber

Insoluble fibers do not dissolve in water. These fibers are better known as roughage and include cellulose, hemicellulose, and lignan. Insoluble fibers help move food through the intestinal tract and soften stools, helping prevent constipation. In addition to promoting regularity, these mighty fibers may help decrease your risk for colon cancer, hemorrhoids, and a condition known as diverticulosis.

Generous quantities of insoluble fiber can be found in whole-grain breads and cereals; wheat bran; brown rice; nuts such as almonds, hazelnuts, and walnuts; seeds such as flaxseeds and sesame seeds; legumes such as lentils, soybeans, white beans, kidney beans, and peanuts; fruits such as avocados, dates, grapes, cherries, and berries; and vegetables such as dark green leafy vegetables, eggplant, onions, and broccoli.

# Fiber's Health Benefits

Fiber is incredibly important to good health. Fiber's special benefits not only promote good health but also may help reduce the risk for some chronic health conditions. Fiber hardly works alone, though. Most foods that include a significant amount of fiber also supply essential nutrients such as complex carbohydrates, vitamins, minerals, antioxidants, and phytonutrients.

## Increase Heart Health

Ever since Dr. Ancel Keys published his ever-popular Seven Countries Study in the 1950s, much attention was given to the fact that people from the Mediterranean region experienced the lowest percentages of mortality from cardiovascular diseases. Something obviously needed to be said about the way these folks ate and lived. The Mediterranean diet consists of a wide variety of foods high in fiber, high in healthy fats, and low in saturated fat, all of which are important for managing risk factors associated with heart disease.

Many components lead to heart health, so why is fiber so special? A fiber-rich diet, especially rich in soluble fiber, has the ability to help lower total blood cholesterol levels—more specifically, LDL (bad) cholesterol. Soluble fiber binds with cholesterol, which keeps it from becoming reabsorbed and instead pulls it out of the body as waste. Lowering your total cholesterol can mean lowering your risk for heart and artery disease. Recent data also suggest that adequate fiber intake can lower blood pressure. And higher-fiber foods will, with any luck, displace your high-fat and processed foods in meals and snacks, lowering your overall fat intake.

The Mediterranean diet differs from many others in that meals revolve around plant foods that are naturally high in fiber, as opposed to animal foods, which can contribute loads of saturated fat and cholesterol—both of which can lead to heart disease. That's not to say that animal foods are not part of this eating style, but they play a much smaller role than plant-based foods. In addition, the animal foods that are included are much lower in saturated fat and cholesterol.

Popular Mediterranean foods and dishes such as lentil soup, hummus, bulgur, and tabbouleh are high in fiber and low in saturated fat and cholesterol, a winning combination for good heart health.

## Manage Your Waistline

We have long known that there is a strong correlation between a healthy body weight and the Mediterranean diet. Many factors may be at work here, but—believe it or not—fiber is one of the main explanations.

Fiber-rich foods such as fruits, vegetables, legumes, and whole grains can help make you feel fuller sooner, helping you eat less. In addition, they can help you feel satisfied for longer, keeping you from snacking when you shouldn't. Fewer calories mean less fat. That might explain why many people use the Mediterranean diet not only for better health but also to drop a few extra pounds.

Keep in mind that fiber alone isn't the magic cure for weight loss. Those healthy, high-fiber foods need to replace foods high in calories, fat, and sugar. As with most of the health benefits associated with fiber, you will get the most benefit if you incorporate your higher-fiber diet with a healthy, well-balanced diet and an active lifestyle.

## Control Your Blood Sugar

With its fiber-rich components, the Mediterranean diet has been shown to protect against type 2 diabetes. Obese or overweight folks are prone to developing type 2 diabetes, so it makes sense that if the Mediterranean diet can help manage waistlines, then it can help protect against type 2 diabetes in that way.

But even more importantly, for people with type 2 diabetes or other blood sugar ailments, a diet high in fiber, especially soluble fiber, can be a major advantage. Fiber seems to help slow the absorption of sugar into the bloodstream, which in turn slows down the rise of glucose or blood sugar. For some people, this can help reduce amounts of medication or the need for medication. However, if you have diabetes or other blood sugar problems, be sure to speak with your doctor and/or a dietitian before using a fiber-rich diet to control your blood glucose levels.

## Reduce Your Colon Cancer Risk

Research shows strong evidence that a diet rich in fiber can help to lower your chance of developing colon and rectal cancers. By speeding up the time it takes for waste to move through your digestive tract, it leaves less time for cancer-causing agents to hang around and come in contact with the intestinal walls. In addition, fiber helps form a bulkier, heavier stool and controls the pH balance, or the level of acidity and alkalinity, within the intestines.

Because most high-fiber diets are lower in saturated fats, this also may provide protection. Saturated fats have a strong correlation with the risk of colon cancer. Your diet needs to be higher in fiber, and it needs to be the whole package (like the Mediterranean diet) to reap all the benefits.

## Support Your Digestive and Bowel Health

Because the Mediterranean diet is rich in fiber, it can help you dodge some uncomfortable and sometimes painful flare-ups from digestive disorders such as diverticulosis. A higher-fiber diet is used as standard therapy for folks who are diagnosed with diverticular disease of the colon, which can lead to symptoms such as abdominal pain, fever, and diarrhea.

Softer and more regular bowel movements also can prevent constipation and the discomfort that comes with it. In addition, softer and bulkier stools can help decrease your chance of developing hemorrhoids.

## Fuel a Healthy Gut

Growing research shows that keeping your gut bacteria, or your microbiome, in balance may play a key role in your overall health. The trillions of microorganisms, or friendly gut bacteria, living in your intestines may be key to helping you maintain a healthy weight, support immunity, protect your joints, and lower your risk of heart disease and cancer. Fiber leaves your stomach undigested and ends up in your colon, where it helps feed those friendly gut bacteria.

# How Much Fiber Do You Need?

Daily fiber needs differ for men and women, and they change as we age. At this time, there is no recommended daily allowance (RDA) for fiber, but there is what is called Adequate Intake (AI). AI is the daily average amount assumed to be adequate for healthy persons.

The U.S. Department of Agriculture's general recommendation for fiber intake is 14 grams for every 1,000 calories. More specifically, it recommends the following amounts:

- Women under 50 years of age: 25 grams per day
- Women 51 years of age and older: 21 grams per day
- Men under 50 years of age: 38 grams per day
- Men 51 years of age and older: 30 grams per day

According to the latest Dietary Guidelines for Americans, 90 percent of women and 97 percent of men do not meet the recommended fiber intakes in the United States.

## Tips to Increase Your Fiber Intake

It isn't as hard as you might think to increase your daily fiber intake. Following some easy tips that coincide with the Mediterranean diet can add plenty of fiber to your daily diet. It is all about healthy habits and making permanent lifestyle changes.

Be careful to ease your body into a higher-fiber diet. You should increase fiber gradually over several weeks to help your body adjust to the change. Too much fiber too quickly could result in some uncomfortable symptoms, such as bloating, gas, and cramping.

Increase your fluid intake with a higher-fiber diet. Fiber acts as a bulking agent, soaking up some of the fluids in your body. Therefore, it is important to drink extra fluid to keep from becoming dehydrated. More importantly, additional fluids will help keep the fiber traveling to where it needs to go.

Follow these simple tips to increase your daily fiber intake:

- Try dried fruits, which are usually higher in fiber than fresh fruit.
- Swap your white bread for one made with 100 percent whole grain. Be sure to check the label to ensure you have a whole-grain product.

- Experiment with popular fiber-rich grains of the Mediterranean such as bulgur. Bulgur is very versatile and can be used as a meat extender or as a meat substitute in plant-based meals. It also can be used in place of rice or couscous in your favorite dishes.

- Try adding legumes, such as fava beans, lentils, or white beans, to your meals a few times a week. They offer loads of fiber and protein. Add them to soups, stews, casseroles, or salads.

- Stock your pantry with brown rice and whole-wheat pasta or couscous instead of their white counterparts.

- Leave the skin or peel on fruits and vegetables when possible, and wash them well before eating. Most of the fiber found in fruits and vegetables is found in the skin and pulp.

- When you feel the urge to snack, grab a piece of fresh or dried fruit, a handful of nuts, or a few tablespoons of seeds.

- Eat whole fruits and vegetables more often than juices. Most of the fiber found in fruits and veggies is removed when the juice is produced.

## Fiber Label Lingo

Fresh produce, dried fruits, nuts, and beans are naturally good sources of fiber, but what about breads, cereals, pastas, crackers, and other grains? Finding those may take a little more knowledge and practice. To take the mystery out of finding high-fiber foods, you need to learn how to decipher the food label:

- **Good Source of Fiber:** This means the food contains 2.5 to 4.9 grams of fiber per serving, or 10% to 19% Daily Value.

- **High in Fiber, Rich in Fiber, or Excellent Source of Fiber:** This means the food contains 5 grams or more of fiber per serving, or 20% Daily Value.

- **More or Added Fiber:** This means the food contains at least 2.5 grams more fiber per serving than the reference food.

## Don't Overdo It

You *can* get too much of a good thing by overdoing your fiber intake. Although enough fiber is vital to good health, too much fiber can cause some uncomfortable side effects such as diarrhea, gas, bloating, and cramping. Excessive amounts of fiber, in the range of 50 grams or more each day, also can reduce the absorption of some very important nutrients, such as zinc, calcium, magnesium, and iron.

The key is to stay in the recommended range of fiber intake for your age and gender. Gradually increase your fiber daily during a period of several weeks to get your body adjusted to it, and drink plenty of fluids. This ensures you get the fiber you need and your body can handle it, without any adverse effects.

The market is flooded with fiber supplements. To get all the benefits fiber provides, don't take the easy way out. Whole foods provide more fiber as well as added essential nutrients, such as vitamins, minerals, antioxidants, and phytonutrients, that are necessary for optimal health. Never replace whole foods or any food group with a simple supplement. Speak with your doctor before starting a fiber supplement.

# How the Mediterranean Diet Delivers High Fiber

People of the Mediterranean lean toward including fiber-rich foods at every meal and snack. Meals revolve around vegetables, nuts, and beans instead of meat, and desserts chiefly consist of fruits or nuts. Whole grains are used instead of refined grains, and processed foods are used very minimally. All these foods add up to a fiber-rich diet.

The following table shares some of the Mediterranean diet foods that are highest in fiber.

### Fiber-Rich Foods

| Vegetables | Fiber |
| --- | --- |
| Artichoke hearts, cooked (½ cup) | 7.2 grams |
| Peas, green, cooked (½ cup) | 4.4 grams |
| Tomatoes, sun-dried (½ cup) | 3.3 grams |
| Red potato, baked, with skin (1 medium) | 2.5 grams |
| Broccoli, cooked (½ cup) | 2.6 grams |
| Spinach, cooked (½ cup) | 2.2 grams |
| Cabbage, cooked (½ cup) | 1.9 grams |
| Carrots, raw, chopped (½ cup) | 1.8 grams |
| Mushrooms, cooked (½ cup) | 1.7 grams |

| Vegetables | Fiber |
|---|---|
| Turnips, cooked (½ cup) | 1.6 grams |
| Tomato, raw (1 medium) | 1.5 grams |
| Onions, raw, chopped (½ cup) | 1.4 grams |
| Cauliflower, cooked (½ cup) | 1.4 grams |
| Eggplant, cooked (½ cup) | 1.25 grams |
| **Fruit** | **Fiber** |
| Avocado (1 medium) | 9.2 grams |
| Raspberries, raw (1 cup) | 8.0 grams |
| Prunes (1 cup) | 7.7 grams |
| Blueberries, raw (1 cup) | 7.6 grams |
| Dates, chopped (½ cup) | 5.9 grams |
| Figs, dried (½ cup) | 5.5 grams |
| Raisins, seedless (1 cup) | 5.4 grams |
| Pear, raw, with skin (1 medium) | 5.1 grams |
| Apple, raw, with skin (1 medium) | 3.3 grams |
| Strawberries, raw (1 cup) | 3.3 grams |
| Apricots, raw, sliced (1 cup) | 3.3 grams |
| **Grains, Cereal, and Pasta** | **Fiber** |
| Whole-wheat pasta, cooked (1 cup) | 6.3 grams |
| Barley, pearled, cooked (1 cup) | 6.0 grams |
| Bulgur, cooked (½ cup) | 4.1 grams |
| Brown rice, long-grain, cooked (1 cup) | 3.5 grams |
| Quinoa, cooked (½ cup) | 2.6 grams |
| Whole-wheat bread (1 slice) | 1.9 grams |
| Couscous, cooked (½ cup) | 1.1 grams |
| Wheat germ (1 tablespoon) | 1.1 grams |

(continues)

## Fiber-Rich Foods (continued)

| Legumes, Nuts, and Seeds | Fiber |
| --- | --- |
| Split peas, cooked (½ cup) | 8.2 grams |
| Lentils, cooked (½ cup) | 7.8 grams |
| Black beans, cooked (½ cup) | 7.5 grams |
| Lima beans, cooked (½ cup) | 6.6 grams |
| Kidney beans, cooked (½ cup) | 6.5 grams |
| Chickpeas, cooked (½ cup) | 6.25 grams |
| White beans, cooked (½ cup) | 5.6 grams |
| Fava beans (or broad beans), cooked (½ cup) | 4.6 grams |
| Almonds (1 ounce/30g) | 3.5 grams |
| Peanuts (1 ounce/30g) | 2.4 grams |
| Walnuts (1 ounce/30g) | 1.9 grams |

*USDA FoodData Central (fdc.nal.usda.gov).*

# Daily Fiber Intake on the Mediterranean Diet

To prove how simple a day in the life on the Mediterranean diet might be, here is a sample daily menu. (See Chapter 24 for more seasonal menu plans that help increase your fiber.)

Breakfast might include sliced tomato or cucumber with a soft cheese such as feta, goat cheese, or mozzarella; fresh fruit; whole-wheat toast, pita bread, or flatbread dipped in olive oil; or low-fat or fat-free plain or Greek yogurt.

Snacks might include fresh fruit; a handful of nuts or seeds; a piece of soft cheese; whole-grain crackers; or low-fat or fat-free plain or Greek yogurt flavored with honey.

Lunch might include bean or lentil soup; a salad made with plenty of greens, fresh vegetables, and olives; and fresh fruit.

Dinner might include a stew made with poultry, fish, or shellfish; a whole grain such as brown rice or couscous; steamed fresh vegetables drizzled with olive oil; fresh fruit; and a small glass of red wine. (Cooking your vegetables too much can reduce their fiber content. When cooking veggies, try steaming them or cooking them quickly in the microwave.)

## Getting Even More Fiber

You can increase your fiber intake by substituting whole-wheat flour in baked goods or adding wheat bran or oat bran to stews, casseroles, muffins, or yogurt. Try using brown rice or whole-grain couscous instead of white rice or substituting whole-wheat pasta for regular pasta in your favorite recipes.

It can be as easy as cooking zucchini with mushrooms, pine nuts, onions, a pinch of mint, and a splash of olive oil. The result is a wonderfully tasty Mediterranean dish, full of extra fiber, healthy fats, and loads of other essential nutrients.

## In This Chapter

Fiber is a type of carbohydrate that is an indigestible part of plants. Fiber-rich foods include fruits, vegetables, whole grains, nuts, seeds, and beans. Evidence suggests that soluble and insoluble fiber help lower the risk of heart disease and cancer, control blood sugar, and promote regularity. The Mediterranean diet delivers loads of fiber-rich foods that contribute to its many health benefits.

# CHAPTER 17

# Nutrients

With all the healthy foods included on the Mediterranean diet, it's not surprising how jam-packed it is with a vast array of nutrients. The Mediterranean diet has been cited in many clinical papers as being not only a heart-healthy but also an all-around-healthy diet.

What is it about nutrients such as vitamins, minerals, antioxidants, and phytonutrients that make this style of eating so much healthier? You need to become familiar with these nutrients to get a better understanding of the complete nutritional package of the Mediterranean diet.

# Nutrients of Mediterranean Foods

Thirteen main food groups are included in the Mediterranean diet: whole grains, fruits, vegetables, low-fat and fat-free dairy foods, seafood, poultry, olives, legumes, nuts and seeds, potatoes, eggs, some lean red meats, and olive oil, as well as red wine. All these foods contribute an abundance of essential nutrients, and study after study proves that the nutrients that make up the Mediterranean diet boost health and longevity.

Curious about the nutritional content of some other favorite Mediterranean foods? Check out the U.S. Department of Agriculture's FoodData Central database at fdc.nal.usda.gov.

How much you need of various vitamins and minerals depends on your age, gender, and current health status. Check out the whole list of dietary reference intakes (DRIs) for all vitamins and minerals at nal.usda.gov/human-nutrition-and-food-safety/dietary-guidance.

Getting vitamins and minerals from your food is so important, and if you follow the Mediterranean diet, you'll get the nutrients your body needs. Do not rely solely on dietary supplements to provide your daily allotment of vitamins and minerals. Dietary supplements offer only what is listed on the bottle and omit phytonutrients, fiber, and other natural substances that have been proven to be health promoting. As a rule of thumb: food before pills. Supplements should *supplement* your diet, not be used as replacements for foods or food groups. They will not make up for a poor diet.

# Vitamins

Vitamins are a group of organic compounds and nutrients that are required in small, for some even tiny, amounts for optimal health. This earned them the name micronutrients. But don't let the *micro* part fool you. They have big jobs and are involved in just about every function the body performs, from helping fat, protein, and carbohydrates supply energy, to regulating body processes, and everything in between. Some of these vitamins can be obtained from synthesis in the body; however, most are essential, and we need to get them from the foods we eat. Contrary to what you may have heard, vitamins do not supply energy directly, but they do regulate and are needed for the breakdown, or metabolism, of carbohydrates, proteins, and fats that directly supply energy to our body. A healthy, balanced diet can provide just about all the vitamins our body needs. Now you can start to appreciate just why our diet and the food we put into our bodies is so incredibly important!

It's easy to get confused about all the vitamins out there, so let's try to simplify it. Thirteen essential vitamins are needed for our body to function properly, and these are subdivided into two groups: fat-soluble and water-soluble vitamins. Their categories explain how they are both carried in food and transported in the body.

## Fat-Soluble Vitamins

Fat-soluble vitamins dissolve in fat, and that's how they are carried through the bloodstream and the body. It's one reason we do need moderate amounts of fat in our diet. Fat-soluble vitamins can be stored in fat tissue and the liver, and concentrations can build up over time. Therefore, you don't want to consume excessive amounts of fat-soluble vitamins for long periods because that can be harmful.

Here are the fat-soluble vitamins:

**Vitamin A:** Vitamin A promotes normal vision and the growth and health of body cells and tissue, regulates our immune system, and works as an antioxidant in the form of carotenoids. Too much vitamin A in the form of supplements can be toxic to your body because excess is stored. However, eating lots of foods rich in beta-carotene, even though it turns into vitamin A, is not toxic because the body converts beta-carotene into vitamin A only when we need it. Vitamin A is found in liver, milk, fortified breakfast cereals, and eggs. Beta-carotene is found in orange, red, yellow, and dark green vegetables; fruits such as carrots and cantaloupe; sweet potatoes; and spinach.

**Vitamin D:** Vitamin D is essential for the absorption of calcium and phosphorus and for depositing them in the bones and teeth to help make them strong. Vitamin D also is responsible for the regulation of cell growth and for protecting the immune system. The body can make its own vitamin D when the skin is exposed to moderate amounts of sunlight for short periods of time. New research is uncovering even more benefits of vitamin D, which include heart health, lowering blood pressure, and longevity. Vitamin D is found in fortified milk, cereals, and juices; eggs; and fish oils (salmon, shrimp, canned sardines, and cod).

**Vitamin E:** Vitamin E aids in the formation and functioning of red blood cells and other tissues, acts as a powerful antioxidant to protect essential fatty acids, and prevents cell damage from free radicals—all of which may help lower the risk for heart disease, stroke, cancer, and other health conditions of aging. Vitamin E is found in vegetable oils; olives and olive oil; almonds; hazelnuts; sunflower seeds; peanuts; whole grains; fortified cereals; green leafy vegetables such as spinach, mustard greens, turnip greens, kale, and chard; and fruits and vegetables such as bell peppers, kiwis, tomatoes, blueberries, and broccoli.

**Vitamin K:** Vitamin K aids in the regulation of blood clotting to help bleeding stop. The body can produce vitamin K from certain bacteria in the intestines, but we also get it from foods. Vitamin K is found in green leafy vegetables such as spinach, chard, kale, and mustard greens; brussels sprouts; green beans; asparagus; cauliflower; broccoli; green peas; carrots; soybeans; black-eyed peas; pine nuts; and pistachios.

## Water-Soluble Vitamins

Water-soluble vitamins dissolve in water and are carried through the body by watery fluids. Most water-soluble vitamins are not stored in the body, at least not in significant amounts. Instead, the body uses what it needs and excretes the rest through urine. Because this group of vitamins isn't stored, you need a constant supply from your diet to ensure you have optimal amounts. There is less worry of toxicity with water-soluble vitamins but more worry of deficiency.

Here are the water-soluble vitamins:

**Vitamin C:** Boosts the immune system, helps in the production of collagen to hold bones and muscles together, keeps blood vessels healthy, helps to absorb iron, aids in wound healing, promotes gum health, helps to protect from infection, and acts as an antioxidant. Sources include citrus fruits, berries, peppers, potatoes, green leafy vegetables, and tomatoes.

**Folate (folic acid):** Essential for cell division and red blood cell production. Helps produce DNA (our genetic makeup), may help protect against heart disease, and can reduce neural tube birth defects in newborns. Sources include dark green leafy vegetables, avocados, peanuts, most beans, lentils, oranges, fortified breakfast cereals, and wheat germ.

**Thiamin ($B_1$):** Needed to convert carbohydrate-containing foods into energy. Helps keep the brain, nervous system, and heart cells healthy. Sources include lean pork, whole grains, legumes, oatmeal, seeds, spinach, lamb, and lean beef.

**Riboflavin ($B_2$):** Helps produce energy from protein, fat, and carbohydrates; assists in the formation of red blood cells; maintains normal vision and healthy skin, nails, and hair. Sources include yogurt and milk, eggs, whole-grain breads and cereals, cheese, green leafy vegetables, oysters, and clams.

**Niacin ($B_3$):** Helps the body utilize sugars and fatty acids for energy; produces energy in all body cells; maintains normal enzyme function; maintains healthy skin, nerves, and digestion. Sources include lean meats and poultry, seafood, nuts, brown rice, milk, eggs, enriched breads and cereals, whole grains, legumes, and green vegetables.

**Pyridoxine ($B_6$):** Helps make nonessential amino acids (building blocks of protein) which are then used to make body cells; maintains normal brain function; and aids in formation of insulin, red blood cells, and antibodies. Sources include lean meats and poultry, legumes, whole grains, seafood, lentils, green leafy vegetables, carrots, peas, corn, bananas, mangos, potatoes, milk, cheese, and eggs.

**Cobalamin ($B_{12}$):** Helps in the formation of red blood cells, helps the body to utilize fatty acids and some amino acids, maintains healthy nerve cells, and is needed to make DNA genetic material. Sources include lean meats and poultry, seafood, eggs, and milk products.

**Pantothenic acid and biotin:** Involved in the metabolism and production of energy from proteins, fats, and carbohydrates and essential for growth. Sources include eggs, seafood, milk products, whole grains, legumes, potatoes, lean beef, and vegetables in the cabbage family (such as broccoli).

# Minerals

Minerals are a mighty bunch of essential nutrients. They are needed to regulate a host of body processes that are continually taking place—basically, they make things happen. Minerals have many jobs, including giving structure to your body by building strong bones, regulating fluid balance, aiding in muscle contractions, and transmitting nerve impulses. In addition, some minerals are used to make hormones and maintain a normal heartbeat. Unlike vitamins, minerals are inorganic and much tougher. They cannot be destroyed by heat or food-handling methods like vitamins can.

Minerals are first absorbed into the intestines. Some pass directly into the bloodstream and then onto cells, with excess being excreted in the urine. Others are carried by attaching to proteins and become a part of the body's structure. Because these types are stored, excess amounts over long periods of time can be harmful.

Not all minerals have a recommended dietary allowance (RDA). Minerals that do have an RDA include copper, iodine, iron, molybdenum, selenium, and zinc. The others have Adequate Intake (AI) levels instead.

Minerals come in two categories: major (calcium, chloride, magnesium, phosphorus, potassium, sodium, and sulfur) and trace (chromium, cobalt, copper, fluoride, iodine, iron, manganese, molybdenum, selenium, and zinc). Both major and trace minerals are essential for many vital bodily functions and processes. Major minerals are needed by the body in greater amounts than trace minerals. It doesn't mean one is any more important than the other, just that the body needs varying amounts to do its job. (A few other minerals, including boron, nickel, arsenic, silicon, and vanadium, have not yet been deemed necessary for health by nutrition experts.)

Minerals are abundant and can be found in a wide variety of foods that are common to the Mediterranean diet. However, we will focus on just a few of the powerhouse players:

**Calcium:** Calcium is the most abundant mineral in the body, with almost 99 percent of it being stored in the tissues of the bones. In addition to giving bones strength, this major mineral helps slow the rate of bone loss as you age, helps your muscles contract and your heart beat, regulates blood pressure, regulates normal nerve function, helps blood clot if you are bleeding, and helps keep teeth strong and healthy. If you don't get enough calcium in your diet, your bones will release stored calcium into your blood, and weakened bones will result. Sources of calcium include milk and most dairy products, canned sardines and salmon with edible bones, broccoli, legumes, almonds, dried figs, dark green leafy vegetables such as spinach and kale, calcium-fortified tofu, and other fortified foods such as orange juice.

**Iron:** A good part of iron can be found in your red blood cells, also known as hemoglobin. It serves as a delivery service, transporting oxygen from your lungs throughout the body to where it is needed. Iron also is necessary for brain development and a healthy immune system. If you don't get enough iron, you don't get enough oxygen to the rest of your body. That can result in anemia, which can show up as fatigue, weakness, headaches, irritability, and the feeling of being cold. Iron is found in a variety of food sources, including lean red meats, poultry, pork, lamb, veal, fish, oysters, clams, egg yolks, legumes, lentils, whole grains, dark green leafy vegetables, dried fruits, nuts and seeds, fortified cereals, and wheat germ.

**Selenium:** Working with vitamin E, selenium acts as a powerful antioxidant to protect cells from damage that may lead to heart disease, cancer, and other chronic health conditions. It aids in cell growth and boosts immune function. Sources of selenium include lean meats, eggs, wheat germ, garlic, whole grains, Brazil nuts, walnuts, peanuts, sunflower seeds, raisins, shellfish (lobster, oysters, shrimp, scallops), and fish (salmon, tuna, mackerel, halibut, flounder, and herring). It also can be found in alfalfa, fennel seed, radishes, horseradish, onions, chives, and some mushrooms.

# Antioxidants

You've seen the word *antioxidants* a lot in this book. Antioxidants are a group of nutrients that counteract the effects of harmful free radicals. Free radicals can come from the environment and include things like cigarette smoke, pollution, and ultraviolet light. But these free radicals are also produced as a by-product of the oxygen that our own body cells burn (oxidation). These free radicals created by oxidation of cells are unstable and can damage body cells, tissues, and DNA, causing all sorts of health issues, including heart and artery disease, cancer, cataracts, age-related disorders such as diabetes and Alzheimer's disease, as well as general age-related deterioration. The cells in our body have their own natural defenses against free radicals, but research has discovered that certain vitamins, minerals, and phytonutrients also can help ward off the effects of and damage from these free radicals—and they are fittingly called antioxidants.

Some of the more common antioxidants include beta-carotene (which forms vitamin A in the body), vitamin C, vitamin E, and selenium.

# Phytonutrients

Foods of the Mediterranean diet are full of phytonutrients. Unlike some of the other nutrients we have discussed (vitamins, minerals, proteins, carbohydrates, and fats) phytonutrients are not essential for human life; however, they have been found to promote good health in a very big way.

There are many classes of phytonutrients, and they can be grouped by color. Many of the foods high in phytonutrients are brightly colored, like fruits and vegetables, and all the color groups boast a wide array of phytonutrients. This is why we have repeated that it is important to eat a variety of colorful fruits and vegetables. The more colors, the more phytonutrients!

Phytonutrients are thought to provide health benefits that go beyond that of vitamins and minerals. For a long time, it has been evident that people, like those of the Mediterranean, who eat an abundance of plant foods, including fruits, vegetables, nuts, seeds, and whole grains, seem to be healthier, display lower incidences of chronic diseases such as cancer and heart disease, and live longer lives. It always has been assumed that these results were the workings of essential vitamins and minerals. But it turns out, that was only part of the story, and there might just be thousands of other substances in these plant foods that are beneficial to human health. The belief is that phytonutrients work synergistically with fiber, vitamins, minerals, and antioxidants to promote health and provide added protection. Many health organizations, including the American Heart Association and the National Cancer Institute, recommend whole foods over supplements to ensure consumption of these beneficial phytonutrients.

Most phytonutrients are either flavonoids, which are a subclass of polyphenols, or carotenoids. Polyphenols are a broad class of phytonutrients that include not only flavonoids but also resveratrol and phenolic acids. Because there are literally thousands of phytonutrients, and more are continually being discovered and classified, we will discuss a few of the more common ones here:

**Beta-carotene (carotenoid):** Beta-carotene is a potent antioxidant that prevents damage from free radicals as well as serves as a precursor for the formation of vitamin A. Beta-carotene is found primarily in yellow and orange fruits and vegetables and green leafy vegetables.

**Lutein (carotenoid):** Lutein may prevent and slow macular degeneration, a condition of the eye which can lead to blindness in the elderly. It also acts as an antioxidant to prevent free radical damage to the macula of the eye, prevent formation of cataracts, reduce risk for heart disease, and protect against many types of cancer. Lutein is found primarily in green leafy vegetables, including artichokes, broccoli, spinach, and kale.

**Lycopene (carotenoid):** Lycopene is a potent antioxidant linked with reduced risk of cancer, especially prostate cancer, and may offer protection against heart attacks. It is found primarily in red fruits and vegetables, with tomato products being the most concentrated sources.

**Anthocyanidins (flavonoid):** Anthocyanidins are linked to improved health of the blood vessels, act as an antioxidant, and may maintain brain function and healthy immune function. They are found primarily in blue, purple, and red fruits and vegetables.

# Protein

So far, we have discussed the micronutrients; now it's time to discover a few of the macronutrients, which consist of protein, carbohydrates, and fat. (See Chapter 15 for a full discussion of fats.)

Protein comes from the foods we eat and is part of many body structures, such as collagen, muscles, bones, organs, tendons, ligaments, hair, nails, teeth, and skin. Protein is used in the body to build and repair tissues, to make enzymes and hormones, to transport nutrients, to help muscles contract, to regulate body processes such as fluid balance, ... and the list goes on. If you don't get enough in the way of carbohydrates, protein also can be metabolized and used for energy.

Twenty-two different amino acids (which we discussed in Chapter 12) make up protein. Nine of these are essential, meaning we must get them from food, and the others come from the body's own amino acid collection. These amino acids are strung together in different combinations and make up all the protein needed by the body for each of its functions.

The Mediterranean diet is far from a high-protein diet. In fact, protein consists of about 15 percent of daily caloric intake, which is in line with what most health experts recommend for a healthy diet. On a typical 2,000-calorie diet for adults, this would equate to 300 calories, or 75 grams of protein. Too much protein can cause a host of health problems, so sticking with a more moderate protein intake is the way to go.

The protein sources common to the Mediterranean diet may be a bit different from what you are used to. They include low to moderate amounts of animal proteins such as lean meats (only small amounts of red meat), dairy products, and eggs, with a larger emphasis on plant protein sources, such as nuts, seeds, whole grains, legumes, and lentils. Fish and seafood are major protein contributors, too.

The following table lists common protein sources in the Mediterranean diet and how much protein they contain per serving.

## Mediterranean Protein Sources

| Food | Protein |
| --- | --- |
| Chicken breast, cooked (½ breast) | 26.6 grams |
| Salmon, cooked (3 ounces/85g) | 21.6 grams |
| Fava beans, cooked (1 cup) | 12.9 grams |
| Yogurt, plain, low-fat (1 cup) | 12.9 grams |
| Lentils, cooked (½ cup) | 8.9 grams |
| Fat-free milk (8 ounces/225g) | 8.4 grams |
| Egg (1 large) | 6.3 grams |
| Sardines (2) | 5.9 grams |
| Bulgur, cooked (1 cup) | 5.6 grams |
| Walnuts (1 ounce/30g) | 4.3 grams |
| Feta cheese (1 ounce/30g) | 4 grams |

*USDA FoodData Central (fdc.nal.usda.gov).*

# Energy-Boosting Mediterranean Carbohydrates

The category of carbohydrates includes not only starches but also sugar and fiber. Starches and sugars are your body's main source of fuel. (You can find more on fiber in Chapter 16.) Carbohydrates can be a big source of calories in the typical diet, but the type of carbohydrate you choose can make all the difference.

Even though starches and sugars are both carbohydrates, they can be very different. Sugars are considered simple carbohydrates because they are made of only one or two sugars. If foods have one unit of sugar, they are called monosaccharides. These are the building blocks to disaccharides, which have two units of sugar. Simple sugars include foods and beverages such as honey, jelly, syrup, table sugar, candy, soft drinks, fruit juices, and, yes, fruit (although fruit contains a naturally occurring sugar called fructose, not an added sugar). Even milk contains a simple, naturally occurring sugar called lactose. When you have a sweet tooth, these are some of the types of carbohydrates you crave!

When three or more of these units or simple sugars are linked together, they become complex carbohydrates (or starches) called polysaccharides. Complex carbohydrates can be found in grains, nuts, seeds, fruits, and vegetables. Foods higher in starchy complex carbohydrates include breads, cereal, rice, pasta, potatoes, legumes, peas, lentils, yams, winter squash, and corn. All grains include starchy carbohydrates, but whole grains are better for you because they contain more fiber and nutrient content. Complex carbohydrates might not satisfy your sweet tooth like simple carbohydrates because starch molecules are larger and, therefore, do not taste as sweet.

No matter which type of carbohydrate is consumed, simple or complex, they all are broken down to their most basic form, which is glucose. Glucose is the type of sugar or carbohydrate that is absorbed and used for energy in the body. Because simple carbohydrates are already broken down and in a single form, they are absorbed much more quickly than complex carbohydrates that are larger and need to be broken down further. The longer time required to break down complex carbohydrates means glucose is released into the bloodstream much slower than with simple carbohydrates, helping regulate blood sugar levels. Even though fruit contains forms of simple sugars, it also contains complex carbohydrates and fiber, and they help slow the absorption of glucose into the bloodstream. In addition, many simple carbohydrates are empty calories, meaning they provide calories, through added sugar, but not much in the way of nutritional value, while complex carbohydrates are quite the opposite, providing fiber and other essential nutrients. Of course, this doesn't apply to foods like fruit and milk, which both contain a natural form of simple sugar and are high on the nutrition content list.

Contrary to popular belief, carbohydrates do not make you fat and are not the lone culprit in causing people to be overweight. Eating too much, whether carbohydrates, proteins, or fats, provides excess calories that are stored as fat in the body. Glucose, or the sugar that complex carbohydrates are broken down into, will not cause your body to make or store fat. Glucose is converted to body fat only if you consume more total calories than your body needs. But remember that your choice of carbohydrates matters most.

Carbohydrates are essential, and your body needs the energy they produce. In fact, glucose is the only source of energy your brain can actually use. The key is choosing complex carbohydrates over simple sugars and refined carbohydrates, especially the empty-calorie versions. Choosing complex over simple and refined carbohydrates makes a world of difference to your health and your weight. So eat carbohydrates in moderation, and properly balance your diet with the other macronutrients: fat and protein.

Carbohydrates are an essential part of any healthy diet, and as we have seen, complex carbohydrates are a large part of the Mediterranean diet. The Mediterranean diet is made of about 45 to 50 percent of total calories from carbohydrates, with the vast majority of these carbohydrates coming from complex sources such as legumes, couscous, potatoes, brown rice, vegetables, barley, and bulgur, just to name a few. These are all complex carbohydrates with loads of fiber and other essential nutrients. When people of the Mediterranean eat carbohydrates, they definitely make them count!

## In This Chapter

Vitamins and minerals are essential for normal body function, and eating a varied and well-balanced diet can help you get all your body needs. Vitamins are separated into water-soluble and fat-soluble categories. Minerals are either major or trace. Antioxidants protect from the damage of free radicals and can help prevent cancer, heart disease, cataracts, and a host of other chronic health conditions. The most common are beta-carotene, vitamins E and C, and selenium. Phytonutrients are not essential nutrients like vitamins and minerals; these compounds found in plants may work with essential nutrients to protect our health even more. Carbohydrates, protein, and fat are macronutrients. Carbohydrates are essential to a healthy diet and should consist mostly of the complex variety. Protein is moderate on the Mediterranean diet, coming more from plant sources than animal sources.

# PART 4

# FLAVORS OF THE MEDITERRANEAN

Fresh, delicious recipes and detailed menu plans can help inspire you to begin a new way of eating. The recipes and menu plans in Part 4 can make implementing the Mediterranean diet in your everyday life easier.

Going to a party? No problem. You'll find plenty of appetizer recipes in Chapter 18.

Need a pizza for a Friday night meal with the family? You'll find a variety of pizza and flatbread recipes in Chapter 20.

Want some desserts that won't expand your waistline? Check out the recipes in Chapter 23.

The recipes in these chapters span all the seasons and use fresh, seasonal ingredients. Use the recipes in season or whenever you like!

And after you've tried some of the recipes, check out our ideas for seasonal menu plans in the last chapter. Let these recipes and menus help you incorporate all the foods you have read about and are eager to try. *Bon appétit!*

# CHAPTER 18

# Appetizers and Snacks

Mediterranean diet appetizers focus on fresh, flavorful, plant-based ingredients. They are a great way to get more nutritious vegetables into your diet and can count as servings of recommended food groups.

Ingredients are king when it comes to creating great flavor in these appetizers. By strategically selecting and combining a few key Mediterranean foods—such as feta cheese, sun-dried tomatoes, figs, dates, balsamic vinegar, and extra-virgin olive oil—even the humblest ingredients are elevated to appetizer greatness!

One central ingredient is freshly ground black pepper, which provides a delightful peppery zing. If you don't already have one, you might want to consider purchasing a high-quality grinder and whole peppercorns and seasoning your Mediterranean diet foods with freshly ground pepper.

# Roasted Red Pepper Tapenade

Roasted red peppers lend a smoky-sweet flavor when blended with salty Kalamata olives in this delicious summer-inspired tapenade.

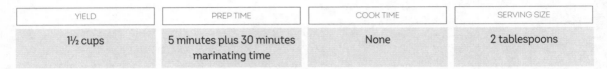

| YIELD | PREP TIME | COOK TIME | SERVING SIZE |
|---|---|---|---|
| 1½ cups | 5 minutes plus 30 minutes marinating time | None | 2 tablespoons |

2 jarred roasted red peppers, finely diced

20 pitted Kalamata olives, finely diced

1 Roma tomato, seeded and finely diced

2 cloves garlic, finely minced (about 1 tsp)

¼ tsp freshly ground black pepper

2 tsp extra-virgin olive oil

1. In a medium bowl, combine roasted red peppers, Kalamata olives, Roma tomato, and garlic. Add black pepper and extra-virgin olive oil, and mix well.

2. Set aside for 30 minutes so flavors can meld.

3. Serve at room temperature with crackers, atop a slice of toasted baguette, as a sandwich spread, in an omelet, in a wrap, on a pizza, or to top chicken or fish.

**Variation:** For an even smokier flavor, roast your own red peppers. Char red peppers over a gas flame or under a broiler until the skin is black all over. Place peppers in a paper bag, fold over the top to seal, and let steam for 10 minutes. When cool enough to handle, peel off the skin and discard, and slice and discard the seeds and juice.

| EACH SERVING HAS | | | |
|---|---|---|---|
| 15 calories 1.5g total fat | 0g saturated fat 0g protein | 1g carbohydrates 0g fiber | 0mg cholesterol 70mg sodium |

# Pesto

Basil is the epitome of summer. Its fresh aroma is irresistible!

| YIELD | PREP TIME | COOK TIME | SERVING SIZE |
|:---:|:---:|:---:|:---:|
| 1 cup | 20 minutes | 6 minutes | 1 tablespoon |

¼ cup pine nuts

3 cloves garlic

1 tsp kosher salt

4 oz (115g) fresh basil leaves (about 3 cups packed)

⅔ cup extra-virgin olive oil

1 cup freshly grated Parmesan cheese

1. In a small skillet over medium heat, toast pine nuts for 5 or 6 minutes until lightly browned.

2. In a food processor, process toasted pine nuts, garlic, and kosher salt until finely chopped.

3. Add basil leaves to the mixture, and process until basil is finely chopped.

4. With the food processor running, slowly add extra-virgin olive oil. Continue to process until smooth.

5. Add Parmesan cheese, and pulse until cheese is incorporated.

**Variation:** For flavor variations, use walnuts instead of pine nuts, or try arugula instead of basil. You can use this pesto in many ways. For example, mix ½ cup pesto with 1 pound (450g) whole-wheat pasta, cooked, and serve with additional Parmesan cheese as a garnish. If the pesto is too thick, add 1 or 2 tablespoons of the pasta cooking water to thin it.

| EACH SERVING HAS | | | |
|:---:|:---:|:---:|:---:|
| 120 calories<br>12g total fat | 2.5g saturated fat<br>2g protein | 1g carbohydrates<br>0g fiber | 5mg cholesterol<br>75mg sodium |

# Melon, Figs, and Prosciutto

Balsamic vinegar becomes sweet when reduced and is a nice contrast to the salty components in this summer dish.

| YIELD | PREP TIME | COOK TIME | SERVING SIZE |
| --- | --- | --- | --- |
| 4 servings | 15 minutes | 9 minutes | ¼ recipe |

½ cup balsamic vinegar

½ cantaloupe, peeled and seeded

4 thin slices prosciutto

4 fresh figs

4 oz (115g) goat cheese, crumbled

1 tbsp extra-virgin olive oil

Freshly ground black pepper

1. In a small saucepan over high heat, cook balsamic vinegar for 9 minutes or until it is reduced to 2 tablespoons and thick. Remove from heat, and let cool.

2. Cut cantaloupe into about 24 thin slices. Place about 6 slices on each plate.

3. Roll up each prosciutto slice from the short end, and place one roll on each plate.

4. Slice each fig lengthwise into 4 pieces, and divide equally among the plates.

5. Crumble 1 ounce (30g) goat cheese over each plate.

6. Drizzle each plate with cooled balsamic vinegar and then extra-virgin olive oil. Sprinkle with black pepper.

| EACH SERVING HAS | | | |
| --- | --- | --- | --- |
| 250 calories<br>14g total fat | 7g saturated fat<br>11g protein | 22g carbohydrates<br>2g fiber | 35mg cholesterol<br>550mg sodium |

# Stuffed Dates

Medjool dates are loved for their size, sweetness, and chewy texture, and these stuffed versions are deliciously sweet and savory. If you think you do not like dates, try these for a perfect fall dish—they are nature's candy bar!

| YIELD | PREP TIME | COOK TIME | SERVING SIZE |
|---|---|---|---|
| 12 dates | 15 minutes | 15 minutes | 1 date |

1 Italian sausage link

12 Medjool dates

3 tbsp finely chopped roasted almonds

½ cup goat cheese

2 tbsp finely chopped fresh parsley

1. In a small skillet over medium heat, cook Italian sausage for 12 to 15 minutes or until cooked through. Remove from heat, and let cool.

2. Slice cooked link in half lengthwise, and cut 1 half-link into 12 half-rounds. (Save the other half-link for another use.)

3. Slit each Medjool date down the center—being careful to not slice all the way through the date or through the ends—and remove the pit.

4. In a small bowl, combine almonds and goat cheese. Divide into 12 portions.

5. Into each date, stuff 1 piece of sausage and 1 portion of goat cheese mixture, mounding the cheese mixture outside the slit. Repeat until all dates are stuffed.

6. Sprinkle with parsley.

**Variation:** You can omit the sausage and use the cheese mixture only, or stuff the dates with whole almonds and add plain goat cheese. You also can use other date varieties in this recipe, but Medjool dates are best.

| EACH SERVING HAS | | | |
|---|---|---|---|
| 170 calories 5g total fat | 2g saturated fat 4g protein | 31g carbohydrates 3g fiber | 10mg cholesterol 150mg sodium |

# Mushroom Crostini

In this fall dish, simple sautéed mushrooms become meaty and earthy, making a delicious topping for crostini.

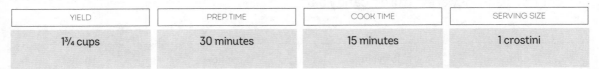

| YIELD | PREP TIME | COOK TIME | SERVING SIZE |
|-------|-----------|-----------|--------------|
| 1¾ cups | 30 minutes | 15 minutes | 1 crostini |

⅛ cup olive oil

3 tbsp minced shallot

8 oz (225g) white button mushrooms, chopped

8 oz (225g) baby portobello mushrooms, chopped

¼ cup white wine

3 cloves garlic, minced

1 tbsp fresh thyme leaves, minced

¼ tsp kosher salt

⅛ tsp freshly ground black pepper

1 baguette

1. Preheat the oven to 375°F (190°C).

2. In a large skillet over medium heat, heat olive oil. When oil is hot, add shallot, and cook for 2 or 3 minutes.

3. Add white button mushrooms, baby portobello mushrooms, white wine, garlic, thyme, kosher salt, and black pepper to the skillet, and cook for about 10 minutes or until all the wine and the liquid the mushrooms gave off as they cook have evaporated.

4. Meanwhile, slice baguette diagonally into ½-inch (1.25cm) slices. Place baguette slices on a shallow baking sheet, and toast in the oven for 4 or 5 minutes or until golden brown. Remove from the oven.

5. Spoon mushroom mixture evenly onto toasted baguette slices, and serve warm.

**Variation:** For added flavor, brush the bread slices with about 2 tablespoons olive oil before toasting. You also can rub the toasted bread with raw garlic after removing it from the oven.

| EACH SERVING HAS | | | |
|---|---|---|---|
| 30 calories 1.5g total fat | 0g saturated fat 1g protein | 3g carbohydrates 0g fiber | 0mg cholesterol 45mg sodium |

# Lemon Cannellini Spread

Lemon zest adds a refreshing zing to this summery white bean spread.

| YIELD | PREP TIME | COOK TIME | SERVING SIZE |
|---|---|---|---|
| 2 cups | 10 minutes | None | ¼ cup |

1 clove garlic, peeled

1 (15-oz/425g) can cannellini beans, drained, liquid reserved

1 tbsp lemon zest

1 tbsp extra-virgin olive oil

2 tsp ground coriander

¼ tsp chopped fresh rosemary leaves

1. In a food processor, pulse garlic until finely chopped.

2. Add cannellini beans, lemon zest, extra-virgin olive oil, ground coriander, and rosemary leaves. Purée, stopping occasionally to scrape the sides of the bowl with a spatula and add reserved liquid as necessary, until the mixture is creamy.

3. Use as a spread on a sliced baguette or as a sandwich spread.

**Variation:** You can use any white bean in this recipe. Also try substituting tarragon for the rosemary.

| EACH SERVING HAS | | | |
|---|---|---|---|
| 60 calories 2g total fat | 0g saturated fat 3g protein | 9g carbohydrates 3g fiber | 0mg cholesterol 140mg sodium |

# Hummus

Savory and creamy, hummus is a great dip or sandwich spread for springtime–
or anytime!

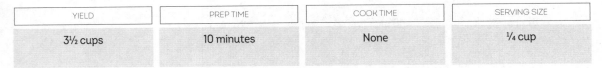

| YIELD | PREP TIME | COOK TIME | SERVING SIZE |
| --- | --- | --- | --- |
| 3½ cups | 10 minutes | None | ¼ cup |

2 cloves garlic, peeled

2 (15-oz/425g) cans chickpeas (garbanzo beans), drained, liquid reserved

2 tbsp freshly squeezed lemon juice

2 tbsp extra-virgin olive oil

2 tbsp tahini

4 tsp ground coriander

2 tsp cumin

½ tsp kosher salt

⅛ tsp freshly ground black pepper

1. In a food processor, pulse garlic until finely chopped.
2. Add chickpeas, lemon juice, extra-virgin olive oil, tahini, ground coriander, cumin, kosher salt, and black pepper. Purée, stopping occasionally to scrape the sides of the bowl with a spatula and add reserved liquid as necessary, until the mixture is creamy.

**Note:** Made from sesame seeds that are ground to a paste, tahini is the consistency of peanut butter. Before using, you might need to stir it vigorously to incorporate the oil that has risen to the top.

**Variation:** Add 2 jarred roasted red peppers for a smoky flavor. Or add a handful of fresh cilantro and lemon zest.

| EACH SERVING HAS | | | |
| --- | --- | --- | --- |
| 80 calories 4g total fat | 0g saturated fat 3g protein | 9g carbohydrates 2g fiber | 0mg cholesterol 200mg sodium |

# Eggplant Rolls

Grilling gives eggplant a wonderful, smoky flavor and beautiful grill marks. These tasty eggplant rolls are the perfect fall dish.

| YIELD | PREP TIME | COOK TIME | SERVING SIZE |
|---|---|---|---|
| 10 rolls | 15 minutes | 7 minutes | 1 roll |

⅛ cup olive oil

2 tbsp Italian seasoning

1 tsp dried mint leaves

½ tsp kosher salt

⅛ tsp freshly ground black pepper

1 medium eggplant

1 (3-oz/85g) block feta cheese

1. In a small bowl, combine olive oil, Italian seasoning, mint leaves, kosher salt, and black pepper.

2. Cut eggplant lengthwise into ⅛-inch (3mm) slices. Brush both sides of eggplant slices with olive oil mixture.

3. On an outdoor grill or stove-top grill pan over medium heat, grill eggplant slices for 5 to 7 minutes, turning halfway through the cook time. Eggplant should be lightly browned and soft.

4. Meanwhile, slice feta cheese block into ¼-inch (0.5cm) slices. Cut each slice in half lengthwise.

5. Place 1 eggplant slice on your work surface. Set 1 piece of feta at one end of eggplant slice, and roll eggplant over feta. Repeat with remaining eggplant and feta. Serve at room temperature.

**Variation:** You can use ricotta cheese instead of feta, mixing the Italian seasoning, mint, kosher salt, and black pepper into the ricotta. Or try brushing the eggplant with plain olive oil and sprinkle only with salt and pepper before grilling.

| EACH SERVING HAS | | | |
|---|---|---|---|
| 60 calories 4.5g total fat | 1.5g saturated fat 2g protein | 4g carbohydrates 2g fiber | 10mg cholesterol 190mg sodium |

# Baked Vegetable Omelet

The Italian frittata is the inspiration for this egg, vegetable, and cheese dish—a savory delight morning or night. A frittata is cooked in a skillet on the stove over very low heat and finished in the oven under the broiler. This is a simpler version but just as delicious.

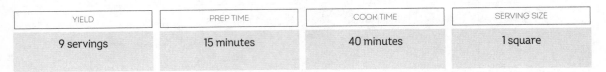

| YIELD | PREP TIME | COOK TIME | SERVING SIZE |
| --- | --- | --- | --- |
| 9 servings | 15 minutes | 40 minutes | 1 square |

1 tbsp olive oil

10 large eggs

¼ cup asparagus, thinly sliced

¼ cup finely chopped red onion

½ cup sun-dried tomatoes, packed in oil

1 cup fresh baby spinach

¼ cup finely chopped red bell pepper

1 cup sliced mushrooms

12 oz (340g) part-skim ricotta cheese, drained

¼ tsp kosher salt

⅛ tsp freshly ground black pepper

1 tbsp finely chopped fresh parsley

1. Preheat the oven to 350°F (175°C). Coat a 9×9-inch (23×23cm) baking dish with olive oil; be sure to coat the sides well.

2. In a large bowl, beat the eggs well.

3. In a separate large bowl, combine asparagus, red onion, sun-dried tomatoes, baby spinach, red bell pepper, mushrooms, ricotta cheese, kosher salt, and black pepper.

4. Pour beaten eggs over vegetable mixture, and mix well.

5. Transfer mixture to the prepared baking dish, and bake for about 40 minutes or until eggs are set in the center.

6. Remove from the oven, run a knife around the edges of the pan, and cut into 9 portions.

7. Garnish each serving with a pinch of parsley. Serve warm or at room temperature.

**Variation:** For a sweeter, more intense vegetable flavor, roast the vegetables. Let them cool before combining them with the eggs in step 4.

| EACH SERVING HAS | | | |
| --- | --- | --- | --- |
| 160 calories 10g total fat | 4g saturated fat 12g protein | 5g carbohydrates 1g fiber | 245mg cholesterol 250mg sodium |

# Crab Cakes

Crab cakes are always a hit in the summer months. Serve these seafood favorites as a main course or as an appetizer.

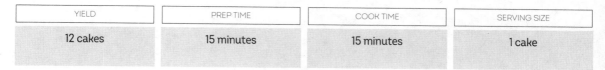

| YIELD | PREP TIME | COOK TIME | SERVING SIZE |
|---|---|---|---|
| 12 cakes | 15 minutes | 15 minutes | 1 cake |

1 large egg, lightly beaten

1 tbsp Dijon mustard

1 tbsp light mayonnaise

2 tbsp finely chopped fresh parsley

2 tbsp finely diced red onion

2 tbsp finely diced red bell pepper

1 tbsp Old Bay Seasoning

1 lb (450g) lump crabmeat

1 cup Italian-style breadcrumbs

2 tbsp olive oil

1. Preheat the oven to 400°F (200°C).

2. In a large bowl, combine egg, Dijon mustard, mayonnaise, parsley, red onion, red bell pepper, and Old Bay Seasoning.

3. Gently add crabmeat and Italian-style breadcrumbs, taking care not to break up the crabmeat.

4. Form ¼ cup crab mixture into a patty 1 inch (2.5cm) thick. Repeat until 12 patties are formed.

5. In a large nonstick skillet over medium heat, heat 1 tablespoon olive oil. When olive oil is hot, add 6 patties and cook for 1 or 2 minutes per side or until slightly browned. (You are just adding color, not cooking the patties all the way through.) Transfer the patties to a baking sheet. Add remaining 1 tablespoon olive oil to the skillet, and fry the remaining 6 patties. Transfer this batch of patties to the baking sheet with the first batch.

6. Bake the patties for 5 to 10 minutes or until golden brown.

**Note:** Be sure to use high-quality lump or jumbo lump crabmeat if you can. Processed crabmeat can contain bits of shell or cartilage, so if that's all you can find, gently pick through the crab and remove any bits that you find.

| EACH SERVING HAS | | | |
|---|---|---|---|
| 100 calories 4g total fat | 1g saturated fat 9g protein | 8g carbohydrates 0g fiber | 50mg cholesterol 340mg sodium |

# Tomato Basil Bocconcini

Sweet summer tomatoes and fresh basil are a match made in culinary heaven. The bocconcini brings a lovely creaminess to complete this summery dish.

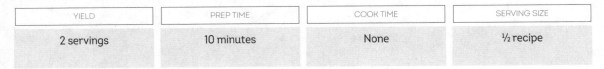

| YIELD | PREP TIME | COOK TIME | SERVING SIZE |
|---|---|---|---|
| 2 servings | 10 minutes | None | ½ recipe |

4 oz (115g) bocconcini
  (about 2 balls)

2 medium tomatoes

15 large fresh basil leaves

2 tsp extra-virgin olive oil

Kosher salt

Freshly ground black pepper

1. Slice each bocconcini ball into 4 slices.

2. Core tomatoes, and cut each into 4 horizontal slices.

3. On each plate, layer 1 tomato slice, 1 basil leaf, and 1 bocconcini slice. Repeat, making 4 stacks on each plate.

4. Drizzle the stacks with extra-virgin olive oil, and sprinkle with a pinch of kosher salt and black pepper.

5. Cut the remaining basil leaves into fine shreds, and use to garnish each serving.

**Variation:** If you cannot find bocconcini in your market, you can use any type of fresh mozzarella.

| EACH SERVING HAS | | | |
|---|---|---|---|
| 210 calories<br>14g total fat | 6g saturated fat<br>15g protein | 7g carbohydrates<br>1g fiber | 35mg cholesterol<br>610mg sodium |

# Lamb Pesto Crostini

Crostini means "little toasts," and these crostini are the perfect springtime starter before a meal, or you can serve them as an entrée paired with a salad.

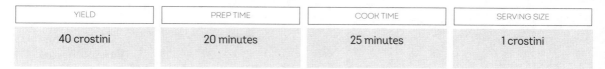

| YIELD | PREP TIME | COOK TIME | SERVING SIZE |
|---|---|---|---|
| 40 crostini | 20 minutes | 25 minutes | 1 crostini |

1 baguette

1½ lb (680g) lamb shoulder

1 tsp Italian seasoning

⅛ tsp kosher salt

⅛ tsp freshly ground black pepper

3 large Roma tomatoes

6 tbsp Pesto (page 223)

1. Preheat the oven to 400°F (200°C).

2. Slice baguette into ⅛-inch (3mm) slices. Arrange slices in a single layer on an ungreased baking sheet, and bake for 3 or 4 minutes per side or until lightly toasted. Remove from the oven, and let cool.

3. Season lamb shoulder on both sides with Italian seasoning, kosher salt, and black pepper. On a grill set to medium heat, cook lamb for 8 to 10 minutes per side or until a meat thermometer shows an internal temperature of 145°F (65°C) in the thickest part. Remove from the grill, place on a plate, cover with aluminum foil, and let rest for 5 minutes.

4. Meanwhile, core Roma tomatoes and slice in half lengthwise. Slice again into half-rounds approximately ⅛ inch (3mm) thick.

5. Slice cooled lamb into slices ⅛ inch (3mm) thick.

6. Spread a little Pesto onto each crostini. Add 1 tomato slice on each, and top with 1 slice of lamb. Repeat until all crostini are topped.

**Variation:** Serve some crostini with lamb and some without—the crostini are delicious with just the pesto and tomato.

| EACH SERVING HAS | | | |
|---|---|---|---|
| 150 calories<br>6g total fat | 2g saturated fat<br>7g protein | 18g carbohydrates<br>1g fiber | 10mg cholesterol<br>240mg sodium |

# Lemon Minted Melon

Cold melon is so refreshing in the summertime. This sweet mint syrup gives it an extra-special twist.

| YIELD | PREP TIME | COOK TIME | SERVING SIZE |
|---|---|---|---|
| 4 servings | 5 minutes | 5 minutes | ¼ melon with 1 tablespoon syrup |

1 medium cantaloupe

⅓ cup sugar

¼ cup water

1 tbsp finely chopped fresh mint, plus more for garnish (optional)

1 tsp lemon zest

1. Cut cantaloupe in half, and remove the seeds. Slice cantaloupe into 12 wedges. Remove the skin from each wedge.

2. In a small saucepan over medium-high heat, combine sugar, water, mint, and lemon zest. Cook for 5 minutes or until sugar has dissolved. Remove from heat, and let cool.

3. Arrange 3 wedges of melon on each plate, and drizzle with 1 tablespoon sweet mint syrup. Repeat with remaining wedges and syrup.

4. Garnish with additional mint leaves, if using.

**Variation:** This recipe works well with any variety of melon, such as honeydew, crenshaw, or canary. When choosing a melon, look for one that is heavy for its size. The blossom end should give slightly when pressed and give off a hint of the melon's aroma.

| EACH SERVING HAS | | | |
|---|---|---|---|
| 120 calories 0g total fat | 0g saturated fat 1g protein | 29g carbohydrates 1g fiber | 0mg cholesterol 25mg sodium |

# Onion Apple Marmalade

When onions are caramelized, they become sweet and delicious, giving this marmalade a delightful earthy sweetness.

| YIELD | PREP TIME | COOK TIME | SERVING SIZE |
|---|---|---|---|
| 1½ cups | 5 minutes | 30 minutes | 2 tablespoons |

1 tbsp olive oil

3 cups diced white onion

1 cup finely diced
 Red Delicious apple

½ tsp kosher salt

2 tbsp sugar

1 tbsp apple cider vinegar

1 tbsp water

1. In a large nonstick skillet over medium heat, heat olive oil.

2. Add white onion, Red Delicious apple, and kosher salt, and cook, stirring occasionally, for 10 minutes.

3. Add sugar, apple cider vinegar, and water to the skillet, and cook, stirring occasionally, for 15 to 20 more minutes or until onions are golden brown.

4. Use marmalade as a topping for crostini or pizza, as a sandwich spread, or on grilled chicken or pork.

| EACH SERVING HAS | | | |
|---|---|---|---|
| 20 calories<br>0.5g total fat | 0g saturated fat<br>0g protein | 4g carbohydrates<br>0g fiber | 0mg cholesterol<br>40mg sodium |

# Parmesan Pepper Crisps

These savory cheese crisps can be served with appetizers, a salad, or a bowl of soup on a cold winter day. Opt for fresh Parmesan cheese rather than a preshredded variety for the best flavor.

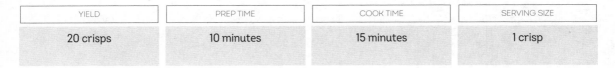

| YIELD | PREP TIME | COOK TIME | SERVING SIZE |
|---|---|---|---|
| 20 crisps | 10 minutes | 15 minutes | 1 crisp |

1 tbsp olive oil

2 cups all-purpose flour, plus additional flour for rolling out dough

1 cup shredded Parmesan cheese

¼ tsp kosher salt

1 tsp freshly ground black pepper

¾ cup warm water

1. Preheat the oven to 400°F (200°C). Coat a baking sheet with olive oil.

2. In a large bowl, combine all-purpose flour, Parmesan cheese, kosher salt, and black pepper.

3. Add warm water, and mix until the dough forms a ball. Turn out dough onto a floured surface, and knead gently for 2 or 3 minutes.

4. Sprinkle the top of the dough with flour, and roll out into a 12×12-inch (30.5×30.5cm) square that's ⅛ inch (3mm) thick.

5. Using a pizza cutter or sharp knife, cut the dough into ¼-inch (0.5cm) strips. Transfer dough strips to the prepared baking sheet.

6. Bake on the top oven rack for 12 to 15 minutes or until slightly golden.

**Variation:** Rosemary would be a great addition to the cheese crisps. Add 1 teaspoon chopped fresh rosemary to the flour, cheese, salt, and pepper mixture in step 2.

| EACH SERVING HAS | | | |
|---|---|---|---|
| 70 calories 2.5g total fat | 1g saturated fat 3g protein | 10g carbohydrates 0g fiber | 5mg cholesterol 105mg sodium |

# Smoked Salmon Bites

Cool, crunchy cucumber is used as the base for flavorful smoked salmon in this great summer dish.

| YIELD | PREP TIME | COOK TIME | SERVING SIZE |
|---|---|---|---|
| 12 salmon bites | 15 minutes | None | 1 salmon bite |

1 cucumber

2 tbsp extra-virgin olive oil

2 tsp freshly squeezed lemon juice

1/8 tsp kosher salt

1/8 tsp freshly ground black pepper

1 clove finely minced garlic

1 tbsp finely chopped red onion

2 tbsp crumbled feta cheese

2 tbsp finely chopped red bell pepper

1 tbsp finely chopped fresh parsley

1 tsp finely chopped fresh basil

1/3 lb (150g) smoked salmon

1. Cut cucumber into 12 1/8-inch (3mm) rounds, and set aside rounds. Peel, seed, and dice the remaining cucumber, enough for 1/4 cup.

2. In a small bowl, combine extra-virgin olive oil, lemon juice, kosher salt, black pepper, garlic, and red onion.

3. Add feta cheese, diced cucumber, red bell pepper, parsley, and basil to the olive oil mixture, and stir to coat.

4. Cut salmon into 12 pieces.

5. Place 1 piece of salmon on each cucumber slice, and top with 1 teaspoon vegetable mixture. Repeat until you have 12 portions.

**Note:** Smoked salmon comes in cold-smoked or hot-smoked. Either type can be used in this recipe. You may see cold-smoked salmon labeled as "nova" or "lox"; it's usually sold in very thin slices. Hot-smoked salmon is sold in large pieces and is flaky like a piece of cooked fish.

**Variation:** Instead of cucumbers, use a toasted slice of baguette, or serve on an endive leaf.

| EACH SERVING HAS | | | |
|---|---|---|---|
| 80 calories 6g total fat | 1.5g saturated fat 5g protein | 1g carbohydrates 0g fiber | 15mg cholesterol 125mg sodium |

# CHAPTER 19

# Soups and Salads

Throughout history, and throughout the Mediterranean, soups have provided warmth, nourishment, and comfort—a meal in a bowl. The basis of most Mediterranean soups is high-quality chicken, beef, or vegetable broth. You can purchase low-sodium broths or make your own so you can control the sodium level. Most soups freeze well and make great meals.

Salads are another traditional, popular Mediterranean dish. Salads can be so much more than just mixed greens. Adding fruits, vegetables, beans, and nuts to greens results in salads that are as delicious for your eyes as they are for your taste buds—not to mention complete meals. From a simple cucumber salad to a more filling shrimp and melon salad, salads allow great versatility and provide loads of nutrition. What you top your salad with should be just as healthy and light as the ingredients in the salad. Make your own dressing with ingredients such as extra-virgin olive oil, vinegar, mustard, shallots, herbs, and spices, and your salad will pop with flavor.

# Tomato Basil Soup

This warm and rich soup uses high-quality canned tomatoes to get the flavor of summer tomatoes anytime, even when they are not in season.

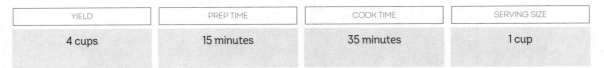

| YIELD | PREP TIME | COOK TIME | SERVING SIZE |
|---|---|---|---|
| 4 cups | 15 minutes | 35 minutes | 1 cup |

1 tbsp olive oil

1 cup diced white onion

2 ribs celery, chopped

1 tbsp minced garlic

1 tbsp dried basil

1 tsp sugar

2 (14.5-oz/410g) cans diced tomatoes, no salt added

½ tsp kosher salt

⅛ tsp freshly ground black pepper

1 tbsp extra-virgin olive oil

1. In a large stockpot over medium heat, heat olive oil. When oil is hot, add white onion, celery, and garlic, and cook for 5 minutes.

2. Add basil, sugar, tomatoes with juice, kosher salt, and black pepper.

3. Bring to a boil, reduce heat to low, and simmer for 20 minutes.

4. Add extra-virgin olive oil.

5. Using an immersion blender, purée the soup in the pot until smooth. Or carefully transfer to a blender to purée. Do not fill the blender more than ½ full per batch because hot liquids expand when blended. Remove the center of the blender lid to allow steam to escape, and place a kitchen towel over the top. Purée for 1 minute or until smooth. Transfer the puréed soup to a large bowl, repeat until you've puréed the rest, and return the puréed soup to the pot.

6. Cook for 10 more minutes before serving.

| EACH SERVING HAS | | | |
|---|---|---|---|
| 140 calories 7g total fat | 1g saturated fat 2g protein | 17g carbohydrates 5g fiber | 0mg cholesterol 350mg sodium |

# Lemon Lentil Soup

The hint of lemon and tangy yogurt add a wonderful flavor dimension to this lentil soup. Using lemon juice and lemon zest is a great way to decrease sodium in soups without sacrificing flavor.

| YIELD | PREP TIME | COOK TIME | SERVING SIZE |
| --- | --- | --- | --- |
| 10 cups | 15 minutes | 30 minutes | 1 cup soup with 2 tablespoons yogurt |

1 tbsp olive oil

1 cup diced white onion

½ cup sliced celery, ¼ in (0.5cm) thick

½ cup diced carrots, ¼ in (0.5cm) thick

8 cups vegetable broth

2 cups red lentils

2 dried bay leaves

1 clove minced garlic

1 tsp dried oregano leaves

¼ tsp freshly ground black pepper

1 tbsp ground coriander

Zest of 1 lemon

1 cup shredded kale

1¼ cups plain Greek yogurt

Sprigs of fresh parsley

1. In a large stockpot over medium heat, heat olive oil. When oil is hot, add white onion, celery, and carrots, and cook, stirring occasionally, for 5 minutes.

2. Add vegetable broth, red lentils, bay leaves, garlic, oregano, black pepper, and ground coriander, and stir to combine. Increase the heat to medium-high, and bring the soup to a boil.

3. Reduce the heat to low, and simmer, stirring occasionally, for 20 minutes.

4. Stir in lemon zest and kale. Cook for 5 minutes or until kale is wilted. Remove and discard bay leaves.

5. Serve 1 cup soup with 2 tablespoons Greek yogurt. Garnish with parsley sprigs.

**Variation:** Add 1 tablespoon finely diced pancetta (unsmoked bacon) or bacon along with the vegetables in step 1.

| EACH SERVING HAS | | | |
| --- | --- | --- | --- |
| 190 calories 3g total fat | 0.5g saturated fat 13g protein | 30g carbohydrates 7g fiber | 0mg cholesterol 150mg sodium |

# Butternut Squash Soup

This sweet butternut squash soup is creamy and delicious. It's comfort in a cup on a chilly winter night.

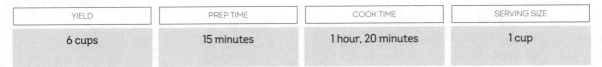

| YIELD | PREP TIME | COOK TIME | SERVING SIZE |
| --- | --- | --- | --- |
| 6 cups | 15 minutes | 1 hour, 20 minutes | 1 cup |

2 medium butternut squash (about 3 lb/1.5kg)

1 tbsp olive oil

1 cup white onion, diced

1 tsp Italian seasoning

4 cups low-sodium chicken broth

1 clove garlic, minced

½ tsp kosher salt

⅛ tsp freshly ground black pepper

1 tbsp honey

1½ tsp peeled and finely grated fresh ginger

1. Preheat the oven to 400°F (200°C).

2. Cut butternut squash in half lengthwise, remove the seeds, and place squash halves on a baking sheet, cut side down. Bake for 30 to 45 minutes or until a knife can be inserted easily.

3. When squash is cool enough to handle, use a spoon to remove the flesh from the skin, and set aside.

4. In a large stockpot over medium heat, heat olive oil. When oil is hot, add white onion, and cook, stirring occasionally, for 5 to 7 minutes. Add Italian seasoning, and stir to combine.

5. To the pot, add squash, 3 cups chicken broth, garlic, kosher salt, black pepper, honey, and ginger. Reduce heat to low, and cook for 20 minutes.

6. Using an immersion blender, purée half of the soup in the pot. Or carefully transfer half of the soup to a blender to purée. Do not fill the blender more than ½ full per batch because hot liquids expand when blended. Remove the center of the blender lid to allow steam to escape, and place a kitchen towel over the top. Purée for 1 minute or until smooth. Transfer the puréed soup to a large bowl, repeat until you've puréed half, and return the puréed soup to the pot.

7. Add remaining 1 cup chicken broth, and cook for 10 more minutes.

| EACH SERVING HAS | | | |
| --- | --- | --- | --- |
| 190 calories 3.5g total fat | 0.5g saturated fat 6g protein | 39g carbohydrates 6g fiber | 0mg cholesterol 230mg sodium |

# Vegetable Orzo Soup

This hearty vegetable soup is easy to make and is a warm treat in the springtime. Orzo, a small, rice-shaped pasta, adds to the soup's heartiness. Although orzo looks like rice, it's made from the same semolina flour as any pasta and is stocked in the pasta aisle.

| YIELD | PREP TIME | COOK TIME | SERVING SIZE |
| --- | --- | --- | --- |
| 5 cups | 20 minutes | 30 minutes | 1 cup |

1 tbsp olive oil

¼ cup chopped celery

½ cup diced white onion

¼ cup sliced carrots

1 (14.5-oz/410g) can diced tomatoes, no salt added

4 cups low-sodium chicken broth

1 cup chopped zucchini

1 cup sliced mushrooms

1 clove garlic, finely minced

½ cup orzo

1 tsp Italian seasoning

½ tsp kosher salt

¼ tsp freshly ground black pepper

Sprigs of fresh parsley

1. In a large stockpot over medium heat, heat olive oil. When oil is hot, add celery, white onion, and carrots. Cook, stirring occasionally, for 5 minutes.

2. Add tomatoes with liquid, chicken broth, zucchini, mushrooms, garlic, orzo, Italian seasoning, kosher salt, and black pepper. Increase the heat slightly, and bring to a gentle boil. Cook, stirring occasionally, for 25 minutes.

3. Garnish with parsley sprigs.

**Variation:** Add 1 link cooked spicy Italian sausage to the soup. Cut it into slices, and add along with the tomatoes in step 2.

| EACH SERVING HAS | | | |
| --- | --- | --- | --- |
| 120 calories<br>4g total fat | 0g saturated fat<br>6g protein | 16g carbohydrates<br>2g fiber | 0mg cholesterol<br>260mg sodium |

# Split Pea Soup

Sweet and smoky, this warm and comforting soup is perfect for wintertime.

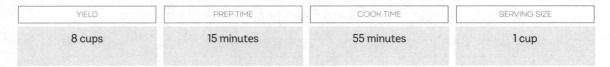

| YIELD | PREP TIME | COOK TIME | SERVING SIZE |
|---|---|---|---|
| 8 cups | 15 minutes | 55 minutes | 1 cup |

1 tbsp olive oil

1 cup diced yellow onion

½ cup diced celery

½ cup diced carrots

1 smoked ham hock

2 cloves garlic, minced

2 tsp ground coriander

1 tsp dried oregano

¼ tsp freshly ground
black pepper

6 cups low-sodium
chicken stock

16 oz (450g) dried split
peas

8 fresh chives, minced

1. In a large stockpot over medium heat, heat olive oil. When oil is hot, add yellow onion, celery, and carrots, and cook for 5 minutes.

2. Add ham hock, garlic, ground coriander, oregano, and black pepper. Stir to combine, and cook for 1 minute.

3. Increase the heat slightly, and add chicken stock and split peas. Bring to a boil, cover, and reduce heat to a simmer. Cook for 40 to 50 minutes or until peas are tender.

4. Remove the ham hock. Or, if desired, shred the meat and return it to the soup after it has been blended.

5. Using an immersion blender, purée half of the soup in the pot. Or carefully transfer half of the soup to a blender to purée. Do not fill the blender more than ½ full per batch because hot liquids expand when blended. Remove the center of the blender lid to allow steam to escape, and place a kitchen towel over the top. Purée for 1 minute or until smooth. Transfer the puréed soup to a large bowl, repeat until you've puréed half, and return the puréed soup to the pot.

6. Garnish with fresh chives.

**Variation:** Add crispy pancetta (unsmoked bacon) or bacon as a garnish along with the chives.

| EACH SERVING HAS | | | |
|---|---|---|---|
| 260 calories<br>4.5g total fat | 1g saturated fat<br>18g protein | 37g carbohydrates<br>15g fiber | 20mg cholesterol<br>240mg sodium |

# Gazpacho

This cold soup is bright-tasting with ripe summer tomatoes–very refreshing on a hot summer day.

| YIELD | PREP TIME | COOK TIME | SERVING SIZE |
|---|---|---|---|
| 3 cups | 20 minutes plus 1 hour cooling time | 5 minutes | ¾ cup |

2 cups ice

8 large tomatoes

½ cup diced celery

½ cup peeled, seeded, and diced cucumber, plus more for garnish

4 scallions, white parts only, sliced

1 clove garlic, minced

1 tbsp freshly squeezed lemon juice

1 tsp lemon zest

½ tsp kosher salt

⅛ tsp freshly ground black pepper

1 tbsp minced fresh parsley

1 tbsp extra-virgin olive oil, plus more for garnish

1. In a medium saucepan over medium-high heat, bring 3 quarts (3 liters) water to a boil.

2. In a large bowl, add 2 cups ice and fill with cold water.

3. Cut a small *X* into the bottom of each tomato. Place 4 tomatoes in the boiling water, and cook for 30 seconds. Using a slotted spoon or tongs, remove tomatoes and immediately transfer them to the ice water. Repeat with the remaining 4 tomatoes.

4. Peel tomatoes starting at the *X*. Roughly chop the peeled tomatoes, and transfer to a food processor.

5. Add celery, cucumber, scallions, garlic, lemon juice, lemon zest, kosher salt, black pepper, parsley, and extra-virgin olive oil to the food processor. Pulse 3 or 4 times to roughly chop. Transfer half of the mixture to a large bowl.

6. Purée the remaining mixture in the food processor. Transfer the puréed ingredients to the bowl, and mix with the roughly chopped ingredients.

7. Refrigerate for at least 1 hour to allow the flavors to meld.

8. Garnish with additional chopped cucumber and a drizzle of extra-virgin olive oil.

| EACH SERVING HAS | | | |
|---|---|---|---|
| 60 calories 4g total fat | 0.5g saturated fat 2g protein | 7g carbohydrates 2g fiber | 0mg cholesterol 260mg sodium |

# Mixed Bean Soup

Hearty, savory, and satisfying, this fall bean soup is warm and filling.

| YIELD | PREP TIME | COOK TIME | SERVING SIZE |
|---|---|---|---|
| 6 cups | 15 minutes plus overnight soaking time | 3 hours | 1 cup |

1 cup dry pinto or
   cranberry beans

1 cup dry white beans

1 tbsp olive oil

1 cup diced white onion

½ cup diced celery

½ cup diced carrots

8 cups low-sodium
   chicken broth

1 tbsp Italian seasoning

⅛ tsp freshly ground
   black pepper

1 smoked ham hock

1. Pick through dried pinto and white beans, and remove any stones.

2. Add beans to a large bowl, and cover with enough cold water that they will remain covered as they double in size. Soak overnight. Remove any bad-looking beans, and drain and rinse beans.

3. In a medium saucepan over medium heat, heat olive oil. When oil is hot, add white onion, celery, and carrots, and sauté for 5 minutes.

4. Add chicken broth, beans, Italian seasoning, black pepper, and ham hock. Increase heat to high, and bring to a rolling boil.

5. Reduce heat to medium, and cook for 2½ to 3 hours or until beans are tender.

6. Remove the ham hock. Or, if desired, shred the meat and return it to the soup.

**Note:** Cranberry beans have a creamy texture and are cream colored with deep red or cranberry-colored markings. As pretty as they are when they're dry, they do not keep the red markings when they're cooked.

**Variation:** You can use any bean in this recipe. Try mixing and matching as many types of beans as you like. Just keep the total at 2 cups.

| EACH SERVING HAS | | | |
|---|---|---|---|
| 200 calories 10g total fat | 3g saturated fat 8g protein | 20g carbohydrates 6g fiber | 10mg cholesterol 910mg sodium |

# Marinated Artichoke Salad

The flavors of an antipasto platter shine in this quick and delicious wintertime salad.

| YIELD | PREP TIME | COOK TIME | SERVING SIZE |
|---|---|---|---|
| 3 cups | 15 minutes plus 30 minutes marinating time | None | ½ cup |

⅓ cup canned artichoke hearts in water, drained

¼ cup pitted and chopped Kalamata olives

⅓ cup chopped jarred roasted red peppers

¼ cup crumbled feta cheese

2 tbsp finely chopped red onion

1 tbsp extra-virgin olive oil

1 tbsp balsamic vinegar

1 clove garlic, finely minced

1 tbsp finely chopped fresh parsley

⅛ tsp kosher salt

⅛ tsp freshly ground black pepper

1. In a large bowl, combine artichoke hearts, Kalamata olives, roasted red peppers, feta cheese, red onion, extra-virgin olive oil, balsamic vinegar, garlic, parsley, kosher salt, and black pepper.

2. Cover and refrigerate for at least 30 minutes to allow flavors to meld.

3. Serve as a small salad or as a side dish with a variety of appetizers.

**Variation:** Add 2 ounces (55g) each of sliced cheese and salami, and serve on a bed of mixed greens.

| EACH SERVING HAS | | | |
|---|---|---|---|
| 90 calories 5g total fat | 1.5g saturated fat 3g protein | 9g carbohydrates 3g fiber | 5mg cholesterol 600mg sodium |

# Roasted Beet Salad

Fall is a great time for roasting beets, which brings out their delicious sweet and earthy flavor.

| YIELD | PREP TIME | COOK TIME | SERVING SIZE |
|---|---|---|---|
| About 4 cups | 30 minutes | 1 hour | 1 cup |

2 large beets

3 tbsp extra-virgin olive oil

1 tbsp finely chopped shallot

1 clove garlic, minced

1 tbsp apple cider vinegar

¼ tsp Dijon mustard

1½ tsp finely chopped fresh mint leaves

2 tsp honey

½ tsp lemon zest

⅛ tsp kosher salt

⅛ tsp freshly ground black pepper

1 cup shredded romaine lettuce

2 oz (55g) feta cheese

2 tbsp chopped pistachios (purchased roasted and salted)

1. Preheat the oven to 400°F (200°C).

2. Remove any greens from beets. Wrap each beet in aluminum foil, and bake for 1 hour or until knife-tender. Remove from the oven, and set aside to cool.

3. When beets are completely cool, use a paring knife to peel. Cut beets into 1-inch (2.5cm) cubes, and place in a medium bowl.

4. In a small bowl, make the dressing by combining extra-virgin olive oil, shallot, garlic, apple cider vinegar, Dijon mustard, mint, honey, lemon zest, kosher salt, and black pepper.

5. Add 2 tablespoons dressing to cubed beets.

6. Toss 1 tablespoon dressing with shredded romaine lettuce.

7. Arrange salad on plates using ¼ cup romaine lettuce, about 1 cup beets, and ½ ounce (14g) feta cheese. Top with ½ tablespoon pistachios.

**Note:** Don't throw away those beet greens! You can use beet greens as you would other dark leafy greens. Wash and tear into 2- or 3-inch (5 to 7.5cm) pieces, and sauté in olive oil and garlic until wilted.

| EACH SERVING HAS | | | |
|---|---|---|---|
| 190 calories 15g total fat | 4g saturated fat 4g protein | 10g carbohydrates 2g fiber | 15mg cholesterol 270mg sodium |

# Golden Couscous Salad

The sweetness of the golden raisins complements the couscous's curry essence in this summer salad that's great as a side dish with grilled lamb or chicken.

| YIELD | PREP TIME | COOK TIME | SERVING SIZE |
| --- | --- | --- | --- |
| 10 cups | 20 minutes plus 30 minutes marinating time | 20 minutes | ½ cup |

1 tbsp olive oil

8 oz (225g) Israeli couscous

2 cups warm water

⅓ cup golden raisins

½ tsp curry powder

¼ cup pine nuts

1 clove garlic, finely minced

½ cup finely chopped red bell pepper

½ cup finely diced celery

4 scallions, finely minced

1 tsp orange zest

1 tbsp extra-virgin olive oil

½ tsp kosher salt

⅛ tsp freshly ground black pepper

1. In a small saucepan over medium heat, heat olive oil. When oil is hot, add couscous, and cook, stirring occasionally, for about 5 minutes or until slightly toasted.

2. Add warm water, golden raisins, and curry powder, and mix well. Bring to a boil. Reduce heat to a simmer, cover, and simmer for 15 minutes or until all liquid is absorbed.

3. Remove from heat, transfer couscous mixture to a large bowl, and cool to room temperature.

4. Meanwhile, in a small skillet over medium heat, toast pine nuts for 5 or 6 minutes or until lightly browned.

5. When couscous has cooled, add garlic, red bell pepper, celery, scallions, orange zest, extra-virgin olive oil, kosher salt, black pepper, and pine nuts, and mix well. Refrigerate for at least 30 minutes to allow the flavors to meld.

**Variation:** Instead of Israeli couscous, which is a small pea–size white couscous that's larger than the couscous you may be familiar with, you can use whole-grain couscous to boost your fiber intake.

| EACH SERVING HAS | | | |
| --- | --- | --- | --- |
| 80 calories 2.5g total fat | 0g saturated fat 2g protein | 12g carbohydrates 1g fiber | 0mg cholesterol 50mg sodium |

# Tuna Salad
*with Capers and Potatoes*

This light, refreshing tuna salad is very different from the mayonnaise-based versions and perfect for warmer months. The capers—immature buds of the caper bush native to the Mediterranean that are picked, dried, and pickled—add a nice briny tang.

| YIELD | PREP TIME | COOK TIME | SERVING SIZE |
|---|---|---|---|
| 4 servings | 15 minutes | 15 minutes | ⅓ cup tuna mixture, 2 ounces (55g) potato, and 1 cup lettuce |

8 oz (225g) new potatoes

4 tbsp balsamic vinaigrette

10 cherry tomatoes, halved

10 Kalamata olives, pitted and halved

1 tbsp minced red onion

2 tbsp capers

1 (6-oz/170g) can solid albacore tuna, in spring water, drained

4 cups mixed lettuce greens

1. In a medium saucepan over medium-high heat, boil potatoes for 15 minutes or until knife-tender. Remove from the water, and cool to room temperature.

2. When potatoes have cooled, slice them ¼ inch (0.5cm) thick.

3. In a small bowl, gently combine 1 tablespoon balsamic vinaigrette with potato slices.

4. In a medium bowl, gently combine cherry tomatoes, Kalamata olives, red onion, capers, tuna, and 2 tablespoons balsamic vinaigrette.

5. In a large bowl, toss mixed lettuce greens with remaining 1 tablespoon balsamic vinaigrette.

6. To serve, place 1 cup lettuce greens on each of 4 plates. Top evenly with sliced potato and ⅓ cup tuna mixture.

| EACH SERVING HAS | | | |
|---|---|---|---|
| 200 calories 10g total fat | 1.5g saturated fat 13g protein | 15g carbohydrates 3g fiber | 15mg cholesterol 510mg sodium |

# Fennel and Apple Salad

Fennel's slight licorice flavor combines nicely with the sweetness of the apples in this bright, refreshing winter salad.

| YIELD | PREP TIME | COOK TIME | SERVING SIZE |
|---|---|---|---|
| 4 cups | 20 minutes | None | 1 cup |

¼ cup extra-virgin olive oil

1 clove garlic, finely minced

1 tbsp freshly squeezed lemon juice

1 tbsp lemon zest

¼ tsp kosher salt

⅛ tsp freshly ground black pepper

4 scallions

2 medium Red Delicious apples

1 bulb fennel

1 cup baby spinach

1. In a large bowl, combine extra-virgin olive oil, garlic, lemon juice, lemon zest, kosher salt, and black pepper.

2. Cut scallions, separating the white parts from the green tops. Finely mince the white parts, and add to the bowl. Cut the green tops diagonally into ⅛-inch (3mm) slices, and add to the bowl. Mix well.

3. Cut Red Delicious apples into slices ⅛ inch (3mm) thick. Cut across the slices to make sticks ⅛ inch (3mm) thick. Immediately toss apple sticks in olive oil mixture to prevent browning, mixing well after each addition. (There is no need to core the apples because you slice from the outer edges toward the core. Discard the core.)

4. Remove green stalks and fronds from fennel bulb. Slice bulb in half through the center of the root, and cut out and discard the hard triangular core. Cut fennel into thin slices, using a mandoline slicer if you have one. Add to the bowl, and toss well.

5. Add baby spinach to the bowl, and toss to coat.

**Variation:** Add ½ cup pomegranate seeds or 1 cup seedless grapes, cut in half.

| EACH SERVING HAS | | | |
|---|---|---|---|
| 210 calories 14g total fat | 2g saturated fat 2g protein | 23g carbohydrates 6g fiber | 0mg cholesterol 170mg sodium |

# Shrimp and Melon Salad

Shrimp and sweet summer melon are a great pairing in this refreshing summer salad.

| YIELD | PREP TIME | COOK TIME | SERVING SIZE |
|---|---|---|---|
| 2 servings | 15 minutes | None | ½ recipe |

2 cups red leaf lettuce, torn into bite-size pieces

⅓ cup cubed cantaloupe, ½-in (1.25cm) cubes

1 scallion, white and green parts, finely chopped

½ Hass avocado, diced

½ lb (225g; 26 to 30 count, about 14) cooked shrimp, tail on

2 tbsp balsamic vinaigrette

1 tbsp finely chopped fresh basil

1. Evenly divide red leaf lettuce between 2 plates.

2. Evenly divide cantaloupe, scallion, and Hass avocado between each plate.

3. Top each plate with about 7 shrimp. Stand shrimp in the center of the salad mixture with their tails pointing up.

4. Drizzle each serving with 1 tablespoon balsamic vinaigrette, and garnish with ½ teaspoon basil.

| EACH SERVING HAS | | | |
|---|---|---|---|
| 250 calories 22g total fat | 3g saturated fat 8g protein | 9g carbohydrates 4g fiber | 55mg cholesterol 200mg sodium |

# Minted Cucumber Salad

The crunch of the cool cucumber and the fresh flavor of mint in this salad will cool you down on a hot summer day.

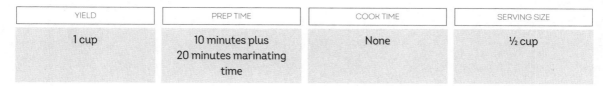

| YIELD | PREP TIME | COOK TIME | SERVING SIZE |
|---|---|---|---|
| 1 cup | 10 minutes plus 20 minutes marinating time | None | ½ cup |

1 tbsp extra-virgin olive oil

⅛ tsp kosher salt

⅛ tsp freshly ground black pepper

1 tbsp finely minced red onion

1 tbsp finely chopped fresh mint leaves

1 English cucumber or regular cucumber

1. In a medium bowl, combine extra-virgin olive oil, kosher salt, black pepper, red onion, and mint.

2. Peel cucumber, slice in half lengthwise, and scoop out the seeds with a small spoon. Cut cucumber halves into ⅛-inch (3mm) slices. Add slices to olive oil mixture, and stir to combine.

3. Let mixture rest for 20 minutes.

4. Serve at room temperature.

**Variation:** Use basil instead of mint and serve on a bed of lettuce greens. Make it a meal by adding ½ cup cooked shrimp.

| EACH SERVING HAS | | | |
|---|---|---|---|
| 70 calories 7g total fat | 1g saturated fat 1g protein | 2g carbohydrates 1g fiber | 0mg cholesterol 120mg sodium |

# Spinach, Orange, and Feta Salad

Used as a salad green, raw spinach has a completely different flavor and texture than cooked spinach, as you will discover in this soon-to-be favorite summer salad.

| YIELD | PREP TIME | COOK TIME | SERVING SIZE |
|---|---|---|---|
| 4 cups | 20 minutes | None | 2 cups |

2 medium oranges

3 tbsp extra-virgin olive oil

1 tbsp white balsamic vinegar

¼ tsp Dijon mustard

1 tsp Italian seasoning

1 tsp minced shallot

1 tbsp freshly squeezed orange juice

1 tsp honey

2 cups packed baby spinach, washed thoroughly

2 oz (55g) feta cheese

¼ cucumber, peeled, seeded, and diced

¼ cup chopped pecans, toasted

¼ cup sliced red onion rings

1. Cut off the tops and bottoms of oranges. Place oranges cut side down on a cutting board, cut off peel and white pith, and slice each orange from top to bottom. Holding the orange over a small bowl to catch the juice, cut out segments, leaving behind the membrane between each section. Set aside orange segments. Squeeze the remaining orange membrane over the small bowl to catch the juice.

2. In a separate small bowl, make dressing by whisking together extra-virgin olive oil, white balsamic vinegar, Dijon mustard, Italian seasoning, shallot, 1 tablespoon orange juice, and honey.

3. In a large bowl, toss baby spinach with 1 tablespoon dressing.

4. Add orange segments, feta cheese, and cucumber, and gently toss to combine.

5. Top with toasted pecans and red onion rings, and drizzle with extra dressing if desired.

**Variation:** Instead of toasted pecans, try toasted almonds, pine nuts, or pistachios. (See the following Classic Mixed Greens Salad with Balsamic Vinaigrette recipe for directions on how to toast nuts.)

| | EACH SERVING HAS | | |
|---|---|---|---|
| 340 calories<br>23g total fat | 6g saturated fat<br>8g protein | 31g carbohydrates<br>7g fiber | 25mg cholesterol<br>390mg sodium |

# Classic Mixed Greens Salad
## with Balsamic Vinaigrette

A fresh, flavorful mixed greens salad can be served alongside any meal and is perfect by itself as a summertime lunch.

| YIELD | PREP TIME | COOK TIME | SERVING SIZE |
|---|---|---|---|
| 4 servings | 15 minutes | None | 1¼ cups salad |

4 cups mixed salad greens

½ cup sliced radishes

½ cup halved cherry tomatoes

¼ cup shredded carrots

¼ cup extra-virgin olive oil

1 tbsp balsamic vinegar

1 tbsp finely minced shallot

¼ tsp Italian seasoning

¼ tsp Dijon mustard

¼ tsp kosher salt

⅛ tsp freshly ground black pepper

½ tsp sugar

¼ cup coarsely chopped walnuts, toasted

1. In a large bowl, toss together mixed salad greens, radishes, cherry tomatoes, and carrots.

2. In a small bowl, whisk together extra-virgin olive oil, balsamic vinegar, shallot, Italian seasoning, Dijon mustard, kosher salt, black pepper, and sugar.

3. Pour dressing over greens mixture, and toss to coat.

4. Evenly divide the salad among 4 plates, and garnish with toasted walnuts.

**Note:** Toasting any nut brings out its full flavor. To toast nuts, place them in a single layer in a small skillet over medium heat. Cook, stirring occasionally, for 5 to 7 minutes or until lightly browned—keep an eye on them because they can burn quickly. Or toast nuts in a preheated 400°F (200°C) oven for 5 to 7 minutes.

**Variation:** This balsamic vinaigrette works well with just about any fruits, vegetables, and meats. Keep it on hand, and you might find yourself drizzling it on a variety of recipes.

| EACH SERVING HAS | | | |
|---|---|---|---|
| 190 calories 19g total fat | 2.5g saturated fat 2g protein | 7g carbohydrates 2g fiber | 0mg cholesterol 160mg sodium |

# Tabbouleh Salad

Bulgur has a nice nutty flavor. Its tender, chewy texture balances nicely with the vegetables and herbs in this fall salad.

| YIELD | PREP TIME | COOK TIME | SERVING SIZE |
|---|---|---|---|
| 3 cups | 15 minutes plus 2½ hours soaking time | None | ½ cup |

½ cup bulgur wheat

1 cup water

½ cup finely chopped fresh parsley

⅓ cup finely diced tomato

¼ cup thinly sliced scallions

1 cup peeled, seeded, and finely diced cucumber

⅓ cup finely chopped fresh mint leaves

1 tbsp extra-virgin olive oil

1 tbsp freshly squeezed lemon juice

1. In a large bowl, cover bulgur wheat with water. Let soak in the refrigerator for 2½ hours or overnight. The bulgur will absorb the water and double in size.

2. Add parsley, tomato, scallions, cucumber, and mint to the bulgur, and mix well.

3. Add extra-virgin olive oil and lemon juice, and mix well.

| EACH SERVING HAS | | | |
|---|---|---|---|
| 70 calories 2.5g total fat | 0g saturated fat 2g protein | 11g carbohydrates 3g fiber | 0mg cholesterol 10mg sodium |

# CHAPTER 20

# Flatbreads, Pizza, Wraps, and More

Flatbreads are versatile and make a quick substitute for traditional pizza crust. This type of bread has been a prominent food in many different cultures. In Persia and central Asia, you would find flatbread in the form of naan; in the Middle East, pita and lavash. No matter what you call it, flatbread can be the basis for a nutrient-rich snack, lunch, or dinner, topped with just about anything, including heart-healthy Mediterranean ingredients.

If you prefer a traditional-crust pizza, you can find a variety of premade doughs, from white, to whole-wheat, to flavored versions like garlic and herb. Making pizza at home allows you to control your toppings and choose healthier, Mediterranean-style options.

Finally, give your wraps and sandwiches a Mediterranean flair by filling them with raw or grilled vegetables, avocados, beans, hummus, herbs, and spices. Top them with a zingy yogurt topping, olive oil, or red wine vinegar. The recipes in this chapter will inspire you to think differently about your toppings and fillings!

# Caramelized Onion Flatbread

This Mediterranean-inspired flatbread topped with sweet caramelized onions will warm you on a crisp fall day.

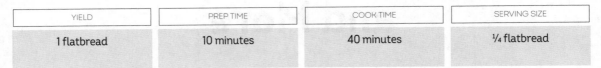

| YIELD | PREP TIME | COOK TIME | SERVING SIZE |
|---|---|---|---|
| 1 flatbread | 10 minutes | 40 minutes | ¼ flatbread |

1 tbsp olive oil

1 large sweet onion, sliced ⅛ in (3mm) thick

1 oz (30g) pancetta (unsmoked bacon), diced

1 (3-oz/85g) flatbread

1 oz (30g) fresh mozzarella, sliced

1 tbsp finely chopped fresh parsley

1. Preheat the oven to 400°F (200°C). Oil a baking sheet.

2. In a large skillet over medium heat, heat olive oil. When oil is hot, add sweet onion, and cook, stirring occasionally, for 20 minutes or until onions are golden brown. Remove from heat.

3. In a small skillet over medium heat, cook pancetta for 10 minutes or until crisp. Remove from heat, and drain pancetta on a paper towel.

4. Place flatbread on the prepared baking sheet, and spread onions over top. Sprinkle pancetta over the onions, and top with sliced mozzarella.

5. Bake for 8 to 10 minutes or until cheese is melted.

6. Garnish with parsley. Cut into 4 pieces.

**Variation:** Use any type of cheese you like. Blue cheese would be great with this recipe. You also could use prosciutto, bacon, or ham instead of the pancetta.

| EACH SERVING HAS | | | |
|---|---|---|---|
| 160 calories<br>9g total fat | 3g saturated fat<br>6g protein | 15g carbohydrates<br>2g fiber | 15mg cholesterol<br>290mg sodium |

# Pear, Provolone, Asiago, and Balsamic Flatbread

Sweet pears; sharp cheese; and sweet, savory balsamic syrup balance each other beautifully in this fall-inspired flatbread.

| YIELD | PREP TIME | COOK TIME | SERVING SIZE |
| --- | --- | --- | --- |
| 1 flatbread | 10 minutes | 10 minutes | ¼ flatbread |

1 red pear

1 (3-oz/85g) flatbread

1½ oz (43g) provolone cheese

1 tbsp Asiago cheese, shredded

1 tbsp balsamic syrup

1. Preheat the oven to 400°F (200°C). Oil a baking sheet.

2. Slice pear in half, and core it. Slice one pear half into very thin slices, less than ⅛ inch (3mm) thick. Reserve other half for another use.

3. Place flatbread on the prepared baking sheet, and top with provolone cheese. Place sliced pears on top of provolone, with the skin sides all facing the same direction. Sprinkle pears with Asiago cheese.

4. Bake for 8 to 10 minutes or until edges are slightly golden.

5. Drizzle top of flatbread with balsamic syrup. Cut into 4 pieces.

**Variation:** Try different cheeses in place of the provolone such as Brie, Gorgonzola, or pecorino Romano. Garnish with 1 teaspoon fresh chopped mint or 1 tablespoon toasted walnuts. Red pears, a different variety from their green or yellow counterparts, make a beautiful presentation in this dish, but feel free to use any type of pear you enjoy.

| EACH SERVING HAS | | | |
| --- | --- | --- | --- |
| 140 calories 4.5g total fat | 2.5g saturated fat 6g protein | 19g carbohydrates 4g fiber | 10mg cholesterol 210mg sodium |

# Mushroom, Artichoke, and Arugula Flatbread

The addition of arugula lends a nice, peppery bite to this fall flatbread.

| YIELD | PREP TIME | COOK TIME | SERVING SIZE |
|---|---|---|---|
| 1 flatbread | 10 minutes | 13 to 15 minutes | ¼ flatbread |

1 tbsp olive oil

¼ cup finely diced onion

1 cup sliced baby portobello mushrooms

¼ tsp dried oregano

⅓ cup artichoke quarters in spring water, drained

1 clove garlic, finely minced

6 Kalamata olives, pitted and halved

2 tbsp white wine

⅛ tsp freshly ground black pepper, plus more for garnish

1 (3-oz/85g) flatbread

½ oz (14g) Parmesan cheese, freshly grated

½ cup fresh arugula leaves

Extra-virgin olive oil

1. Preheat the oven to 400°F (200°C). Oil a baking sheet.

2. In a large sauté pan over medium heat, heat olive oil. When oil is hot, add onion, baby portobello mushrooms, and oregano, and cook, stirring occasionally, for 5 minutes.

3. Add artichokes, garlic, Kalamata olives, white wine, and black pepper, and cook for 2 minutes or until wine has evaporated.

4. Place flatbread on the prepared baking sheet, and evenly distribute warm mushroom mixture over the top. Sprinkle with ¼ ounce (7g) Parmesan cheese.

5. Bake for 8 to 10 minutes or until edges are slightly golden.

6. Top with arugula and remaining ¼ ounce (7g) Parmesan cheese. Garnish with additional black pepper and a drizzle of extra-virgin olive oil. Cut into 4 pieces.

| EACH SERVING HAS | | | |
|---|---|---|---|
| 140 calories 7g total fat | 1.5g saturated fat 5g protein | 14g carbohydrates 2g fiber | 5mg cholesterol 290mg sodium |

# Tomato Basil Pizza

Fresh, juicy, summer tomatoes and sweet, aromatic basil are a perfect match. Fresh mozzarella adds a creamy, smooth richness.

| YIELD | PREP TIME | COOK TIME | SERVING SIZE |
|---|---|---|---|
| 1 pizza | 15 minutes | 10 minutes | ⅛ pizza |

16 oz (450g) purchased pizza dough

1 tbsp Pesto (page 223)

2 large Roma tomatoes, sliced ¼ in (0.5cm) thick

3 oz (85g) fresh mozzarella, sliced ¼ in (0.5cm) thick

1 tbsp fresh basil, thinly sliced

⅛ tsp freshly ground black pepper

1. Preheat the oven according to the pizza dough package directions. Oil a baking sheet.

2. Place pizza dough on a well-floured surface, and roll out to 12 inches (30.5cm) round. Transfer to the prepared baking sheet.

3. Brush pizza dough with Pesto and then layer sliced Roma tomatoes and mozzarella over top.

4. Bake for 10 minutes or until edges are slightly browned.

5. Sprinkle with fresh basil and black pepper. Cut into 8 pieces.

**Variation:** Try this pizza with ⅓ cup sun-dried tomatoes instead of fresh Romas. Or sprinkle with 2 tablespoons toasted pine nuts.

| EACH SERVING HAS | | | |
|---|---|---|---|
| 160 calories<br>5g total fat | 1g saturated fat<br>7g protein | 25g carbohydrates<br>1g fiber | 5mg cholesterol<br>260mg sodium |

# Butternut Squash and Goat Cheese Pizza

Sweet butternut squash and tangy goat cheese pair beautifully on this wintertime pizza. Opt for fresh butternut squash already peeled and cubed, if your market offers it, to save some prep time.

| YIELD | PREP TIME | COOK TIME | SERVING SIZE |
|---|---|---|---|
| 1 pizza | 10 minutes | 20 minutes | ⅛ pizza |

16 oz (450g) purchased pizza dough

1 tbsp olive oil

1 cup peeled, seeded, and diced butternut squash, ⅛-in (3mm) cubes

¼ cup diced onion

¼ tsp kosher salt

⅛ tsp freshly ground black pepper

1 clove garlic, finely minced

1 tsp chopped fresh thyme leaves

1 tbsp white wine

2 oz (55g) goat cheese

2 tbsp chopped walnuts, toasted

1 tbsp finely chopped fresh parsley

1. Preheat the oven according to the pizza dough package directions. Oil a baking sheet.

2. Place pizza dough on a well-floured surface, and roll out to 12 inches (30.5cm) round. Transfer to the prepared baking sheet.

3. In a large sauté pan over medium heat, heat olive oil. When oil is hot, add butternut squash, onion, kosher salt, and black pepper. Cook, stirring occasionally, for 8 minutes.

4. Add garlic, thyme, and white wine, and cook for 2 more minutes. Remove from heat.

5. Spread warm squash mixture evenly over pizza dough. Crumble goat cheese over top.

6. Bake for 8 to 10 minutes in the center of the oven or until edges are slightly golden.

7. Garnish with walnuts and parsley. Cut into 8 pieces.

**Variation:** Try using ½ teaspoon fresh rosemary instead of 1 tablespoon fresh parsley. Gorgonzola instead of goat cheese would also be a nice substitution.

| EACH SERVING HAS | | | |
|---|---|---|---|
| 190 calories<br>7g total fat | 2g saturated fat<br>6g protein | 27g carbohydrates<br>1g fiber | 5mg cholesterol<br>290mg sodium |

# Veggie Wrap

Roasting summer vegetables brings out their natural sweetness and intensifies the flavor.

| YIELD | PREP TIME | COOK TIME | SERVING SIZE |
|---|---|---|---|
| 4 wraps | 30 minutes | 50 minutes | ½ wrap |

1 red bell pepper

1 orange bell pepper

2 tbsp olive oil

½ tsp kosher salt

⅛ tsp freshly ground black pepper

1 tsp dried mint leaves

1 tsp ground coriander

1 tbsp Italian seasoning

2 medium zucchini, sliced lengthwise, ¼ in (0.5cm) thick

1 medium eggplant, sliced lengthwise, ¼ in (0.5cm) thick

1 red onion, sliced into ¼-in (0.5cm) rings

1 cup Hummus (page 228)

4 lavash-style soft flatbreads

4 oz (115g) feta cheese, crumbled

1 cup grated cucumber

1. Preheat the oven broiler. Oil a baking sheet.

2. Cut off tops and bottoms of red and orange bell peppers. Slice down one side of each pepper, open, and remove ribs and seeds. Place on the prepared baking sheet, skin side up, and press to flatten. Broil peppers 2 inches (5cm) from the broiler for 8 to 10 minutes or until tops are charred. Remove from the oven, cover with aluminum foil, and set aside.

3. Preheat the oven to 400°F (200°C). Oil a rimmed baking sheet.

4. In a small bowl, combine olive oil, kosher salt, black pepper, mint, ground coriander, and Italian seasoning. Brush zucchini, eggplant, and red onion slices on both sides with oil mixture, and spread in a single layer on the prepared baking sheet. Bake for 30 to 40 minutes or until tender and lightly browned.

5. Meanwhile, peel off charred skin from bell peppers, using a knife tip to scrape it away from the flesh if needed, and discard. Slice peppers into thin strips.

6. Spread ¼ cup Hummus onto each flatbread. Top each with ¼ of zucchini, eggplant, peppers, and onions, and sprinkle 1 ounce (30g) feta cheese over top. Roll flatbreads, and slice in half. Serve with grated cucumber.

| EACH SERVING HAS | | | |
|---|---|---|---|
| 250 calories<br>11g total fat | 3.5g saturated fat<br>8g protein | 30g carbohydrates<br>5g fiber | 15mg cholesterol<br>590mg sodium |

# Chicken Almond Wrap

This Mediterranean twist on chicken salad will become a fast favorite. A yogurt dressing with a hint of bright lemon zest completes the dish.

| YIELD | PREP TIME | COOK TIME | SERVING SIZE |
|-------|-----------|-----------|--------------|
| 3 wraps | 20 minutes plus 30 minutes marinating time | 20 minutes | ½ wrap |

8 oz (225g) boneless, skinless chicken breast

1 tsp olive oil

½ tsp kosher salt

¼ tsp freshly ground black pepper

¼ cup plain Greek yogurt

1 clove garlic, finely minced

1 tsp spicy brown mustard

1 tsp honey

1 tsp lemon zest

1 tsp extra-virgin olive oil

½ cup finely diced celery

1 tbsp finely minced red onion

1 tsp finely chopped fresh mint

½ cup halved red grapes

1 cup finely shredded savoy cabbage

¼ cup slivered almonds, toasted

3 lavash-style flatbreads

1½ cups lettuce spring mix

1. Coat chicken with olive oil, and sprinkle with ¼ teaspoon kosher salt and ⅛ teaspoon black pepper.

2. On an outdoor grill or stove-top grill pan over medium heat, cook chicken for 8 to 10 minutes per side or until a meat thermometer shows an internal temperature of 165°F (75°C) in the thickest part of the breast. Remove from heat, and let rest for 5 minutes.

3. In a small bowl, combine Greek yogurt, garlic, spicy brown mustard, honey, lemon zest, and extra-virgin olive oil. Mix well.

4. Dice chicken into ½-inch (1.25cm) cubes.

5. In a large bowl, combine chicken, celery, red onion, mint, red grapes, savoy cabbage, remaining ¼ teaspoon salt, remaining ⅛ teaspoon pepper, and almonds. Mix well.

6. Add yogurt mixture to chicken mixture, and mix well. Refrigerate for 30 minutes to allow flavors to meld.

7. Place 1 cup chicken mixture on each flatbread, and top with ½ cup lettuce spring mix. Roll flatbreads, and slice in half.

| EACH SERVING HAS | | | |
|---|---|---|---|
| 290 calories 14g total fat | 3g saturated fat 11g protein | 31g carbohydrates 3g fiber | 15mg cholesterol 580mg sodium |

# Chicken Tzatziki Pita

This chicken, fresh veggie, and cool tzatziki pita is a delicious summer meal. Tzatziki is a common condiment in Greece and Turkey; it can be used as a dip with pita wedges, too.

| YIELD | PREP TIME | COOK TIME | SERVING SIZE |
|---|---|---|---|
| 2 pita sandwiches | 10 minutes | 20 minutes | 1 half-pita sandwich |

1 tsp olive oil

¼ tsp Italian seasoning

¼ tsp kosher salt

⅛ tsp freshly ground black pepper

8 oz (225g) boneless, skinless chicken breast

½ cup plain Greek yogurt

¼ cup peeled, seeded, and finely chopped cucumber

1 small clove garlic, finely minced

1 pita, cut in half

1 small tomato, thinly sliced

6 rings red onion, thinly sliced

1 tbsp finely chopped fresh parsley

1. In a medium bowl, combine olive oil, Italian seasoning, ⅛ teaspoon kosher salt, and black pepper. Add chicken, and turn to coat.

2. On an outdoor grill or stove-top grill pan over medium heat, cook chicken for 8 to 10 minutes per side or until a meat thermometer shows an internal temperature of 165°F (75°C) in the thickest part of the breast. Remove from heat, and let rest.

3. In a small bowl, make tzatziki sauce by combining remaining ⅛ teaspoon salt, Greek yogurt, cucumber, and garlic.

4. Slice chicken into ¼-inch (0.5cm) slices.

5. Spread 1 tablespoon tzatziki sauce in each pita half's pocket. Evenly divide chicken, tomato, and red onion between pita halves. Garnish with parsley.

**Variation:** Instead of grilling the chicken, you can bake it. Preheat the oven to 375°F (190°C), place the chicken on a baking sheet, and cook for about 30 minutes.

| EACH SERVING HAS | | | |
|---|---|---|---|
| 320 calories<br>10g total fat | 5g saturated fat<br>33g protein | 22g carbohydrates<br>2g fiber | 75mg cholesterol<br>500mg sodium |

# Prosciutto and Roasted Vegetable Panini

Prosciutto has the flavor of very mild ham with just a hint of salt. Paired with roasted vegetables and melted cheese, it is amazing.

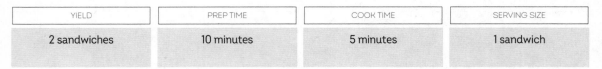

| YIELD | PREP TIME | COOK TIME | SERVING SIZE |
|---|---|---|---|
| 2 sandwiches | 10 minutes | 5 minutes | 1 sandwich |

4 slices potato bread

2 tsp olive oil

2 oz (55g) provolone cheese

2 oz (55g) prosciutto

⅔ cup roasted vegetables

1. Brush one side of each slice of potato bread with olive oil. Place 2 pieces of bread in the panini press, oiled side down.

2. Place 1 slice provolone cheese on each slice of bread in the press. Top each slice with half of the prosciutto and half of the roasted vegetables. Cover with the remaining slices of bread, oiled side up this time.

3. Cook for 3 minutes or until golden brown.

**Note:** If you do not have a panini press, cook the sandwiches in a nonstick skillet over medium heat for 3 minutes per side or until golden brown.

**Variation:** You can omit the provolone and roasted vegetables and use mozzarella and fresh tomato slices instead.

| EACH SERVING HAS | | | |
|---|---|---|---|
| 450 calories 20g total fat | 7g saturated fat 23g protein | 48g carbohydrates 5g fiber | 40mg cholesterol 1450mg sodium |

# CHAPTER 21

# Main Dishes

Fish receives extra recognition in the Mediterranean diet: at least two servings or more each week are recommended to get the omega-3 fatty acids you need for good health. Fish and shellfish can be grilled, panfried, baked, or cooked in a stew. Many varieties are available at your local market, flash-frozen and individually packaged. The recipes in this chapter are easy to make and will help you find tasty ways to include more fish in your weekly menu plans.

Pasta, especially whole-grain pasta, is so versatile that your pantry should never be without it. With a basic tomato sauce, pesto, or a little drizzle of a good-quality extra-virgin olive oil combined with shaved Parmesan and freshly ground black pepper, you have the basis of a delicious meal. Pasta is typically made from semolina flour, a refined flour; brown rice, quinoa, and whole-wheat pastas are preferred on the Mediterranean diet for their higher protein, fiber, vitamin, and mineral content. Try a few to find a brand and type you like.

Chicken is the most commonly consumed poultry in Mediterranean cooking. It is easy to cook and goes well with a wide range of other ingredients. If you have had trouble producing a moist chicken breast, you likely are overcooking it. Cook to an internal temperature of 165°F (75°C), and you will end up with moist and juicy meat every time.

# Seafood Stew

This light and flavorful stew features tender fish or other seafood in a savory broth with a hint of spiciness from the red pepper flakes–perfect for a fall dish.

| YIELD | PREP TIME | COOK TIME | SERVING SIZE |
|---|---|---|---|
| 8 cups | 20 minutes | 50 minutes | 1 cup |

1 small bulb fennel

3 tbsp olive oil

4 cloves garlic, thinly sliced

1 large onion, thinly sliced

1 tbsp frozen orange juice concentrate, thawed

1 (14-oz/400g) can diced tomatoes

½ tsp red pepper flakes

1 cup dry white wine

5 cups bottled clam juice (or seafood stock)

2 lb (1kg) seafood (any firm whitefish or any shellfish, such as cod, halibut, sole, tilapia, shrimp, clams, or mussels)

1. Remove green stalks and fronds from fennel bulb. Slice bulb in half through the center of the root, and cut out and discard the hard triangular core. Cut fennel into thin slices, using a mandoline slicer if you have one.

2. In a large saucepan over medium heat, heat olive oil. When oil is hot, add garlic, onion, and fennel, and cook for 5 to 10 minutes or until vegetables begin to brown.

3. Add orange juice concentrate, tomatoes, red pepper flakes, white wine, and clam juice. Bring to a boil, reduce heat to a simmer, and cook for 30 minutes.

4. Meanwhile, cut seafood into bite-size pieces.

5. Increase the heat to medium. Add fish, if using (if using shellfish, do not add yet), and cook for 2 minutes.

6. Add shellfish, if using, and cook for 5 minutes or until shells begin to open. Discard any that do not open.

| EACH SERVING HAS | | | |
|---|---|---|---|
| 210 calories<br>7g total fat | 1g saturated fat<br>22g protein | 9g carbohydrates<br>2g fiber | 85mg cholesterol<br>440mg sodium |

# Pan-Seared Orange Scallops

In this summery seafood dish, orange adds a sweet flavor that intensifies the natural sweetness of the scallops.

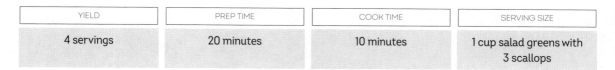

| YIELD | PREP TIME | COOK TIME | SERVING SIZE |
| --- | --- | --- | --- |
| 4 servings | 20 minutes | 10 minutes | 1 cup salad greens with 3 scallops |

3 medium oranges

⅛ cup white balsamic vinegar

1 clove garlic, finely minced

1 tsp Dijon mustard

¼ tsp kosher salt

½ cup extra-virgin olive oil

2 tbsp olive oil

2 tbsp all-purpose flour

1 lb (450g) U10 sea scallops

½ tsp chopped fresh oregano leaves

4 cups packed mixed salad greens

1 avocado, peeled and diced

1. Zest 1 orange to yield ¼ teaspoon zest. Set aside zest and zested orange. Juice remaining 2 whole oranges to yield ½ cup juice.

2. Cut off the top and bottom of the zested orange. Place orange cut side down on a cutting board, cut off remaining peel and white pith, and slice around orange from top to bottom. Holding orange over a bowl to catch any juice, cut out segments, leaving behind the membrane between each section. Set aside orange segments.

3. In a small bowl, make salad dressing by combining orange zest, white balsamic vinegar, garlic, Dijon mustard, ⅛ teaspoon kosher salt, and ¼ cup orange juice. Slowly whisk in extra-virgin olive oil. Set aside.

4. In a large nonstick skillet over medium heat, heat 2 tablespoons olive oil.

5. Meanwhile, place all-purpose flour in a shallow dish, and dredge the tops and bottoms of scallops in flour, shaking off any excess.

6. When olive oil is hot, add half of scallops, one at a time, and cook for 2 or 3 minutes. Do not move the scallops as they cook so they develop a brown crust. Turn over scallops when golden brown, and cook for 2 or 3 more minutes or until the sides are all white with no translucence in the middle. Transfer scallops to a plate, and cover with foil. Repeat with remaining scallops, adding more olive oil if needed.

*(continues)*

# *Pan-Seared Orange Scallops*

7. To the hot skillet, add the remaining ¼ cup orange juice and remaining ⅛ teaspoon salt. Cook for 1 or 2 minutes or until liquid is reduced by half and resembles a glaze. Remove from heat, and stir in oregano.

8. In a large bowl, add mixed salad greens, reserved orange segments, and avocado. Add salad dressing, and toss to combine.

9. Evenly divide salad mixture among 4 plates. Top each with 3 scallops, and drizzle with skillet sauce.

**Note:** The scallops called for in this recipe are U10, which refers to the number of scallops in 1 pound (450g). The *U* means "under," so U10 means under 10 scallops per 1 pound (450g). The larger the number, the smaller the scallop.

| EACH SERVING HAS | | | |
|---|---|---|---|
| 560 calories 43g total fat | 6g saturated fat 22g protein | 26g carbohydrates 7g fiber | 35mg cholesterol 360mg sodium |

# Sole Florentine

Sole is a mild-flavored whitefish that pairs well with spinach and summertime tomatoes.

| YIELD | PREP TIME | COOK TIME | SERVING SIZE |
|---|---|---|---|
| 4 servings | 15 minutes | 30 minutes | 1 fillet |

½ cup diced tomatoes

1 clove garlic, minced

1 tbsp minced shallot

1 cup chopped fresh spinach

¼ tsp kosher salt, plus more for garnish

1 tbsp olive oil

4 (4-oz/115g) sole fillets

Freshly ground black pepper

1 tbsp finely chopped fresh parsley

1 lemon, cut into 4 wedges

1. Preheat the oven to 350°F (175°C). Oil a 9×9-inch (23×23cm) baking dish.

2. In a small bowl, combine tomatoes, garlic, shallot, spinach, kosher salt, and olive oil.

3. Place 1 sole fillet on a cutting board. Spoon 1 tablespoon tomato-spinach mixture on the bottom half of the fillet. Roll the fillet over the tomato-spinach mixture, and place the rolled fillet seam side down in the baking dish. Repeat with the remaining fillets and tomato-spinach mixture, placing the rolled fillets against each other in the baking dish to prevent unrolling.

4. Pour any additional tomato-spinach mixture over the tops of the fillets.

5. Bake for 25 to 30 minutes or until fish flakes easily.

6. Garnish with additional salt and black pepper, parsley, and lemon wedges.

| EACH SERVING HAS | | | |
|---|---|---|---|
| 140 calories<br>5g total fat | 1g saturated fat<br>22g protein | 2g carbohydrates<br>0g fiber | 55mg cholesterol<br>220mg sodium |

# Almond-Crusted Barramundi

Ground almonds and breadcrumbs lend a pleasing crunch to this baked fish dish. Barramundi is a firm whitefish native to northern Australia and southeast Asia. It is very rich in omega-3 fatty acids.

| YIELD | PREP TIME | COOK TIME | SERVING SIZE |
|---|---|---|---|
| 4 servings | 15 minutes | 15 minutes | 1 fillet |

⅓ cup whole almonds

1 clove garlic

¼ tsp freshly ground black pepper

1 tbsp Dijon mustard

2 tbsp honey

1 tbsp olive oil

Zest of 1 lemon

2 tbsp Italian-seasoned breadcrumbs

4 (3-oz/85g) barramundi fillets (or any firm whitefish such as snapper, mullet, or halibut)

1 lemon, cut into 4 wedges

1. Preheat the oven to 375°F (190°C). Oil a 9×13-inch (23×33cm) baking dish.

2. In a food processor, pulse almonds, garlic, and black pepper until finely chopped. (Be careful not to overmix, or you will make almond butter.)

3. In a small bowl, combine Dijon mustard, honey, olive oil, and lemon zest.

4. In a separate small bowl, combine Italian-seasoned breadcrumbs and almond mixture.

5. Coat each barramundi fillet in the Dijon mustard mixture and then pat almond mixture onto the fillets, coating each side well. Place coated fillets in the prepared baking dish, and bake for 15 minutes or until fish flakes easily.

6. Serve with lemon wedges.

**Note:** You can make your own breadcrumbs using stale bread. Leave the bread uncovered on a baking sheet for a day to dry completely and then process in a food processor until fine. For this recipe's Italian-seasoned breadcrumbs, add a pinch each of garlic powder, oregano, basil, and kosher salt to the breadcrumbs, and stir well.

| EACH SERVING HAS | | | |
|---|---|---|---|
| 310 calories 14g total fat | 1.5g saturated fat 27g protein | 20g carbohydrates 3g fiber | 40mg cholesterol 270mg sodium |

# Salmon Fennel Bundles

Fennel gives this salmon dish a light anise flavor, and steaming the fish in a foil packet yields a very moist fillet. You can prepare the packets ahead of time and cook them when ready.

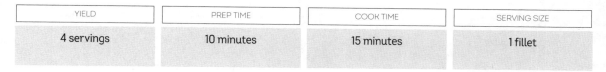

| YIELD | PREP TIME | COOK TIME | SERVING SIZE |
|---|---|---|---|
| 4 servings | 10 minutes | 15 minutes | 1 fillet |

2 tbsp freshly squeezed lemon juice

¼ cup olive oil

¼ tsp dried basil

⅛ tsp kosher salt

⅛ tsp freshly ground black pepper

2 tbsp dry white wine

1 bulb fennel

4 (6-oz/170g) salmon fillets, skin removed

4 tsp capers

1. Preheat the oven to 350°F (175°C). Cut 4 pieces of aluminum foil approximately 12 inches (30.5cm) long each.

2. In a small bowl, combine lemon juice, olive oil, basil, kosher salt, black pepper, and white wine.

3. Remove green stalks and fronds from fennel bulb. Slice bulb in half through the center of the root, and cut out and discard the hard triangular core. Cut fennel into thin slices, using a mandoline slicer if you have one.

4. In the center of each piece of aluminum foil, place ¼ of the sliced fennel. Set 1 salmon fillet on top of each fennel portion. Spoon about 2 tablespoons lemon mixture over each salmon fillet, and add 1 teaspoon capers on top of each fillet. Seal each packet tightly.

5. Bake for 15 minutes. Remove from the oven, and let rest for 5 minutes before opening.

| EACH SERVING HAS | | | |
|---|---|---|---|
| 390 calories 25g total fat | 3.5g saturated fat 35g protein | 5g carbohydrates 2g fiber | 95mg cholesterol 250mg sodium |

# Spicy Tomato Sauce
*with Linguine*

Red pepper flakes give this pasta dish's tomato sauce a spicy kick. This recipe uses pantry ingredients so it can be made at any time; it also freezes well.

| YIELD | PREP TIME | COOK TIME | SERVING SIZE |
|---|---|---|---|
| About 3½ cups | 10 minutes | 25 minutes | ½ cup |

1 tbsp olive oil

½ cup diced onion

1 tsp kosher salt

2 cloves garlic, finely minced

1 tbsp tomato paste

1 tsp balsamic vinegar

2 (14.5-oz/410g) cans diced tomatoes, no salt added

1 tsp Italian seasoning

¼ tsp red pepper flakes

¼ tsp freshly ground black pepper

8 oz (225g) uncooked linguine

Freshly shaved Parmesan cheese

1. In a large saucepan over medium heat, heat olive oil. When oil is hot, add onion and ½ teaspoon kosher salt, and cook, stirring occasionally, for 5 minutes.

2. Stir in garlic, tomato paste, and balsamic vinegar, and sauté for 1 minute.

3. Add tomatoes with liquid, Italian seasoning, red pepper flakes, and black pepper. Simmer, stirring occasionally, for 20 minutes.

4. Meanwhile, fill a large saucepan ⅔ full of water, add remaining ½ teaspoon salt, and bring to a boil over medium-high heat. Add linguine, and cook according to the package directions. Drain pasta.

5. Serve ½ cup pasta with ½ cup sauce. Garnish with Parmesan cheese.

**Variation:** Add your favorite protein such as shrimp or chicken.

| | EACH SERVING HAS | | |
|---|---|---|---|
| 200 calories<br>3g total fat | 0g saturated fat<br>6g protein | 36g carbohydrates<br>2g fiber | 0mg cholesterol<br>200mg sodium |

# Angel Hair Pasta

*with Pesto, Mushrooms, and Arugula*

Peppery arugula adds a nice contrast to the sweet basil pesto in this summery angel hair pasta dish.

| YIELD | PREP TIME | COOK TIME | SERVING SIZE |
|---|---|---|---|
| 6 cups | 15 minutes | 10 minutes | 1 cup |

½ tsp kosher salt

8 oz (225g) uncooked angel hair pasta (may be labeled "capellini")

1 tbsp olive oil

½ cup diced onion

8 oz (225g) baby portobello mushrooms, sliced

⅓ cup Pesto (page 223)

3 cups arugula

Freshly shaved Parmesan cheese

1. Fill a large saucepan ⅔ full of water, add kosher salt, and bring to a boil over medium-high heat. Add angel hair pasta, and cook according to the package directions. Drain pasta.

2. In a large skillet over medium heat, add olive oil. When oil is hot, add onion, and cook for 4 minutes or until soft.

3. Add baby portobello mushrooms, and cook for 5 minutes or until the liquid released from the mushrooms has evaporated. Remove from heat.

4. In a large bowl, toss the cooked pasta with Pesto.

5. Add arugula to the skillet with the mushroom mixture, and toss well. Arugula should be slightly wilted.

6. Place pasta on a large serving platter or on individual plates, top with arugula-mushroom mixture, and garnish with Parmesan cheese.

**Variation:** Instead of arugula, you could use the same amount of baby spinach leaves.

| EACH SERVING HAS | | | |
|---|---|---|---|
| 260 calories<br>11g total fat | 2g saturated fat<br>8g protein | 32g carbohydrates<br>2g fiber | 5mg cholesterol<br>50mg sodium |

# Lamb Patties and Pasta

These savory lamb patties are a great alternative to beef. They're great with pasta, as in this recipe, but they are also nice stuffed in pitas and they freeze well, too.

| YIELD | PREP TIME | COOK TIME | SERVING SIZE |
| --- | --- | --- | --- |
| 4 servings | 20 minutes | 15 minutes | 3 patties with 1 cup pasta |

1 lb (450g) ground lamb

¾ cup finely chopped yellow onion

1 tbsp finely minced garlic

1¼ tsp kosher salt

½ tsp freshly ground black pepper

8 oz (225g) uncooked linguine

1 tbsp pine nuts

8 oz (225g) white button mushrooms

¼ cup sun-dried tomatoes, sliced into strips

1 cup fresh baby spinach

1 cup arugula

4 oz (115g; about 1 cup) Manchego cheese, shredded

1. In a medium bowl, combine lamb, ½ cup yellow onion, garlic, ½ teaspoon kosher salt, and ¼ teaspoon black pepper.

2. Form lamb mixture into 12 patties 2 inches (5cm) in diameter and ¾ inch (2cm) thick.

3. Heat a large nonstick skillet over medium heat. Add patties, and cook for 3 or 4 minutes per side until lightly browned and cooked through. Transfer patties to a plate, and cover with foil. Retain the pan and pan juice.

4. Fill a large saucepan ⅔ full of water, add ½ teaspoon salt, and bring to a boil over medium-high heat. Add linguine, and cook according to the package directions. Drain pasta.

5. Meanwhile, in a small skillet over medium heat, toast pine nuts for 3 or 4 minutes or until lightly browned. Remove from the pan, and set aside.

6. Wash white button mushrooms, and discard the stems. Slice mushrooms into slices ⅛ inch (3mm) thick.

7. Return the large nonstick skillet to medium heat. When the pan is warm, add the remaining ¼ cup onion, sliced mushrooms, sun-dried tomatoes, remaining ¼ teaspoon salt, and remaining ¼ teaspoon pepper. Cook, stirring occasionally, for 4 minutes.

8.  Add baby spinach and arugula, remove from heat, and mix well. Greens should be slightly wilted.

9.  Add pine nuts and pasta, and mix well.

10. Place 1 cup pasta mixture and 3 lamb patties on each plate. Garnish with Manchego cheese.

**Variation:** Manchego is a Spanish sheep's milk cheese. If you can't find it, you can substitute pecorino or Parmesan. Also feel free to use only spinach instead of both spinach and arugula.

EACH SERVING HAS

| 660 calories | 15g saturated fat | 42g carbohydrates | 135mg cholesterol |
| 38g total fat | 38g protein | 4g fiber | 865mg sodium |

# Lamb Shanks

This is a classic, hearty spring dish with a rich, meaty sauce. It is delicious alongside couscous, rice, polenta, or mashed potatoes.

| YIELD | PREP TIME | COOK TIME | SERVING SIZE |
|---|---|---|---|
| 4 servings | 20 minutes | 2¼ hours | 1 shank with ½ cup sauce |

4 (4-oz/115g) lamb shanks

¼ cup all-purpose flour

¼ cup plus 2 tbsp olive oil

2 stalks celery, sliced ¼ in (0.5cm) thick

1½ cups sliced carrots (about 2 or 3 large), ¼ in (0.5cm) thick

2 cups chopped onion

⅓ cup tomato paste

6 cloves garlic, finely minced

½ tsp dried oregano

½ tsp dried rosemary

¼ tsp freshly ground black pepper

2 cups dry red wine

4 cups beef broth

2 bay leaves

1. Preheat the oven to 325°F (190°C).

2. Dredge lamb shanks in all-purpose flour, and shake off excess.

3. In a large, 8-quart (7.5-liter) ovenproof pot over medium heat, heat ¼ cup olive oil. When oil is hot, add shanks, in batches if necessary, and cook for 3 or 4 minutes per side or until browned. Transfer browned shanks to a plate, discard oil, and clean the pot.

4. Add remaining 2 tablespoons oil to the clean pot, and return to medium heat. Add celery, carrots, and onion, and cook for 10 minutes.

5. Add tomato paste, garlic, oregano, rosemary, and black pepper. Cook, stirring occasionally, for 3 minutes.

6. Add red wine, beef broth, and bay leaves, and stir well. Add lamb shanks, and bring to a boil.

7. Remove from heat, cover the pot, and bake for 2 hours or until tender.

8. Skim off any oil from the surface. Remove bay leaves.

9. Serve 1 shank and ½ cup sauce per plate.

| EACH SERVING HAS | | | |
|---|---|---|---|
| 550 calories 37g total fat | 10g saturated fat 26g protein | 26g carbohydrates 4g fiber | 80mg cholesterol 170mg sodium |

# Crispy Turkey Cutlets

These turkey cutlets have a nice crunch from the breadcrumb coating, which is laced with Parmesan cheese. It's the perfect comfort food during the cold winter months.

| YIELD | PREP TIME | COOK TIME | SERVING SIZE |
|---|---|---|---|
| 4 servings | 20 minutes | 15 minutes | 4 ounces (115g) |

½ cup freshly grated Parmesan cheese

½ cup Italian-seasoned breadcrumbs

⅛ tsp kosher salt

⅛ tsp freshly ground black pepper

2 eggs

1 lb (450g) boneless, skinless turkey breast

2 tbsp olive oil

1 tbsp finely chopped fresh parsley

1 lemon, cut into 4 wedges

1. In a small bowl, combine Parmesan cheese, Italian-seasoned breadcrumbs, kosher salt, and black pepper. Pour onto a large plate.

2. In a shallow dish, beat eggs.

3. Slice turkey breast into 4 equal-size pieces.

4. Cover 1 piece with 2 layers of plastic wrap, place on a cutting board, and pound with a meat mallet (or heavy skillet) until turkey is ¼ inch (0.5cm) thick. Set aside, and repeat with remaining pieces.

5. Dip each turkey piece into beaten eggs and then coat each side in breadcrumb mixture.

6. In a large skillet over medium heat, heat olive oil. When oil is hot, add 2 breaded turkey breasts, and cook for 2 minutes per side or until golden brown and a meat thermometer shows an internal temperature of 165°F (75°C) in the thickest part of the breast. Reduce the heat if the pieces brown too quickly and turkey is still pink inside. Repeat with remaining breasts.

7. Garnish each serving with parsley and a lemon wedge.

| EACH SERVING HAS | | | |
|---|---|---|---|
| 320 calories | 4g saturated fat | 12g carbohydrates | 160mg cholesterol |
| 14g total fat | 37g protein | 1g fiber | 580mg sodium |

# Chicken Piccata

This classic chicken dish has a refreshing hint of lemon and piquant capers, perfect for spring.

| YIELD | PREP TIME | COOK TIME | SERVING SIZE |
|---|---|---|---|
| 4 servings | 20 minutes | 20 minutes | 4 ounces (115g) chicken, ¼ cup sauce, ¼ cup spinach |

4 (4-oz/115g) boneless, skinless chicken breasts

¼ cup all-purpose flour

¼ tsp kosher salt

¼ tsp freshly ground black pepper

1 tbsp olive oil

1 cup finely diced white onion

2 tbsp white wine or chicken broth

1 tbsp freshly squeezed lemon juice

½ cup low-sodium chicken broth

1 clove garlic, finely minced

3 tbsp capers

1 cup baby spinach leaves

1 tbsp finely chopped fresh parsley

1. Cover 1 chicken breast with 2 layers of plastic wrap, place on a cutting board, and pound with a meat mallet (or heavy skillet) until chicken is ½ inch (1.25cm) thick. Set aside, and repeat with remaining breasts.

2. On a large, shallow plate, combine all-purpose flour, kosher salt, and black pepper.

3. Dredge each chicken breast in flour mixture, and shake off any excess.

4. In a large skillet over medium heat, heat olive oil. When oil is hot, add chicken breasts, and cook for 4 to 6 minutes per side or until slightly golden in color and a meat thermometer shows an internal temperature of 165°F (75°C) in the thickest part of the breast. Reduce the heat if the breasts brown too quickly and chicken is still pink inside. Transfer chicken to a plate, and cover with aluminum foil to keep warm.

5. Add white onion to the skillet, and cook for 1 minute. Add white wine, lemon juice, chicken broth, garlic, and capers, and cook for 5 to 7 minutes or until the liquid has reduced by half and thickened slightly.

6. Place baby spinach leaves on a platter, top with chicken, and pour pan sauce evenly over the top. Garnish with parsley.

| EACH SERVING HAS | | | |
|---|---|---|---|
| 390 calories 22g total fat | 4.5g saturated fat 19g protein | 29g carbohydrates 3g fiber | 45mg cholesterol 890mg sodium |

# CHAPTER 22

# Side Dishes

You can make a powerfully nutritious side dish—and even a complete meal—by combining vegetables, legumes, and grains. The various flavors and textures these foods offer enable you to put together a wide range of new combinations without a lot of effort. Make it a point each month to try a new vegetable recipe, such as those in this chapter—you might just find a new favorite!

Beans, both dried and canned, are a must for a Mediterranean pantry. Serve them cold in a salad; purée them into a creamy dip; or add them to soups, stews, casseroles, or even your favorite steamed veggie dish. Some versatile beans to keep on hand include chickpeas (garbanzo beans), red kidney beans, and cannellini beans, although any type of bean you enjoy should be in your pantry. On days when you have some free time, soak a pot of dried beans before you go to bed. The next day, drain the water and cook the beans. Toss in any leftover vegetables or meat during the last hour of cooking.

Whole grains and seeds pair well with many different foods and make a great base for vegetables, herbs, and spices. Cook a batch of bulgur, barley, polenta, or quinoa, and add a little onion, garlic, or any vegetable you have on hand for a simple and healthy dish.

# Zucchini and Walnuts

Zucchini takes on a new life with walnuts and sweet mint in this fragrant, delicious mixture, perfect for a summer day.

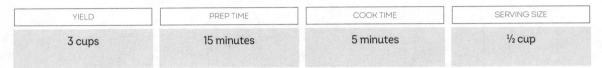

| YIELD | PREP TIME | COOK TIME | SERVING SIZE |
|-------|-----------|-----------|--------------|
| 3 cups | 15 minutes | 5 minutes | ½ cup |

2 large zucchini (about 2¼ cups sliced)

1 tbsp olive oil

½ cup finely diced onion

1 cup sliced baby portobello mushrooms

¼ tsp kosher salt

⅛ tsp freshly ground black pepper

3 tbsp finely chopped walnuts, toasted

2 tsp finely chopped mint leaves

1. Slice zucchini in half lengthwise. Cut each half lengthwise again so you have 4 pieces. Slice each piece across into ¼-inch (0.5cm) slices.

2. In a large skillet over medium heat, heat olive oil. When oil is hot, add onion and cook, stirring occasionally, for 1 minute.

3. Add baby portobello mushrooms, zucchini, kosher salt, and black pepper. Cook, stirring occasionally, for 3 minutes.

4. Add walnuts and mint, and cook for 1 minute. Remove from heat and serve.

**Variation:** Use any type of mushroom you have available. Also try using other nuts such as pecans, cashews, or almonds.

| EACH SERVING HAS | | | |
|---|---|---|---|
| 70 calories<br>5g total fat | 0.5g saturated fat<br>1g protein | 4g carbohydrates<br>1g fiber | 0mg cholesterol<br>85mg sodium |

# Two-Cheese Risotto

Classic risotto is rich, creamy, and has an almost soup-like consistency. This cheesy version is the perfect comfort food on a cold winter day.

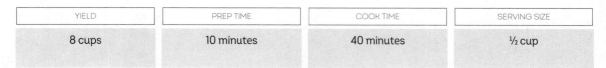

| YIELD | PREP TIME | COOK TIME | SERVING SIZE |
| --- | --- | --- | --- |
| 8 cups | 10 minutes | 40 minutes | ½ cup |

3 tbsp olive oil

1 cup finely chopped onion

2 cloves garlic, finely chopped

8 cups low-sodium chicken broth

16 oz (450g) arborio rice

½ cup white wine

1 cup freshly grated Parmesan cheese

¼ cup freshly grated Asiago cheese

½ tsp kosher salt

1. In a small skillet over medium heat, heat 1 tablespoon olive oil. When oil is hot, add onion and sauté for 8 minutes.

2. Add garlic, and cook for 2 minutes. Remove from heat.

3. In a large saucepan over low heat, bring chicken broth to a simmer.

4. In a 6-quart (5.5-liter) saucepan over medium heat, heat remaining 2 tablespoons oil. When oil is hot, add arborio rice. Cook, stirring constantly with a wooden spoon or heat-safe spatula to prevent sticking, for 7 minutes.

5. Add white wine to hot rice, and stir until wine has evaporated.

6. Add 1 ladle of warm broth (about ½ cup) to rice, and constantly stir until the rice has absorbed all the liquid. Repeat, adding 1 ladle of broth each time and stirring constantly. Continue until rice will not absorb any more liquid. This will take 20 to 25 minutes.

7. Add sautéed onion mixture to rice, and stir gently to incorporate.

8. When rice has a thick, creamy, soup-like consistency, remove from heat.

9. Add Parmesan cheese, Asiago cheese, and kosher salt, and stir to combine.

*(continues)*

# *Two-Cheese Risotto*

**Note:** It is essential to use arborio rice when you are making risotto. Arborio rice is a high-starch, short-grained rice. If you use any other kind of rice, the risotto will not achieve its creamy consistency.

**Variation:** Sauté 8 ounces (225g) sliced mushrooms along with the onions.

| EACH SERVING HAS | | | |
|---|---|---|---|
| 175 calories<br>5g total fat | 1.5g saturated fat<br>7g protein | 25g carbohydrates<br>1g fiber | 10mg cholesterol<br>180mg sodium |

# Sautéed Spinach and Mushrooms

Garlic permeates the spinach and mushrooms in this delicious summer side dish that is a perfect base for fish or chicken.

| YIELD | PREP TIME | COOK TIME | SERVING SIZE |
|---|---|---|---|
| 2 cups | 10 minutes | 6 minutes | ½ cup |

1 tbsp olive oil

4 cloves garlic, finely minced

8 oz (225g) mushrooms, sliced

⅛ tsp kosher salt

¼ tsp freshly ground black pepper

10 cups spinach leaves

1 oz (30g) freshly grated Parmesan cheese

1. In a large skillet over medium heat, heat olive oil. When oil is hot, add garlic, mushrooms, kosher salt, and black pepper, and cook for 5 minutes.

2. Add spinach to the skillet, and stir constantly for 1 minute or until spinach is wilted.

3. Remove from heat, and stir in Parmesan cheese.

| EACH SERVING HAS | | | |
|---|---|---|---|
| 100 calories<br>6g total fat | 2g saturated fat<br>6g protein | 10g carbohydrates<br>4g fiber | 5mg cholesterol<br>270mg sodium |

# Rosemary Garlic Potatoes

Flavored with the piney, floral taste of rosemary, these aromatic potatoes taste delicious and make the perfect winter side dish!

| YIELD | PREP TIME | COOK TIME | SERVING SIZE |
|-------|-----------|-----------|--------------|
| 2 cups | 10 minutes | 30 minutes | ½ cup |

2 tbsp olive oil

1 tsp finely minced fresh rosemary leaves

2 cloves garlic, finely minced

¼ tsp kosher salt

⅛ tsp freshly ground black pepper

1 lb (450g) red potatoes, skin on, scrubbed well

1. Preheat the oven to 400°F (200°C).

2. In a large bowl, combine olive oil, rosemary, garlic, kosher salt, and black pepper.

3. Cut red potatoes into quarters, toss in olive oil mixture, and transfer to a baking sheet.

4. Bake, stirring occasionally, for 30 minutes or until golden brown.

| EACH SERVING HAS | | | |
|---|---|---|---|
| 140 calories 7g total fat | 1g saturated fat 2g protein | 19g carbohydrates 2g fiber | 0mg cholesterol 125mg sodium |

# Curried Cauliflower

This sweet and savory winter dish combines curry-spiced cauliflower, crunchy almonds, and sweet golden raisins.

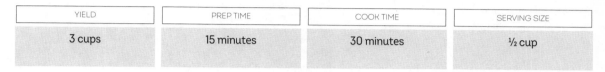

| YIELD | PREP TIME | COOK TIME | SERVING SIZE |
|---|---|---|---|
| 3 cups | 15 minutes | 30 minutes | ½ cup |

**1 medium head cauliflower**

**2 tbsp olive oil**

**½ tsp kosher salt**

**⅛ tsp freshly ground black pepper**

**2 cloves garlic, finely minced**

**1 tsp curry powder**

**1 medium red onion, thinly sliced**

**¼ cup golden raisins**

**2 tbsp water**

**¼ cup slivered almonds, toasted**

1. Preheat the oven to 350°F (175°C).

2. Slice cauliflower in half, cut out the triangular core at the base of the head, and separate into florets. Cut large pieces, if necessary, so all pieces are approximately the same size.

3. In a large bowl, combine olive oil, kosher salt, black pepper, garlic, and curry powder.

4. Add cauliflower, red onion, and golden raisins to olive oil mixture, and mix thoroughly.

5. Transfer cauliflower mixture to a 9×9-inch (23×23cm) baking dish. Add water.

6. Bake, stirring occasionally, for 30 minutes or until cauliflower is tender.

7. Remove from the oven, and sprinkle with almonds.

| EACH SERVING HAS | | | |
|---|---|---|---|
| 120 calories<br>7g total fat | 1g saturated fat<br>3g protein | 14g carbohydrates<br>3g fiber | 0mg cholesterol<br>190mg sodium |

# Lemon Kale Ribbons

Garlic and red pepper flakes provide a nice kick to leafy green kale and tangy lemon in this vegetable dish that is perfect for summer.

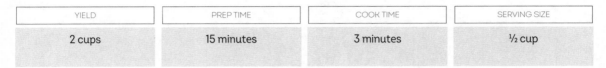

| YIELD | PREP TIME | COOK TIME | SERVING SIZE |
| --- | --- | --- | --- |
| 2 cups | 15 minutes | 3 minutes | ½ cup |

8 oz (225g) fresh kale, rinsed

2 tbsp olive oil

1 tbsp finely minced shallot

4 cloves garlic, finely sliced

⅛ tsp red pepper flakes

1 tbsp freshly squeezed lemon juice

¼ tsp kosher salt

⅛ tsp freshly ground black pepper

1. Cut away the tough center stalks of the kale leaves. Slice leaves into ¼-inch (0.5cm) strips.

2. In a large skillet over medium heat, heat olive oil. When oil is hot, add shallot, garlic, and red pepper flakes, and cook for 1 minute.

3. Add kale, and cook, stirring constantly, for 2 minutes.

4. Remove from heat. Add lemon juice, kosher salt, and black pepper, and mix well.

**Variation:** Cook a slice of pancetta or bacon and then cook the shallots and garlic in the reserved olive oil to add flavor. Crumble the crispy pancetta or bacon and use as a garnish.

| EACH SERVING HAS | | | |
| --- | --- | --- | --- |
| 100 calories 7g total fat | 1g saturated fat 2g protein | 7g carbohydrates 1g fiber | 0mg cholesterol 150mg sodium |

# Minted Peas
*with Pancetta*

Peas and pancetta get a spring pick-me-up with the addition of refreshing fresh mint.

| YIELD | PREP TIME | COOK TIME | SERVING SIZE |
|---|---|---|---|
| 1½ cups | 5 minutes | 6 minutes | ½ cup |

1½ oz (43g) pancetta (unsmoked bacon), diced

2 tbsp finely diced shallots

10 oz (285g) frozen peas, thawed

1 tbsp finely sliced fresh mint leaves

⅛ tsp kosher salt

⅛ tsp freshly ground black pepper

1. In a large skillet over medium heat, cook pancetta for 3 minutes or until lightly browned.

2. Add shallots, and cook for 1 minute.

3. Add peas, and cook, stirring occasionally, for 2 minutes or until warmed through.

4. Remove from heat. Add mint, kosher salt, and black pepper, and stir well.

**Variation:** Substitute bacon if pancetta is not available.

| EACH SERVING HAS | | | |
|---|---|---|---|
| 140 calories 7g total fat | 2g saturated fat 7g protein | 14g carbohydrates 4g fiber | 10mg cholesterol 300mg sodium |

# Pickled Asparagus

This crisp and tangy asparagus is delicious eaten alone or added to a spring or summer salad.

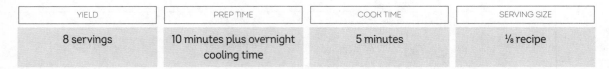

| YIELD | PREP TIME | COOK TIME | SERVING SIZE |
|---|---|---|---|
| 8 servings | 10 minutes plus overnight cooling time | 5 minutes | ⅛ recipe |

1 lb (450g) fresh asparagus

2 cups ice

1½ cups water

1½ cups distilled white vinegar

3 tbsp sugar

3 tsp kosher salt

1 heaping tsp pickling spices

1 tsp red pepper flakes

Sprig of fresh dill

1 clove garlic, sliced

1. Wash asparagus, and trim off the tough ends.

2. In a large bowl, add 2 cups ice and fill with cold water.

3. Fill a large saucepan ¾ full of water, and bring to a boil over high heat. Add asparagus, and blanch for 1 minute. Using a slotted spoon or tongs, remove asparagus and immediately transfer it to the ice water.

4. In a small saucepan over medium heat, combine water, distilled white vinegar, sugar, kosher salt, pickling spices, red pepper flakes, and dill. Cook, stirring occasionally, for 4 minutes or until sugar is dissolved. Remove from heat, and cool completely.

5. Pack asparagus and garlic slices into a canning jar or any glass container that can be covered tightly. Pour in vinegar mixture. Chill overnight in the refrigerator, and keep refrigerated. Consume within 1 week.

**Variation:** Add a few small whole or sliced peppers such as banana peppers along with the asparagus.

| EACH SERVING HAS | | | |
|---|---|---|---|
| 40 calories 0g total fat | 0g saturated fat 1g protein | 7g carbohydrates 1g fiber | 0mg cholesterol 720mg sodium |

# Bean and Vegetable Patties

The cornmeal in this fall recipe adds a pleasing sweetness and a crispy texture. This recipe can be made as an entrée or appetizer. For an appetizer, make smaller patties and serve with garlic aioli (a strongly flavored garlic mayonnaise).

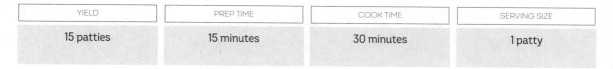

| YIELD | PREP TIME | COOK TIME | SERVING SIZE |
| --- | --- | --- | --- |
| 15 patties | 15 minutes | 30 minutes | 1 patty |

1 (15-oz/425g) can red kidney beans, rinsed and drained

1 large red bell pepper, seeded and chopped

2 stalks celery, roughly chopped

1 small zucchini, roughly chopped

¼ cup fresh parsley leaves

1 clove garlic

½ red onion, roughly chopped

1 tsp kosher salt

¼ tsp freshly ground black pepper

4 tbsp olive oil

¾ cup cornmeal

1 cup all-purpose flour

¼ cup freshly grated Parmesan cheese, plus more for garnish

2 eggs, beaten

Diced fresh tomatoes

Extra-virgin olive oil

1. Preheat the oven to 350°F (175°C).

2. In a food processor, pulse red kidney beans until processed but still chunky.

3. Add red bell pepper, celery, zucchini, parsley, garlic, red onion, kosher salt, black pepper, and 3 tablespoons olive oil. Pulse several times, pausing to scrape down the sides of the bowl, until ingredients are blended and vegetables are chunky and uniform in size but not puréed.

4. In a large bowl, combine cornmeal, all-purpose flour, and Parmesan cheese.

5. Add bean mixture and beaten eggs to cornmeal mixture. Mix well.

6. Form bean mixture into 15 ¼-cup patties ½ inch thick.

7. In a large skillet over medium heat, heat remaining 1 tablespoon olive oil. When oil is hot, add 5 or 6 patties to the pan. Do not overcrowd the pan. Cook patties for 3 minutes per side or until golden brown. Transfer cooked patties to an ungreased baking sheet, and repeat with the remaining mixture. You may need to add another 1 tablespoon olive oil to the skillet between batches.

8. Bake for 15 minutes. Patties will rise and become lighter as they cook.

9. Serve with fresh diced tomatoes, a drizzle of extra-virgin olive oil, and freshly grated Parmesan cheese.

*(continues)*

# *Bean and Vegetable Patties*

**Note:** When forming the patties in step 6, you may want to coat the measuring cup in olive oil lightly to help the mixture release from the cup.

**Variation:** Experiment with different beans in this recipe as you like. Try using chickpeas (garbanzo beans) or black-eyed peas, for example.

| EACH SERVING HAS | | | |
| --- | --- | --- | --- |
| 140 calories 5g total fat | 1g saturated fat 5g protein | 19g carbohydrates 3g fiber | 30mg cholesterol 240mg sodium |

# Panzanella

Panzanella, or bread salad, is popular in the Tuscany region of Italy, as a way to use up stale or leftover bread. This salad pops with savory goodness from the balsamic vinegar, roasted red peppers, and artichoke hearts.

| YIELD | PREP TIME | COOK TIME | SERVING SIZE |
| --- | --- | --- | --- |
| 9 cups | 15 minutes plus 30 minutes marinating time | 15 minutes | 1 cup |

1 French baguette

Nonstick cooking spray or mister with olive oil

1 (13.75-oz/390g) can artichoke hearts packed in water, drained

1 large stalk celery, diced (1 cup)

½ cup chopped roasted red peppers

¼ cup finely diced red onion

⅓ cup chopped sun-dried tomatoes packed in oil

¼ cup chopped fresh parsley

⅔ cup balsamic vinaigrette

1. Preheat the oven to 350°F (175°C).

2. Slice French baguette into 1-inch (2.5cm) cubes. Transfer to a baking sheet, and lightly spray with nonstick cooking spray or mist with olive oil.

3. Bake for 10 to 15 minutes. Remove from the oven, and cool. (This helps prevent the bread from getting soggy when combined with remaining ingredients.)

4. Cut artichoke hearts into bite-size pieces.

5. In a large bowl, combine celery, roasted red peppers, red onion, sun-dried tomatoes, parsley, artichoke hearts, and bread cubes.

6. Pour balsamic vinaigrette over bread mixture, and toss to combine. Let rest at room temperature for 30 minutes to distribute flavor, or refrigerate overnight.

**Variation:** Substitute 1 large fresh tomato, cored and chopped; ½ cucumber, peeled, seeded, and diced; and ¼ cup chopped fresh basil for the artichoke hearts, celery, roasted red peppers, red onion, sun-dried tomatoes, and parsley.

| EACH SERVING HAS | | | |
| --- | --- | --- | --- |
| 300 calories 17g total fat | 2g saturated fat 7g protein | 35g carbohydrates 3g fiber | 0mg cholesterol 650mg sodium |

# Golden Chard

Chard has a mild flavor that is enhanced with sweet golden raisins and a touch of honey in this summer recipe.

| YIELD | PREP TIME | COOK TIME | SERVING SIZE |
|-------|-----------|-----------|--------------|
| 2 cups | 10 minutes | 10 minutes | ½ cup |

1 lb (450g) chard (about 1 bunch)

1 slice pancetta (unsmoked bacon), diced

1 tbsp olive oil

2 tbsp finely diced shallots

½ tsp kosher salt

¼ tsp freshly ground black pepper

⅓ cup golden raisins

1 tbsp honey

1. Cut away the large stems from chard leaves, and set aside stems. Slice leaves crosswise into ¼-inch (0.5cm) ribbons. Chop stems crosswise into ¼-inch (0.5cm) pieces and keep separate from leaves.

2. In a large nonstick skillet over medium heat, cook pancetta until crisp.

3. Add olive oil, shallots, chard stems, kosher salt, and black pepper, and cook, stirring occasionally, for 5 minutes.

4. Add chard leaves, golden raisins, and honey, and cook, stirring frequently, for 1 to 3 minutes or until chard is soft. Remove from heat immediately.

**Variation:** Swiss chard, with white stems, is the most common chard sold in markets, but varieties with yellow, orange, or red stems also work well in this recipe. The more color, the more phytonutrients! To add a smoky flavor, you can use bacon in a 1:1 replacement for the pancetta.

| EACH SERVING HAS | | | |
|------------------|--|--|--|
| 130 calories 6g total fat | 1.5g saturated fat 2g protein | 18g carbohydrates 2g fiber | 5mg cholesterol 410mg sodium |

# Sweet Polenta
## *with Sun-Dried Tomatoes*

Polenta is ground cornmeal. This recipe adds canned corn, which gives extra sweetness to the polenta. Use this dish as a side for chicken, seafood, or lamb.

| YIELD | PREP TIME | COOK TIME | SERVING SIZE |
|---|---|---|---|
| 12 pieces | 5 minutes plus 3 hours cooling time | 30 minutes | 1 piece |

4 cups water

1 tsp kosher salt

1 cup cornmeal

1 (15-oz/425g) can corn, no added salt, drained

⅓ cup chopped sun-dried tomatoes packed in oil

2 tbsp olive oil

1. In a medium saucepan over high heat, bring water and kosher salt to a boil.

2. Add cornmeal very slowly, whisking constantly to avoid lumps. Reduce heat to low (you may need to remove the pan from the heat temporarily to prevent splattering until the mixture cools), and continue to whisk to prevent lumps. As cornmeal cooks, it will begin to solidify. It should pull away from the pan cleanly around the 20-minute mark.

3. Add corn and sun-dried tomatoes. Stir with a spatula, and cook for 5 minutes.

4. You can serve the polenta at this point, spooned out like mashed potatoes, or chill it and then sauté it at a later time. If you plan to chill and sauté at a later time, grease a 9×12-inch (23×30.5cm) pan with 1 tablespoon olive oil. Evenly spread warm polenta into the pan, and refrigerate for 3 or 4 hours or overnight.

5. Cut cooled polenta into 12 equal portions, and transfer to a baking sheet.

6. Lightly dust the top and bottom of each piece of polenta with all-purpose flour.

*(continues)*

# *Sweet Polenta*
## *with Sun-Dried Tomatoes*

7. In a large nonstick skillet over medium heat, heat remaining 1 tablespoon olive oil. When oil is hot, add 6 to 8 polenta squares, depending on the size of your skillet. Do not overcrowd the skillet. Cook for 4 minutes per side or until golden. You may need to add additional olive oil between batches.

8. Remove polenta from the skillet, and serve.

**Note:** Freshly cooked polenta is creamy, like mashed potatoes or a thick, hot cereal. The formed and sliced version of polenta that is sautéed is thick and firm.

**Variation:** If you plan to serve the polenta immediately after cooking, when it is creamy, add ½ cup freshly grated Parmesan or Romano cheese and stir to combine.

| EACH SERVING HAS | | | |
| --- | --- | --- | --- |
| 90 calories<br>3g total fat | 0g saturated fat<br>2g protein | 14g carbohydrates<br>2g fiber | 0mg cholesterol<br>200mg sodium |

# Quinoa Pilaf

Quinoa is technically a seed but looks, and cooks, like a grain or rice. It has a fluffy texture and a nice crunch when you bite into it. This dish is good served either hot or cold for a fall-time delight.

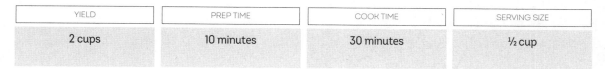

| YIELD | PREP TIME | COOK TIME | SERVING SIZE |
|---|---|---|---|
| 2 cups | 10 minutes | 30 minutes | ½ cup |

1 cup water

½ cup quinoa

1 tbsp olive oil

1 garlic clove, minced

⅓ cup chopped yellow bell pepper

¼ cup chopped scallions, green and white parts

1 cup diced canned tomatoes, with juice

½ tsp kosher salt

⅛ tsp freshly ground pepper

4 tbsp crumbled feta cheese

4 tbsp chopped fresh parsley

1. In a small saucepan over medium-high heat, bring water to a boil. Add quinoa, and return to a boil. Reduce heat to low, cover, and cook for 15 to 20 minutes or until water is absorbed.

2. In a medium skillet over medium heat, heat olive oil. When oil is hot, add garlic and yellow bell pepper, and sauté for 2 minutes.

3. Add scallions, and cook for 1 minute.

4. Add tomatoes with juice, cooked quinoa, kosher salt, and black pepper, and stir to combine. Cook for 2 minutes or until heated through.

5. Top each serving with 1 tablespoon feta cheese and parsley.

**Variation:** Try any combination of vegetables, such as zucchini and cucumbers, or even dried fruit.

| EACH SERVING HAS | | | |
|---|---|---|---|
| 150 calories<br>7g total fat | 2g saturated fat<br>5g protein | 18g carbohydrates<br>2g fiber | 10mg cholesterol<br>510mg sodium |

# Barley and Vegetable Sauté

Barley is a plump, moist grain that takes on the sweet flavors of the vegetables it is cooked with, as you will find in this warming fall recipe.

| YIELD | PREP TIME | COOK TIME | SERVING SIZE |
| --- | --- | --- | --- |
| 4 cups | 20 minutes | 20 minutes | ½ cup |

2 tbsp olive oil

1 cup diced onion

1 cup peeled and cubed sweet potato (about 1 medium), ¼-in (0.5cm) cubes

2 cups pearl barley, cooked according to package directions

1 cup quartered and sliced zucchini, ⅛ in (3mm) thick

1 stalk celery, sliced ⅛ in (3mm) thick

2 cloves garlic, minced

1 cup halved grape tomatoes

¼ tsp minced fresh sage

½ tsp minced fresh rosemary leaves

¾ tsp kosher salt

½ tsp freshly ground black pepper

¼ cup chopped walnuts, toasted

2 tbsp chopped fresh parsley

1. In a large nonstick skillet over medium heat, heat olive oil. When oil is hot, add onion and sweet potato, and cook for 10 minutes or until sweet potatoes are tender.

2. Add cooked barley, stir to combine, and cook for 1 or 2 minutes or until barley is warmed through.

3. Add zucchini, celery, garlic, grape tomatoes, sage, rosemary, kosher salt, and black pepper, and cook for 5 minutes.

4. Garnish with walnuts and parsley, and serve.

**Variation:** Use any variety of vegetables such as carrots, bell peppers, corn, or leeks.

| EACH SERVING HAS | | | |
| --- | --- | --- | --- |
| 130 calories 6g total fat | 1g saturated fat 2g protein | 19g carbohydrates 3g fiber | 0mg cholesterol 200mg sodium |

# CHAPTER 23

# Desserts

In the Mediterranean, fruit is the dessert of choice. It can be as simple as sliced or dried fruit paired with cheese at the end of a meal, or something that takes a little more time to prepare. Try to use fruit in new ways by incorporating it into different recipes. Fruit can add another layer of flavor or remake a dish into something completely new.

Nuts naturally pair well with fruit and are a great snack on their own. This chapter includes several recipes that help you incorporate nuts in your diet.

Nuts are best when they are toasted to bring out all their nutty goodness. To toast nuts, place them in a single layer in a small skillet and set over medium heat. Cook, stirring occasionally, for 5 to 7 minutes or until lightly browned—keep an eye on them because they can burn quickly. Or toast nuts in a preheated 400°F (200°C) oven for 5 to 7 minutes.

# Cinnamon Apple and Nut Phyllo Rolls

These sweet and crunchy rolls pair a filling similar to apple pie with a phyllo dough crust. Fall is the perfect time to find apples at their best.

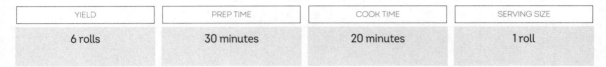

| YIELD | PREP TIME | COOK TIME | SERVING SIZE |
|---|---|---|---|
| 6 rolls | 30 minutes | 20 minutes | 1 roll |

Juice of 1 lemon

2 red apples, peeled, cored, and cut into ⅛-in (3mm) cubes

½ cup dark brown sugar, firmly packed

¼ cup walnuts, toasted

1 tsp ground cinnamon

6 sheets frozen phyllo dough, thawed according to package directions

4 tbsp olive oil

Confectioners' sugar

1. Preheat the oven to 350°F (175°C). Oil a baking sheet.

2. In a small bowl, combine lemon juice and red apples.

3. Add dark brown sugar, walnuts, and ground cinnamon, and mix well.

4. Lay out the stacked sheets of phyllo dough, and pull off 1 sheet at a time to work with. (Lay a damp towel over the rest to keep them from drying out while you work.) With the sheet of phyllo dough in front of you lengthwise, brush with olive oil.

5. Place ¼ cup apple-nut mixture 2 inches (5cm) from the short end of the sheet of dough. Spread apple mixture along the short end so it is about 1½ inches (3.75cm) wide by 5 inches (12.5cm) long and centered between the dough's top and bottom edges. Fold the dough's long edges toward the middle. Brush with more oil, and roll the dough, starting at the end with the apple mixture, to create a log. Transfer to the prepared baking sheet, and repeat with the remaining phyllo dough sheets. Brush the tops with oil.

6. Bake for 15 to 20 minutes or until golden brown.

7. Garnish with confectioners' sugar.

**Variation:** Use any type of fruit instead of apples, or try almonds or pecans instead of walnuts.

| EACH SERVING HAS | | | |
|---|---|---|---|
| 270 calories<br>14g total fat | 2g saturated fat<br>2g protein | 38g carbohydrates<br>3g fiber | 0mg cholesterol<br>95mg sodium |

# Vanilla Panna Cotta

Real vanilla bean flavors the cream and milk in this simple spring dessert.

| YIELD | PREP TIME | COOK TIME | SERVING SIZE |
|---|---|---|---|
| 4 servings | 15 minutes plus 2 hours cooling time | 10 minutes | 4 ounces (115g) |

1¾ cups reduced-fat milk, chilled

2½ tsp unflavored gelatin granules

¼ cup sugar

¼ cup heavy whipping cream

½ vanilla bean

1 cup fresh berries

1. Pour ¼ cup reduced-fat milk into a small bowl. Sprinkle gelatin granules over milk, stir, and let rest for 10 minutes.

2. In a medium pan over low heat, add remaining 1½ cups milk, sugar, and heavy whipping cream.

3. Cut vanilla bean lengthwise, and scrape out the seeds using the blade of a small knife. Add seeds and pod to milk mixture, and cook for 10 minutes. Do not allow to boil.

4. Add gelatin mixture to warm milk mixture, and whisk to combine. Cook for 1 or 2 minutes, and remove from heat. Remove and discard vanilla bean pod.

5. Evenly divide mixture into 4 (1-cup) ramekins that have been sprayed with nonstick cooking spray. Refrigerate 2 hours or overnight.

6. To serve, run a knife around the inside of the ramekin to loosen panna cotta. Dip the bottom of the ramekin in a bowl of hot water for a few seconds and then invert the ramekin onto a plate to release panna cotta.

7. Serve with a side of fresh berries.

**Variation:** Add citrus zest or other spices like cinnamon. You can omit the heavy cream and use only milk, but the little bit of cream enhances the texture.

| EACH SERVING HAS | | | |
|---|---|---|---|
| 160 calories 8g total fat | 5g saturated fat 5g protein | 18g carbohydrates 0g fiber | 30mg cholesterol 50mg sodium |

# Poached Summer Fruit

Wine, cinnamon, and ginger add zest to the pears, peaches, and plums in this sweet summer fruit dish.

| YIELD | PREP TIME | COOK TIME | SERVING SIZE |
| --- | --- | --- | --- |
| 4 portions | 30 minutes plus 2 hours cooling time | 10 minutes | ¼ recipe |

1 (750ml) bottle white wine

1 cup sugar

1 cinnamon stick

Zest of 1 lemon

Juice of 1 lemon

1 (½ in/1.25cm) slice fresh ginger

2 pears, peeled, cored, and halved

2 peaches, peeled, pitted, and halved

2 plums, peeled, pitted, and halved

1. In a medium saucepan over medium heat, combine white wine, sugar, cinnamon stick, lemon zest, lemon juice, and ginger. Bring to a boil, and cook for about 5 minutes or until sugar is dissolved. Reduce heat to a simmer.

2. Add pears, peaches, and plums to the simmering liquid, and gently turn fruit with a large spoon. Cook for 5 minutes.

3. Remove fruit from the poaching liquid, and let both cool. Reserve some of the poaching liquid to drizzle over the fruit when serving if desired.

4. Place cooled fruit and poaching liquid in the refrigerator for 2 hours. (Fruit also can be served warm if you prefer.)

5. Serve ½ pear, ½ peach, and ½ plum per plate. You can slice the fruit and fan them out on the plate for a lovely presentation. Drizzle a spoonful of the poaching liquid over each serving if desired.

**Note:** Cinnamon is reputed to have many health benefits, including anticlotting and antimicrobial properties and blood sugar regulation. Ground cinnamon is an excellent source of manganese and a good source of fiber, vitamin K, calcium, and iron.

**Variation:** Use red wine instead of white, which will add a nice pink color to the fruit.

| EACH SERVING HAS | | | |
| --- | --- | --- | --- |
| 190 calories<br>0g total fat | 0g saturated fat<br>1g protein | 45g carbohydrates<br>5g fiber | 0mg cholesterol<br>0mg sodium |

# Mixed Berry Torte

Sweet berries and creamy, orange-kissed ricotta make a delicious summer treat.

| YIELD | PREP TIME | COOK TIME | SERVING SIZE |
|---|---|---|---|
| 12 slices | 30 minutes plus 2 hours cooling time | 20 minutes | 1 slice |

⅓ cup granulated sugar

½ cup unsalted butter, softened

2 cups all-purpose flour

4 tbsp orange liqueur or orange juice

1 cup ricotta cheese

1 tbsp orange zest

1 tbsp honey

2 tbsp confectioners' sugar, plus more for garnish

1 pint fresh blueberries, washed and dried

8 oz (225g) fresh strawberries, washed, dried, stemmed, and sliced

1. Preheat the oven to 350°F (175°C).

2. In a food processor, pulse together granulated sugar, unsalted butter, all-purpose flour, and orange liqueur several times or until a dough ball forms. Remove dough from the processor and flatten into a disc shape.

3. Evenly press dough into the bottom of a 10-inch (25.5cm) tart pan with a removable bottom. Using a fork, prick the dough all over.

4. Bake for 15 to 20 minutes or until slightly golden brown. Remove from the oven, and let cool to room temperature.

5. Meanwhile, combine ricotta cheese, orange zest, honey, and confectioners' sugar. Spread mixture evenly over the top of the cooled crust.

6. Arrange blueberries on top of ricotta mixture.

7. Chill for 2 hours before serving. Garnish with more confectioners' sugar.

**Variation:** Use any kind of berries, and create a beautiful arrangement.

| EACH SERVING HAS | | | |
|---|---|---|---|
| 250 calories 11g total fat | 7g saturated fat 5g protein | 32g carbohydrates 2g fiber | 30mg cholesterol 20mg sodium |

# Berry Sorbet

Sorbet is sweet, refreshing, and very easy to make with ripe summer berries.

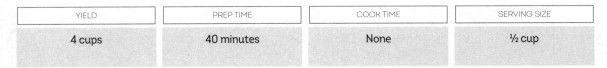

| YIELD | PREP TIME | COOK TIME | SERVING SIZE |
|---|---|---|---|
| 4 cups | 40 minutes | None | ½ cup |

2 cups raspberries, washed, dried, and chopped

1 cup strawberries, washed, dried, stemmed, and finely diced

1 cup sugar

2 tbsp orange liqueur or orange juice

1 cup water

1. In a large bowl, combine raspberries, strawberries, sugar, orange liqueur, and water.

2. Pour mixture into an ice-cream maker. Follow the manufacturer's guidelines, and let run for 30 minutes or until frozen.

**Variation:** If you do not have an ice-cream maker, you can freeze the sorbet mixture for about 8 hours. You will have to scrape it with a fork several times during the freezing process to prevent it from freezing solid. The finished sorbet will have larger ice crystals, making the texture and consistency different—more similar to an Italian ice—but still delicious.

| EACH SERVING HAS | | | |
|---|---|---|---|
| 140 calories<br>0g total fat | 0g saturated fat<br>1g protein | 32g carbohydrates<br>2g fiber | 0mg cholesterol<br>0mg sodium |

# Fruit and Cheese Plate

Fruit is the perfect accompaniment to cheese and acts as a flavor catalyst. The toasted walnuts and almonds and the pomegranate seeds make a crunchy and sweet contrast to the savory cheese.

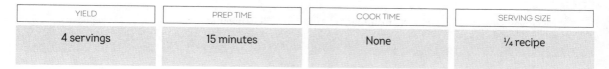

| YIELD | PREP TIME | COOK TIME | SERVING SIZE |
|---|---|---|---|
| 4 servings | 15 minutes | None | ¼ recipe |

4 Medjool dates, pitted

1 oz (30g) walnuts, toasted

1 oz (30g) almonds, toasted

1 pear, cored and sliced

3 oz (85g) Manchego cheese

3 oz (85g) fontina cheese

1 tbsp honey

¼ cup pomegranate seeds

1. On a platter, arrange Medjool dates, walnuts, almonds, pear slices, Manchego cheese, and fontina cheese.

2. Drizzle honey over pear slices, and sprinkle pomegranate seeds over the top.

**Note:** Fontina is a classic Italian cheese made from cow's milk. It can be semisoft to firm, and the flavors can vary depending on where the cheese came from and how long it was aged. It can be eaten on its own, used in recipes, or even used as a fondue because it melts well.

**Variation:** Any type of cheese will do in place of fontina. If you do not have fresh fruit on hand, try using a chutney.

| EACH SERVING HAS | | | |
|---|---|---|---|
| 330 calories<br>21g total fat | 8g saturated fat<br>16g protein | 22g carbohydrates<br>4g fiber | 45mg cholesterol<br>370mg sodium |

# Baked Stuffed Peaches

Sweet summer peaches are filled with a mixture of crunchy oats and nuts—like a peach pie without the crust (and all the work!).

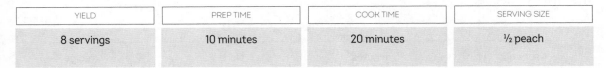

| YIELD | PREP TIME | COOK TIME | SERVING SIZE |
|---|---|---|---|
| 8 servings | 10 minutes | 20 minutes | ½ peach |

4 medium fresh peaches, halved and pitted

¾ cup rolled oats

½ cup unsweetened coconut

¼ cup chopped pistachios

3 tbsp brown sugar, firmly packed

2 egg yolks

½ tsp vanilla extract

2 tbsp butter, at room temperature

1 tbsp honey

¼ tsp kosher salt

1. Preheat the oven to 400°F (200°C). Butter a 9×13-inch (23×33cm) baking dish.

2. Scoop out ¼ of the flesh from the center of each peach half to make room for the filling. Set peaches aside.

3. In a medium bowl, combine rolled oats, coconut, pistachios, brown sugar, egg yolks, vanilla extract, butter, honey, and kosher salt.

4. Divide oat mixture evenly among peach halves, and place peach halves side by side in the prepared baking dish.

5. Bake for 15 to 20 minutes or until oat mixture is golden brown. Serve hot or cold.

**Variation:** Replace the coconut with the same amount of any dried fruit, such as cranberries, blueberries, or cherries. Substitute almonds or walnuts for the pistachios.

| EACH SERVING HAS | | | |
|---|---|---|---|
| 175 calories 10g total fat | 5g saturated fat 3g protein | 20g carbohydrates 3g fiber | 60mg cholesterol 65mg sodium |

# Lemon Ricotta Muffins

Fresh lemon permeates sweet ricotta cheese to create the perfect spring muffins.

| YIELD | PREP TIME | COOK TIME | SERVING SIZE |
|---|---|---|---|
| 12 muffins | 15 minutes | 20 minutes | 1 muffin |

½ cup butter, softened

1 cup granulated sugar

½ cup reduced-fat milk

1 cup ricotta cheese

1 tsp vanilla extract

1 egg, beaten

Zest of 1 lemon

Juice of 1 lemon

1¾ cups all-purpose flour

¼ cup cornmeal

2 tsp baking powder

½ tsp kosher salt

Confectioners' sugar
(optional)

1. Preheat the oven to 350°F (175°C). Spray a 12-cup muffin pan with nonstick cooking spray, or line with paper liners.

2. In a large bowl, and using a mixer on medium speed, cream butter and granulated sugar for 2 minutes.

3. Add reduced-fat milk, ricotta cheese, vanilla extract, egg, lemon zest, and lemon juice. Mix on medium speed for 1 or 2 minutes or until well combined.

4. In a small bowl, combine all-purpose flour, cornmeal, baking powder, and kosher salt.

5. Add flour mixture to milk mixture, and gently fold until just combined.

6. Evenly divide batter among muffin cups, filling each with about ¼ cup batter.

7. Bake for 20 minutes or until golden brown.

8. Sprinkle with confectioners' sugar, if using.

**Variation:** Replace the lemon with any other citrus fruit.

| EACH SERVING HAS | | | |
|---|---|---|---|
| 260 calories<br>10g total fat | 6g saturated fat<br>5g protein | 36g carbohydrates<br>5g fiber | 45mg cholesterol<br>210mg sodium |

# Baklava

In this rich, traditional Middle Eastern dessert, sweet and flaky phyllo dough is laced with honey and walnuts. Finely chop the walnuts in a food processor for the best results.

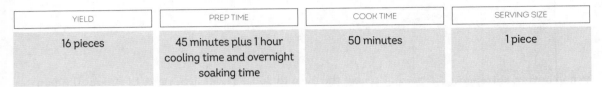

| YIELD | PREP TIME | COOK TIME | SERVING SIZE |
|-------|-----------|-----------|--------------|
| 16 pieces | 45 minutes plus 1 hour cooling time and overnight soaking time | 50 minutes | 1 piece |

1 lb (450g) walnuts

1¼ cups sugar

1 tsp ground cinnamon

¼ tsp ground cloves

14 sheets phyllo dough, thawed according to package directions

1¼ cups butter, melted

¾ cup water

3 oz (85g) orange blossom honey

1 tbsp freshly squeezed lemon juice

1 cinnamon stick

1. Lightly butter the bottom and sides of a 9×13-inch (23×33cm) baking pan.

2. In a medium bowl, combine walnuts, ¼ cup sugar, ground cinnamon, and ground cloves.

3. Lay out the stacked sheets of phyllo dough, and pull off 1 sheet at a time to work with. (Lay a damp towel over the rest to keep them from drying out while you work.) Using a pastry brush, brush 1 sheet with melted butter. Fold sheet in half, and place in the prepared baking pan. Repeat with 4 more sheets of dough, working with 1 sheet at a time, for 5 sheets total.

4. Spread ⅓ of the nut mixture evenly on top of the layered phyllo dough in the pan.

5. Repeat the procedure twice more, using 2 layered sheets of phyllo dough at a time (4 sheets total), ending with a top layer of nuts.

6. Repeat step 3 five more times so you end up with 5 more buttered, folded sheets of phyllo dough on top of nut mixture.

7. Trim the edges of the phyllo dough with a sharp knife to make a clean cut around the edges of the pan.

8. Chill for about 1 hour. This allows the butter to firm up the mixture prior to cutting.

9. Preheat the oven to 350°F (175°C).

10. Remove baklava from the refrigerator. Cut 4 equal rows down the shortest width of the pan from top to bottom. Then, cut horizontally down the center or side to create 8 squares. Finally, slice each square diagonally to get 16 triangles.

11. Bake for 45 to 50 minutes or until golden brown.

12. Meanwhile, in a small saucepan over medium-high heat, combine remaining 1 cup sugar, water, orange blossom honey, lemon juice, and cinnamon stick. Bring to a boil, reduce heat to low, and simmer for 10 minutes. Remove from heat, and cool to lukewarm. Remove and discard cinnamon stick.

13. Remove baklava from the oven, and pour syrup over the top while still hot. Let stand at room temperature overnight for the syrup to absorb.

**Variation:** Add different nuts such as almonds and flavorings such as orange zest to your syrup.

| EACH SERVING HAS | | | |
|---|---|---|---|
| 390 calories 28g total fat | 7g saturated fat 6g protein | 33g carbohydrates 2g fiber | 25mg cholesterol 85mg sodium |

# Almond Cookies

Crispy and sweet with a delicate crumb, these almond-flavored cookies are a tasty treat any time of year.

| YIELD | PREP TIME | COOK TIME | SERVING SIZE |
|---|---|---|---|
| 30 cookies | 20 minutes plus 2 hours chilling time | 20 minutes | 1 cookie |

¾ cup raw almonds

1 cup unsalted butter, softened

½ cup sugar

2 cups all-purpose flour

½ tsp baking powder

1. Preheat the oven to 350°F (175°C). Oil 2 baking sheets.

2. In a food processor, pulse almonds until finely ground.

3. In a large bowl, and using a mixer on medium speed, cream unsalted butter and sugar for 2 minutes.

4. In a medium bowl, combine all-purpose flour, baking powder, and almonds.

5. Add flour mixture to the creamed sugar, and mix on low for about 30 seconds. Increase the speed to medium, and mix for 1 or 2 more minutes or until well combined.

6. Scoop 1-tablespoon cookies onto the prepared baking sheets, and chill for 1 or 2 hours.

7. Bake for 15 to 20 minutes or until slightly golden brown.

**Variation:** Add 1 teaspoon lemon, lime, or orange zest.

| EACH SERVING HAS | | | |
|---|---|---|---|
| 120 calories 8g total fat | 4g saturated fat 2g protein | 11g carbohydrates 1g fiber | 15mg cholesterol 10mg sodium |

# Walnut Cake

Light and sweet with a tender crumb, this cake is excellent any time, but especially in the winter with a cup of hot coffee.

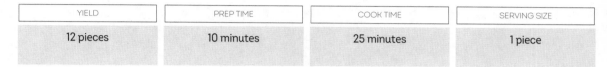

| YIELD | PREP TIME | COOK TIME | SERVING SIZE |
|---|---|---|---|
| 12 pieces | 10 minutes | 25 minutes | 1 piece |

1½ cups all-purpose flour

½ cup granulated sugar

2½ tsp baking powder

¼ tsp kosher salt

1 egg

¼ cup olive oil

¾ cup reduced-fat milk

¾ cup walnuts, chopped

Confectioners' sugar

1. Position a rack in the center of the oven, and preheat the oven to 350°F (175°C). Lightly oil and flour the bottom of an 8×8-inch (20×20cm) baking pan.

2. In a large bowl, combine all-purpose flour, granulated sugar, baking powder, and kosher salt.

3. In a medium bowl, beat together egg, olive oil, and reduced-fat milk.

4. Add egg mixture to flour mixture, and mix until incorporated.

5. Add walnuts, and mix well.

6. Pour batter into the prepared pan. Bake for 20 to 25 minutes or until a toothpick inserted into the center of the cake comes out clean.

7. Remove from the oven, and cool on a wire rack.

8. Transfer cake to a serving platter, and dust with confectioners' sugar. Serve warm or at room temperature.

**Variation:** Add ½ cup dried cranberries or raisins.

| EACH SERVING HAS | | | |
|---|---|---|---|
| 200 calories 10g total fat | 1.5g saturated fat 4g protein | 25g carbohydrates 1g fiber | 0mg cholesterol 125mg sodium |

# Orange Rice Pudding

Sweet orange and cinnamon accent creamy rice and make this rice pudding a wonderful winter dessert.

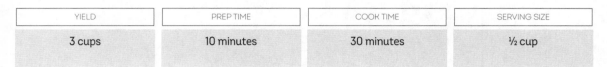

| YIELD | PREP TIME | COOK TIME | SERVING SIZE |
| --- | --- | --- | --- |
| 3 cups | 10 minutes | 30 minutes | ½ cup |

1 cup short-grain white rice

2½ cups reduced-fat milk

1 tsp vanilla extract

1 tsp ground cinnamon

¼ tsp kosher salt

1 large orange

1 tbsp orange liqueur or orange juice

1. In a medium saucepan over medium-high heat, combine short-grain white rice, reduced-fat milk, vanilla extract, ground cinnamon, and kosher salt. Bring to a boil, reduce heat to a simmer, and cook for about 15 minutes.

2. Meanwhile, cut off the top and bottom of orange. Place orange cut side down on a cutting board, cut off peel and white pith, and slice orange from top to bottom. Holding the orange over a bowl to catch the juice, cut out orange segments, leaving behind the membrane between each section. Set aside segments. Squeeze the juice from the remaining orange membranes into the rice mixture.

3. Stir cooked rice, cover, and cook for 15 more minutes or until all liquid has been absorbed.

4. Stir in orange liqueur, and add orange segments. Serve warm or cold.

**Variation:** Add ½ cup golden raisins and ½ cup toasted coconut.

| EACH SERVING HAS | | | |
| --- | --- | --- | --- |
| 190 calories 2g total fat | 1.5g saturated fat 6g protein | 35g carbohydrates 2g fiber | 10mg cholesterol 120mg sodium |

# Fig and Apricot Compote

The sweet-and-sour spice mix in this recipes makes this compote a great spread for any type of bread or cracker.

| YIELD | PREP TIME | COOK TIME | SERVING SIZE |
|-------|-----------|-----------|--------------|
| 3 cups | 10 minutes | 60 minutes | ¼ cup |

8 oz (225g) dried figs, stems removed

6 oz (170g) dried apricots

3 oz (85g) crystallized ginger

2 cinnamon sticks

1 cup sugar

Juice of 1 lemon

1 tsp apple cider vinegar

2 cups water

1. In a food processor, pulse figs until finely chopped. Transfer to a medium saucepan.

2. Add apricots and crystallized ginger to the food processor, and pulse until finely chopped. (Do not overload the food processor because fruit is sticky; you want evenly diced fruit.) Transfer apricots and ginger to the pan with figs.

3. Add cinnamon sticks, sugar, lemon juice, apple cider vinegar, and water to the pan, and stir to combine. Set over medium heat, and bring to a boil.

4. Reduce heat to low, and simmer, stirring occasionally, for 45 to 60 minutes or until most liquid has evaporated.

**Variation:** Try any other type of dried fruit, like cherries, blueberries, or raisins.

| EACH SERVING HAS | | | |
|------------------|---|---|---|
| 170 calories<br>0g total fat | 0g saturated fat<br>1g protein | 45g carbohydrates<br>3g fiber | 0mg cholesterol<br>15mg sodium |

# CHAPTER 24

# Seasonal Menu Plans

Now that you have a firm grasp on what foods are included in the Mediterranean diet and why, it is time to put it all together. It you want to stay on track with your new style of Mediterranean eating, menu planning can help. Planning ahead ensures that you are prepared, stay on track, always have healthy Mediterranean foods on hand, make fewer trips to the market, and increase the variety of foods you eat each day. After you plan your menus for the week—using the Mediterranean Diet Pyramid from Chapter 3 as a guide— you can create your grocery list and make shopping a breeze.

To help you get started, we have created one week of menu plans for each season that incorporate foods of the Mediterranean and many of the recipes in Part 4. These menus are designed to be convenient. They enable you to stock up on ingredients you need for the upcoming week so you can use them throughout the week in various ways.

Use the menus as is, or make changes so they fit your tastes and lifestyle, and before you know it, you naturally will be including more foods from the Mediterranean diet and developing a heart-healthy diet plan.

Chapter 14 gives you ideas for wine pairings if you so desire.

We share many of Part 4's recipes in the following seasonal menus. The remaining menu items are meal suggestions you can fix yourself. Some of the recipes are used in multiple meal plans because the growing seasons vary in different regions. Labeling the menu plans by season is only a guide to help you learn to eat a variety of Mediterranean foods throughout the year.

# Seven-Day Summer Menu Plan

Summer offers an abundance of fresh fruits and vegetables at their peak flavor—summer melons, berries, and tomatoes come to mind. In-season foods tend to be fresher, last longer, and cost less. One way to learn what is in season in your area is to visit your local farmers market. And because it's summertime, grill some fish, lean meats, and veggies. The leftovers can be used for sandwiches and salads throughout the week.

## Day 1

**Breakfast:** Whole-grain waffle with fresh blueberries and low-fat Greek yogurt

**Lunch:** Spinach, Orange, and Feta Salad (page 254); Caramelized Onion Flatbread (page 258)

**Snack:** A handful of walnuts and grapes

**Dinner:** Pan-Seared Orange Scallops (page 269); Minted Cucumber Salad (page 253); steamed zucchini, tomatoes, and onions drizzled with extra-virgin olive oil

**Snack:** Tomato Basil Bocconcini (page 232)

## Day 2

**Breakfast:** Oatmeal with nuts, honey, and fresh raspberries

**Lunch:** Gazpacho (page 245); Smoked Salmon Bites (page 237)

**Snack:** Strawberries

**Dinner:** Grilled lamb chops with Pesto (page 223); Golden Couscous Salad (page 249)

**Snack:** Lemon Minted Melon (page 234)

# Day 3

**Breakfast:** Scrambled egg wrap with tomatoes, feta, and spinach; fat-free milk

**Lunch:** Grilled chicken; Zucchini and Walnuts (page 282); couscous; Classic Mixed Greens Salad with Balsamic Vinaigrette (page 255)

**Snack:** Sliced watermelon

**Dinner:** Prosciutto and Roasted Vegetable Panini (page 266); Baked Stuffed Peaches (page 306)

**Snack:** Pear, Provolone, Asiago, and Balsamic Flatbread (page 259)

# Day 4

**Breakfast:** Low-fat Greek yogurt mixed-berry parfait with granola

**Lunch:** Shrimp and Melon Salad (page 252)

**Snack:** A handful of almonds and grapes

**Dinner:** Hummus (page 228); Veggie Wrap (page 263); Berry Sorbet (page 304)

**Snack:** Strawberries with balsamic reduction

# Day 5

**Breakfast:** Fresh raspberries with melted fontina cheese on toast

**Lunch:** Chicken Tzatziki Pita (page 265); Pickled Asparagus (page 290)

**Snack:** Fresh cherries and a handful of walnuts

**Dinner:** Angel Hair Pasta with Pesto, Mushrooms, and Arugula (page 275)

**Snack:** Lemon Ricotta Muffin (page 307)

## Day 6

**Breakfast:** Blueberry yogurt smoothie

**Lunch:** Tomato Basil Pizza (page 261); Poached Summer Fruit (page 302) with yogurt

**Snack:** A handful of walnuts

**Dinner:** Crab Cakes (page 231); Lemon Kale Ribbons (page 288); Roasted Red Pepper Tapenade (page 222)

**Snack:** Sliced watermelon

## Day 7

**Breakfast:** Baked Vegetable Omelet (page 230); fat-free milk

**Lunch:** Melon, Figs, and Prosciutto (page 224)

**Snack:** Strawberries and almonds

**Dinner:** Grilled halibut; Golden Chard (page 294); quinoa; Mixed Berry Torte (page 303)

**Snack:** Eggplant dip with celery, carrots, and red bell pepper

# Seven-Day Fall Menu Plan

Fall is a transitional time when we have the bounty of leftovers from summer fruits and vegetables that survive until the temperatures drop too low. Fall vegetables like kale and root vegetables are a heartier fare and require a little more preparation. Roasting vegetables helps draw out and concentrate their flavors.

## Day 1

**Breakfast:** Baked Vegetable Omelet (page 230); fat-free milk

**Lunch:** Mushroom, Artichoke, and Arugula Flatbread (page 260)

**Snack:** Nectarine

**Dinner:** Grilled chicken apple sausage; Barley and Vegetable Sauté (page 298); baked acorn squash

**Snack:** Dried cherries and pecans

## Day 2

**Breakfast:** Oatmeal with cinnamon apples

**Lunch:** Chicken Almond Wrap (page 264)

**Snack:** Red and green grapes

**Dinner:** Split Pea Soup (page 244); Classic Mixed Greens Salad with Balsamic Vinaigrette (page 255); Parmesan Pepper Crisps (page 236)

**Snack:** Stuffed Dates (page 225)

## Day 3

**Breakfast:** Whole-grain waffle with orange segments and low-fat yogurt

**Lunch:** Tuna Salad with Capers and Potatoes (page 250)

**Snack:** A handful of almonds and dried apricots

**Dinner:** Two-Cheese Risotto (page 283); Cinnamon Apple and Nut Phyllo Rolls (page 300)

**Snack:** Hummus (page 228) with Parmesan Pepper Crisps (page 236)

## Day 4

**Breakfast:** Apple cinnamon yogurt smoothie

**Lunch:** Mixed Bean Soup (page 246); Mushroom Crostini (page 226)

**Snack:** A handful of cashews

**Dinner:** Caramelized Onion Flatbread (page 258); Classic Mixed Greens Salad with Balsamic Vinaigrette (page 255)

**Snack:** Figs, olives, and mozzarella

## Day 5

**Breakfast:** Scrambled egg wrap with roasted red peppers and onions; fat-free milk

**Lunch:** Eggplant Rolls (page 229); Quinoa Pilaf (page 297)

**Snack:** Orange

**Dinner:** Bean and Vegetable Patties (page 291); steamed broccoli; Baklava (page 308)

**Snack:** Olives; crusty bread dipped in extra-virgin olive oil

## Day 6

**Breakfast:** Yogurt parfait with diced pears and blueberries

**Lunch:** Grilled chicken breast; patty pan squash sautéed with garlic; Tabbouleh Salad (page 256)

**Snack:** Apple

**Dinner:** Seafood Stew (page 268); crusty bread; Classic Mixed Greens Salad with Balsamic Vinaigrette (page 255)

**Snack:** Toasted almonds and pomegranate seeds

## Day 7

**Breakfast:** Pear, Provolone, Asiago, and Balsamic Flatbread (page 259)

**Lunch:** Roasted Beet Salad (page 248); Onion Apple Marmalade (page 235) on crusty bread

**Snack:** Orange

**Dinner:** Lamb Shanks (page 278); garlic mashed potatoes; sautéed spinach

**Snack:** Eggplant dip with whole-wheat pita wedges

# Seven-Day Winter Menu Plan

Cold winter days are a good time to make use of kitchen staples. A well-stocked pantry can help you whip up a delicious meal regardless of the weather outside. Do not be afraid to use frozen vegetables when fresh are not as readily available. Or cook dried beans and pastas with canned ingredients like artichoke hearts, tomatoes, and corn. Dried ingredients like raisins, sun-dried tomatoes, figs, and dates are wonderful to use in winter, too.

## Day 1

**Breakfast:** Poached egg on toast; blood orange sections; fat-free milk

**Lunch:** Lemon Lentil Soup (page 241); Parmesan Pepper Crisps (page 236); Classic Mixed Greens Salad with Balsamic Vinaigrette (page 255)

**Snack:** Low-fat Greek yogurt; almonds; apple wedges

**Dinner:** Roasted chicken; Rosemary Garlic Potatoes (page 286); broccoli rabe

**Snack:** Orange Rice Pudding (page 312)

## Day 2

**Breakfast:** Yogurt parfait with diced pears

**Lunch:** Marinated Artichoke Salad (page 247); ½ turkey sandwich

**Snack:** Dried fruit and walnuts

**Dinner:** Salmon Fennel Bundles (page 273); couscous; baby carrots

**Snack:** Lemon Ricotta Muffin (page 307)

# Day 3

**Breakfast:** Oatmeal with toasted almonds and orange segments; fat-free milk

**Lunch:** Tomato Basil Soup (page 240); Classic Mixed Greens Salad with Balsamic Vinaigrette (page 255)

**Snack:** Low-fat yogurt and apple wedges

**Dinner:** Lamb Patties without pasta (page 276); Sweet Polenta with Sun-Dried Tomatoes (page 295); roasted brussels sprouts

**Snack:** Olive tapenade on a toasted baguette slice

# Day 4

**Breakfast:** Tangerine segments and melted fontina cheese on toast

**Lunch:** Fennel and Apple Salad (page 251); roasted chicken

**Snack:** Cashews; low-fat mozzarella cheese; olives

**Dinner:** Crispy Turkey Cutlets (page 279); Curried Cauliflower (page 287); red kidney beans

**Snack:** Walnut Cake (page 311)

# Day 5

**Breakfast:** Oatmeal with almonds, pears, and honey

**Lunch:** Caramelized Onion Flatbread (page 258); spaghetti squash with chickpeas and feta

**Snack:** Orange sections drizzled with extra-virgin olive oil

**Dinner:** Butternut Squash Soup (page 242); ½ cheese panini; Classic Mixed Greens Salad with Balsamic Vinaigrette (page 255)

**Snack:** Olives; crusty bread dipped in extra-virgin olive oil

## Day 6

**Breakfast:** Whole-grain waffle with sliced apples; low-fat yogurt

**Lunch:** Tuna salad wrap with avocado slices

**Snack:** Pear

**Dinner:** Spicy Tomato Sauce with Linguine (page 274); chicken apple sausage; sautéed zucchini

**Snack:** Stuffed Dates (page 225)

## Day 7

**Breakfast:** Baked Vegetable Omelet (page 230); blood orange sections; fat-free milk

**Lunch:** Turkey panini; watercress salad; cup of minestrone soup

**Snack:** Low-fat Greek yogurt and walnuts

**Dinner:** Butternut Squash and Goat Cheese Pizza (page 262)

**Snack:** Fig and Apricot Compote (page 313); Onion Apple Marmalade (page 235) on crusty bread

# Seven-Day Spring Menu Plan

Spring emerges with delicate leafy greens, tender asparagus, and artichokes. You can even grow your own leafy greens. You just need to protect the young plants from a late frost by covering them if the temperature dips too low. These spring menus are lighter but still satisfying.

## Day 1

**Breakfast:** Baked Vegetable Omelet (page 230); fat-free milk

**Lunch:** Prosciutto and Roasted Vegetable Panini (page 266); avocado slices

**Snack:** Low-fat Greek yogurt and kumquats

**Dinner:** Chicken Piccata (page 280); Sautéed Spinach and Mushrooms (page 285); white kidney beans; Vanilla Panna Cotta (page 301)

**Snack:** Tangelo and a handful of pecans

## Day 2

**Breakfast:** Low-fat Greek yogurt parfait with apple and granola

**Lunch:** Vegetable Orzo Soup (page 243); ½ turkey sandwich

**Snack:** Dried apricots and a handful of walnuts

**Dinner:** Sole Florentine (page 271); Rosemary Garlic Potatoes (page 286); roasted peppers; Almond Cookies (page 310)

**Snack:** Hummus (page 228) with celery and carrot sticks

## Day 3

**Breakfast:** Oatmeal with walnuts and honey

**Lunch:** Chicken Almond Wrap (page 264); steamed asparagus

**Snack:** Low-fat yogurt and apple wedges

**Dinner:** Panzanella (page 293) with turkey; Orange Rice Pudding (page 312)

**Snack:** Fruit and Cheese Plate (page 305)

## Day 4

**Breakfast:** Frozen blueberry yogurt smoothie

**Lunch:** Tuna Salad with Capers and Potatoes (page 250)

**Snack:** Blood orange segments drizzled with extra-virgin olive oil and chopped pistachios

**Dinner:** Appetizer quartet: Lamb Pesto Crostini (page 233); Roasted Red Pepper Tapenade (page 222); Onion Apple Marmalade (page 235); Pickled Asparagus (page 290)

**Snack:** Hummus (page 228) with carrots, radishes, and celery sticks

## Day 5

**Breakfast:** Scrambled egg wrap with feta, mushrooms, and spinach; tangerine segments; fat-free milk

**Lunch:** Lemon Lentil Soup (page 241); ½ cheese panini

**Snack:** Cashews; dried cherries and blueberries

**Dinner:** Spicy Tomato Sauce with Linguine (page 274); Classic Mixed Greens Salad with Balsamic Vinaigrette (page 255)

**Snack:** Olives; crusty bread dipped in extra-virgin olive oil

## Day 6

**Breakfast:** Whole-grain waffle with apple slices and low-fat yogurt

**Lunch:** Mushroom, Artichoke, and Arugula Flatbread (page 260)

**Snack:** Dried dates and apricots with walnuts

**Dinner:** Almond-Crusted Barramundi (page 272); Minted Peas with Pancetta (page 289); quinoa; Almond Cookies (page 310)

**Snack:** Roasted Red Pepper Tapenade (page 222) with whole-wheat pita

## Day 7

**Breakfast:** Broiled pink grapefruit with brown sugar and low-fat Greek yogurt

**Lunch:** Spinach, Orange, and Feta Salad (page 254); cup of vegetable soup

**Snack:** Apple wedges with Manchego cheese

**Dinner:** Lamb Patties and Pasta (page 276); Classic Mixed Greens Salad with Balsamic Vinaigrette (page 255)

**Snack:** Lemon Cannellini Spread (page 227) with toasted whole-wheat flatbread

# Glossary

**alpha linolenic acid (ALA)**   Omega-3 fatty acids found in plant sources.

**amino acids**   The building blocks that make up protein.

**antioxidants**   A group of nutrients that counteract effects of harmful free radicals.

**body mass index (BMI)**   An index calculated using height and weight to determine a person's healthy weight range.

**capers**   Immature buds plucked from a small bush native to the Mediterranean and Middle East.

**carbohydrates**   An organic compound consisting of carbon, hydrogen, and oxygen. A component of food that provides calories and energy to the body.

**cardiovascular disease**   A class of diseases that involve the heart and/or the blood vessels, including the arteries and veins.

**cholesterol**   A soft waxy substance found among the lipids or fats in the bloodstream and in the cells of the body. Dietary cholesterol is found in animal foods.

**complete protein**   A protein that provides the body with an adequate proportion of all nine essential amino acids needed for optimal health.

**complex carbohydrates (starches)**   Three or more simple sugars that are linked together. Also called *polysaccharides*.

**coronary artery disease**   *See* coronary heart disease (CHD).

**coronary heart disease (CHD)**   A narrowing of the small blood vessels that supply both blood and oxygen to the heart.

**DASH diet**   Stands for "Dietary Approaches to Stop Hypertension." A heart-healthy diet to help people manage high blood pressure.

**diabetes**   A group of diseases that are evident by high levels of blood glucose or blood sugar due to defects in either the production or action of insulin (a hormone in the body) or both.

**Dietary Guidelines for Americans**   Science- and evidence-based nutritional and fitness goals that promote health and are meant to help reduce the risk of chronic disease.

**Dietary Reference Intakes (DRI)**   Daily nutrient recommendations for Americans based on age and gender that are set by the Institute of Medicine's Food and Nutrition Board (FNB). Expressed as recommended daily allowance (RDA) or Adequate Intake (AI).

**disaccharides**   *See* simple carbohydrates (simple sugars).

**diverticulosis**    A condition of the colon in which tiny pouches, or diverticula, form on the colon walls. When these pouches become infected or inflamed, the condition is known as diverticulitis.

**docosahexaenoic acid (DHA)**    An omega-3 fatty acid exclusively found in fish and seafood.

**eicosapentaenoic acid (EPA)**    An omega-3 fatty acid exclusively found in fish and seafood.

**empty-calorie foods**    Foods high in calories but low in nutritional content.

**enriched**    When nutrients that were removed during processing are added back to a food.

**fat-soluble vitamins**    Vitamins that dissolve in fat and are carried through the bloodstream and the body through fat (vitamins A, D, E, and K).

**free radicals**    Highly reactive atoms or groups of atoms with an unpaired electron. They can come from the environment, such as cigarette smoke, pollution, and ultraviolet light, or be the by-product of the body using oxygen. Free radicals cause damage to body cells.

**fructose**    The natural sugar found in fruit.

**glucose**    A simple sugar found in some foods that the body uses as a source of energy. It also circulates in the blood as blood glucose or blood sugar.

**gluten**    A mixture of proteins found in wheat, rye, barley, and other foods. It's what gives bread the elasticity and structure that allows it to rise.

**glycemic index (GI)**    A numerical scale that indicates how fast a single food raises blood glucose (blood sugar).

**healthy fats**    Fats that are unsaturated, such as monounsaturated, polyunsaturated, and omega-3 fatty acids. These fats help reduce the risk for heart disease.

**heme iron**    The form of most iron found in animal-based foods.

**high-density lipoproteins (HDL)**    Referred to as "good" cholesterol. Rids the body of dietary cholesterol, which lowers your risk for heart disease.

**hydrogenation**    The process by which liquid vegetable oil is made more solid by the addition of hydrogen.

**hypertension**    The medical term for high blood pressure.

**incomplete protein**    A protein that does not include all nine essential amino acids or does not include all nine in adequate amounts. Found in most plant proteins.

**insoluble fiber**  A type of fiber found in plants that the body cannot digest and does not break down as it passes through the digestive tract. Helps promote regularity.

**ketogenic diet**  A diet that severely restricts carbohydrates and is high in protein and fat. These diets trigger short-term weight loss. *See also* ketosis.

**ketosis**  An abnormal accumulation of ketones in the body that occurs when the person's diet lacks enough carbohydrates, the body's main source of energy, and results in an excessive breakdown of fats.

**lactose**  The natural sugar found in dairy products such as milk.

**lavash**  A flatbread of Middle Eastern origin.

**legumes**  A category of plants that have pods (or fruits) and include beans, peas, lentils, and peanuts.

**lipids**  A general term that refers to all fats, cholesterol, and fatlike substances.

**low-density lipoproteins (LDL)**  Referred to as "bad" cholesterol. Causes cholesterol buildup in artery walls, which increases the risk for heart disease and stroke.

**Mediterranean Diet Pyramid**  A visual representation of the most current nutritional research on the healthy, traditional Mediterranean diet.

**metabolism**  The process by which the body uses or burns calories for energy.

**micronutrients**  *See* vitamins; minerals.

**minerals**  Inorganic compounds essential to the body for various functions. Minerals come in two categories: major and trace. Major minerals are needed by the body in greater amounts than trace minerals.

**monosaccharides**  *See* simple carbohydrates (simple sugars).

**monounsaturated fats**  Fats that are missing one hydrogen pair on their chemical chain. They are typically liquid at room temperature but solidify when chilled. Considered a heart-healthy fat.

**nonheme iron**  The type of most iron found in plant-based foods.

**nutrient-dense foods**  Foods that contain vitamins, minerals, fiber, and other essential nutrients yet are low in calories.

**Nutrition Facts Panel**  The box on food labels that provides required nutritional information.

**omega-3 fatty acids**   A group of essential polyunsaturated fatty acids that are considered heart healthy and health-promoting. Our body cannot produce them, so we must get them from the foods we eat.

**omega-6 fatty acids**   A group of essential polyunsaturated fatty acids. Although they are essential, the amount we should consume has been controversial.

**orzo**   Small, rice-shaped pasta.

**pancetta**   A pork product similar to bacon except pancetta is not smoked.

**phytochemicals**   *See* phytonutrients.

**phytonutrients**   Naturally occurring compounds found in plant-based foods that offer potential health benefits.

**plant sterols/stanols**   Substances found naturally in fruits, vegetables, and plant oils that have been found to lower LDL cholesterol.

**polysaccharides**   *See* complex carbohydrates (starches).

**polyunsaturated fats**   Fats that have more than one missing hydrogen pair on their chemical chain. These fats are typically liquid at room temperature and when chilled. They are considered a healthy fat.

**probiotics**   Live microorganisms (usually bacteria) that are similar to beneficial microorganisms found in our gut. They are good bacteria that may treat and prevent certain illnesses and support general health. An example is the live bacterial cultures found in yogurt.

**proteins**   A macronutrient found both in the foods we eat and in many structures of the body.

**refined grains**   Whole grains that have been processed or milled and have had the bran and germ removed.

**saturated fats**   Fats with a chemical structure that is saturated with hydrogen. They are solid at room temperature and can increase total and bad cholesterol, raising one's risk for heart disease, stroke, and cancer.

**simple carbohydrates (simple sugars)**   Single sugar units or pairs of sugar units linked together.

**soluble fiber**   A type of fiber in plant foods that dissolves easily in water and takes on a soft, gel-like form in the intestines. Helps lower cholesterol and regulate blood sugar.

**smoke point**    The temperature at which an oil will smoke when heated.

**trans fats**    Fats that raise total and bad cholesterol, lower good cholesterol, and increase the risk for heart disease and stroke. Produced when liquid fats are put through the hydrogenation process.

**triglycerides**    The main form of fat in foods. Excess calories from any type of food source are processed in the body and changed to triglycerides for storage as fat in the body.

**vitamins**    Organic compounds and a group of nutrients that are required in small amounts for optimal health.

**water-soluble vitamins**    Vitamins that dissolve in water and are carried through the body by watery fluids (eight B vitamins plus vitamin C).

**whole grains**    Grains that are made of the entire seed of the grain, containing the three key parts: bran, germ, and endosperm.

# Resources

The following websites can help you further your knowledge, keep you up-to-date with new findings, and open the door to discovering more about the Mediterranean diet and good health.

This information was reliable and correct at the time of this writing. We assume no responsibility for any recent changes in contact information that may have occurred since the initial printing of this book.

**Academy of Nutrition and Dietetics**
eatright.org

**American Cancer Society**
cancer.org

**American Diabetes Association**
diabetes.org

**American Heart Association**
heart.org

**American Institute for Cancer Research**
aicr.org

**ConsumerLab.com**
consumerlab.com

**Fats of Life**
fatsoflife.com

**Mediterranean Diet**
mediterraneandiet.com

**Oldways**
oldwayspt.org

**Oldways Whole Grains Council**
wholegrainscouncil.org

**The Olive Oil Source**
oliveoilsource.com

**Produce for Better Health Foundation**
pbhfoundation.org

**Tufts University Health and Nutrition Letter**
healthletter.tufts.edu

**USDA Dietary Guidelines for Americans**
dietaryguidelines.gov

**USDA MyPlate**
myplate.gov

**USDA Nutrition.gov**
nutrition.gov

**The Vegetarian Resource Group**
vrg.org

**Women's Heart Foundation**
womensheart.org

# Index

# A

AA (arachidonic acid), 188

AARP (American Association of Retired Persons), 32

Agatston, Arthur, 59

almonds, 146–147, 149
  Almond Cookies, 310
  Almond-Crusted Barramundi, 272
  Chicken Almond Wrap, 264

Alzheimer's disease, 40

American Association of Retired Persons (AARP), 32

American Heart Association (AHA) diet, 56–57

*American Journal of Clinical Nutrition*, 32

Angel Hair Pasta with Pesto, Mushrooms, and Arugula, 275

anthocyanidins (flavonoid), 214

antioxidants, 212

appetizers
  Baked Vegetable Omelet, 230
  Crab Cakes, 231
  Eggplant Rolls, 229
  Hummus, 228
  Lamb Pesto Crostini, 233
  Lemon Cannellini Spread, 227
  Lemon Minted Melon, 234
  Melon, Figs, and Prosciutto, 224
  Mushroom Crostini, 226
  Onion Apple Marmalade, 235
  Parmesan Pepper Crisps, 236
  Pesto, 223
  Roasted Red Pepper Tapenade, 222
  Smoked Salmon Bites, 237
  Stuffed Dates, 225
  Tomato Basil Bocconcini, 232

apples, 114
  Cinnamon Apple and Nut Phyllo Rolls, 300
  Fennel and Apple Salad, 251
  Onion Apple Marmalade, 235

arachidonic acid (AA), 188

*Archives of Internal Medicine*, 32

artichokes, 121–122

arugula, 127
  Angel Hair Pasta with Pesto, Mushrooms, and Arugula, 275
  Mushroom, Artichoke, and Arugula Flatbread, 260

Atkins, Robert, 58

Atkins diet, 58–59

avocados, 110

# B

Baked Stuffed Peaches, 306

Baked Vegetable Omelet, 230

Baklava, 308

barley
  Barley and Vegetable Sauté, 298
  flour, 103
  hulled, 99

basil, 168–169
  Angel Hair Pasta with Pesto, Mushrooms, and Arugula, 275
  Lamb Pesto Crostini, 233
  Pesto, 223
  Tomato Basil Bocconcini, 232
  Tomato Basil Pizza, 261
  Tomato Basil Soup, 240

beans, 48, 147
  Bean and Vegetable Patties, 291
  cannellini beans, 153

fazolia beans, 153
Lemon Cannellini Spread, 227
Mixed Bean Soup, 249
white kidney beans, 153
beets, Roasted Beet Salad, 248
berries
Berry Sorbet, 304
Mixed Berry Torte, 303
strawberries, 113
beta-carotene (carotenoid), 214
biotin, 211
blood pressure, 33, 39–40
body mass index (BMI), 36
bowel health, fiber and, 199
brain health, Alzheimer's disease, 40
breads, 257
Caramelized Onion Flatbread, 258
Mushroom, Artichoke, and Arugula
Flatbread, 260
Pear, Provolone, Asiago, and Balsamic
Flatbread, 259
bulgur, 99
Tabbouleh Salad, 256
butter and margarine, 70
olive oil substitution ratios, 91
butternut squash
Butternut Squash and Goat Cheese Pizza,
262
Butternut Squash Soup, 242

## C

calcium, 212
cancer, 36–37
cannellini beans, 153
Lemon Cannellini Spread, 227

Caramelized Onion Flatbread, 258
carbohydrates, 216
complex, 216
sugars, 216
cardiovascular disease, 32
risk factors
cholesterol, 33
high blood pressure, 33
triglycerides, 33
cardiovascular health, 32
benefits, 33–34
cardiovascular disease, 32
risk factors, 33
heart disease, 32
carotenoids
beta-carotene, 214
lutein, 214
lycopene, 214
carrots, 126
cheese
Butternut Squash and Goat Cheese Pizza,
262
cheese and yogurt group, Mediterranean
Diet Pyramid, 49
Fruit and Cheese Plate, 305
Lemon Ricotta Muffins, 307
nutritional properties, 164
Parmesan Pepper Crisps, 236
Pear, Provolone, Asiago, and Balsamic
Flatbread, 259
Spinach, Orange, and Feta Salad, 254
Tomato Basil Bocconcini, 232
Two-Cheese Risotto, 283
chicken
Chicken Almond Wrap, 264
Chicken Piccata, 280
Chicken Tzatziki Pita, 265

cholesterol
    benefits, 33–34
    dietary cholesterol, 191
    fiber and, 196
    high-density lipoprotein (HDL), 33
    low-density lipoprotein (LDL), 33
    monounsaturated fats and, 84
Cinnamon Apple and Nut Phyllo Rolls, 300
Classic Mixed Greens Salad with Balsamic
    Vinaigrette, 255
classifications, olive oil
    extra-virgin, 86–87
    lite, 88
    pure, 87–88
    refined, 87–88
    virgin, 87
cobalamin (vitamin $B_{12}$), 211
colon cancer, fiber and, 199
complex carbohydrates, 216
cooking techniques
    olive oil, 89–91
    whole grains, 103–104
couscous, 100
    Golden Couscous Salad, 249
Crab Cakes, 231
Crispy Turkey Cutlets, 279
Curried Cauliflower, 287

**D**

dairy
    nutritional properties, 164
        cheese, 164
        milk, 165
        yogurt, 165
    replacement options, 70

DASH (Dietary Approaches to Stop
    Hypertension) diet, 57
dates, 112
    Stuffed Dates, 225
dementia, Alzheimer's disease, 40
depression, 37
desserts
    Almond Cookies, 310
    Baked Stuffed Peaches, 306
    Baklava, 308
    Berry Sorbet, 304
    Cinnamon Apple and Nut Phyllo Rolls,
      300
    Fig and Apricot Compote, 313
    fruit, 115
    Fruit and Cheese Plate, 305
    Lemon Ricotta Muffins, 307
    Mixed Berry Torte, 303
    nuts, 154
    Orange Rice Pudding, 312
    Poached Summer Fruit, 302
    Vanilla Panna Cotta, 301
    Walnut Cake, 311
DHA (docosahexaenoic acid), 133
diabetes, 38
    risks, 39
    type 1, 39
    type 2, 38
Dietary Approaches to Stop Hypertension
    (DASH) diet, 57
dietary cholesterol, 191
diets, popular, compared to the
    Mediterranean diet
        American Heart Association (AHA) diet,
        56–57
        Atkins diet, 58–59

DASH (Dietary Approaches to Stop Hypertension) diet, 57
Ornish diet, 60
Sonoma diet, 62–63
South Beach diet, 59–60
Zone diet, 61–62
diet versus lifestyle, 29
digestive health, fiber and, 199
docosahexaenoic acid (DHA), 133
dried fruit, 116

**E**

eggplant, 122–123
Eggplant Rolls, 229
eggs, 49, 162
nutritional properties, 162–163
eicosapentaenoic acid (EPA), 133
enriched grains, 96
exercise, 26
extra-virgin olive oil, 86–87

**F**

fall menu plan, 318–320
fats, 21, 28
beneficial
monounsaturated, 186–187
omega-3 fatty acids, 187–188
omega-6 fatty acids, 188–189
polyunsaturated, 187
comparisons, 85
harmful
dietary cholesterol, 191
saturated, 189–190
trans, 190–191

health benefits, 184
intake recommendations, 185
Mediterranean Diet Pyramid group, 47
monounsaturated, 84–85
nutrition label, 76
olive oil
extra-virgin, 86–87
health benefits, 84
history and production, 82
lite, 88
nutritional properties, 85
pure, 87
refined, 87
uses, 83
virgin, 87
polyunsaturated, 85
replacing, 192
saturated, 85
solid versus liquid, 185
transitioning to healthy, 192
fat-soluble vitamins
vitamin A, 209
vitamin D, 209
vitamin E, 209
vitamin K, 210
fatty acids, 186
omega-3s, 187–188
omega-6s, 188–189
fazolia beans, 153
fennel
Fennel and Apple Salad, 251
Salmon Fennel Bundles, 273
fiber, 196
excess, 201
food labels, fiber wording, 201–202

health benefits, 197
  bowel health, 199
  colon cancer risk, 199
  digestive health, 199
  gut health, 199
  heart health, 197–198
  type 2 diabetes, 198
  weight management, 198
increasing intake, 200–201, 204
insoluble, 196–197
intake recommendations, 200
label information, 201
soluble, 196
supplements, 202
figs, 111
  Fig and Apricot Compote, 313
  Melon, Figs, and Prosciutto, 224
fish. *See also* seafood
  Almond-Crusted Barramundi, 272
  cooking techniques, 139
  fish oil supplements, 140–141
  health benefits, 132–133
  increasing intake, 142
  mercury levels, 141
  nutritional properties, 133–134
  salmon, 136, 138
  Salmon Fennel Bundles, 273
  sardines, 138–139
  Seafood Stew, 268
  selection tips, 134–135
  Smoked Salmon Bites, 237
  Sole Florentine, 271
  tuna, 137
  Tuna Salad with Capers and Potatoes, 250
fish and seafood group, Mediterranean Diet Pyramid, 48. *See also* seafood
fish oil supplements, 140–141

flatbreads, 257. *See also* pizza
  Caramelized Onion Flatbread, 258
  Mushroom, Artichoke, and Arugula Flatbread, 260
  Pear, Provolone, Asiago, and Balsamic Flatbread, 259
flavonoids
  anthocyanidins (flavonoid), 214
  wine, 175
flours, 101–102
  barley, 103
  spelt, 102
  whole-rye, 103
  whole-wheat, 102
folate (folic acid), 210
food journal, 64
food labels, 75
  "-free" claims, 78
  Nutrition Facts, 75–76
    fat, 76
    fiber, 76
    fiber wording, 201–202
    health claims, 78–79
    ingredient list, 77
    nutrient content claims, 78–79
    percent Daily Value (%DV), 77–78
    servings per container, 76
    sodium, 76
    sugar, 77
    whole grains, 98
food list, essential Mediterranean diet foods, 72–74, 94
food pairings, wine, 178
fruit
  alternatives to fresh, 115
  apples, 114
  as dessert, 115

avocados, 110
berries, 113
dates, 112
dried, 116
figs, 111
grapes, 113
health benefits, 108
increasing intake, 117
Mediterranean Diet Pyramid group, 47
nutritional properties, 108
olives, 109
oranges, 114
pomegranates, 111
strawberries, 113
fruit juice, 116

## G

garlic, 170
Gazpacho, 245
Golden Chard, 294
Golden Couscous Salad, 249
grains
adding, 71
enriched, 96
Mediterranean Diet Pyramid group, 47
refined, 95
grapes, 113
greens, 127
arugula, 127
kale, 127
mustard greens, 128
romaine lettuce, 128
spinach, 127
Swiss chard, 128
gut health, fiber and, 199
Guttersen, Connie, 62

## H

HDL (high-density lipoprotein), 33
HDL cholesterol, monounsaturated fats
and, 84
health benefits of the Mediterranean diet, 23
Alzheimer's disease, 40
brain health, 40
cancer and, 36–37
cardiovascular health, 32
cholesterol, 33–34
depression, 37
diabetes, 38
risks, 39
type 1, 39
type 2, 38
hypertension, 39–40
Parkinson's disease, 41
rheumatoid arthritis (RA), 41
weight management, 34
BMI, 36
obesity, 35
heart disease, 32
heart health, fiber and, 197–198
herbs, 48, 168. *See also* spices
basil, 168–169
dried herbs, 168
mint, 170
nutritional properties, 169
seasoning blends, 168
thyme, 171
usage tips, 171
high-density lipoprotein (HDL), 33
HDL cholesterol, monounsaturated fats
and, 84
honey, 74
hulled barley, 99

Hummus, 228
hydration, 27
hypertension, 39–40

### I-J

insoluble fiber, 196–197
International Olive Oil Council (IOOC), 87
iron, 212

### K

kale, 127
    Lemon Kale Ribbons, 288
Keys, Ancel, 20–21

### L

LA (linoleic acid), 188
labels, reading, 64
lamb
    Lamb Patties and Pasta, 276
    Lamb Pesto Crostini, 233
    Lamb Shanks, 278
LDL (low-density lipoprotein), 33
    LDL cholesterol, monounsaturated fats
      and, 84
legumes, 48
    cannellini beans, 153
    fazolia beans, 153
    health benefits, 147
    increasing intake, 154
    lentils, 152
    nutritional properties, 148
    peanuts, 152–153
    preparation tips, 149
    storage, 149
    white kidney beans, 153

lemons
    Lemon Cannellini Spread, 227
    Lemon Kale Ribbons, 288
    Lemon Lentil Soup, 241
    Lemon Minted Melon, 234
    Lemon Ricotta Muffins, 307
lentils, 147, 152
    Lemon Lentil Soup, 241
lifestyle, 25
    hydration, 27
    physical activity, 26
    stress, 26
    versus diet, 29
    whole-life approach, 28
linoleic acid (LA), 188
lite olive oil, 88
low-density lipoprotein (LDL), 33
    LDL cholesterol, monounsaturated fats
      and, 84
lutein (carotenoid), 214
lycopene (carotenoid), 214

### M

macronutrients
    carbohydrates, 216
      complex, 216
      sugars, 216
    protein, 214–215
main dishes
    Almond-Crusted Barramundi, 272
    Angel Hair Pasta with Pesto, Mushrooms,
      and Arugula, 275
    Chicken Piccata, 280
    Crispy Turkey Cutlets, 279
    Lamb Patties and Pasta, 276
    Lamb Shanks, 278

Pan Seared Orange Scallops, 269
Salmon Fennel Bundles, 273
Seafood Stew, 268
Sole Florentine, 271
Spicy Tomato Sauce with Linguine, 274
Marinated Artichoke Salad, 247
meal planning, 64
meal prep, 64
meat, 50, 158
    cooking tips, 161–162
    cuts, 160
    grades, 160
    Lamb Patties and Pasta, 276
    Lamb Shanks, 278
    nutritional properties, 159–160
    red meat, 70, 158
    shopping tips, 161–162
Mediterranean diet
    health benefits, 23
    history, 20–21
    key components, 22
    transitioning to, 23–25
    weight management, 63–65
Mediterranean Diet Pyramid, 44–46
    changes, 44
    cheese and yogurt group, 49
    fish and seafood group, 48
    meats and sweets group, 50
    plant group
        beans, nuts, legumes, and seeds, 48
        fats, 47
        fruits and vegetables, 47
        grains, 47
        herbs and spices, 48
        olive oil/olives, 47
    poultry and eggs group, 49
    wine, 50

Mediterranean Foods Alliance (MFA), 79
melon
    Lemon Minted Melon, 234
    Melon, Figs, and Prosciutto, 224
    Shrimp and Melon Salad, 252
menu plans
    fall, 318–320
    spring, 323–325
    summer, 316–318
    winter, 321–323
mercury levels in fish and seafood, 141
micronutrients
    antioxidants, 212
    minerals, 211–212
    phytonutrients, 213–214
    vitamins, 208
        fat-soluble, 209–210
        water-soluble, 210–211
milk, nutritional properties, 165
minerals, 211
    calcium, 212
    iron, 212
    selenium, 212
mint, 170
    Lemon Minted Melon, 234
    Minted Cucumber Salad, 253
    Minted Peas with Pancetta, 289
Mixed Bean Soup, 246
Mixed Berry Torte, 303
monounsaturated fats, 84, 186–187
movement, 26
mushrooms, 125
    Angel Hair Pasta with Pesto, Mushrooms, and Arugula, 275
    Mushroom, Artichoke, and Arugula Flatbread, 260

Mushroom Crostini, 226
Sautéed Spinach and Mushrooms, 285
mustard greens, 128
MyPlate (USDA), 51–52
myths, debunked, 28

# N

National Institutes of Health (NIH), 32
*New England Journal of Medicine*, 32
niacin (vitamin B₃), 210
nutrients, 208
  antioxidants, 212
  carbohydrates, 216
    complex, 216
    sugars, 216
  minerals, 211
    calcium, 212
    iron, 212
    selenium, 212
  phytonutrients, 213
    anthocyanidins (flavonoid), 214
    beta-carotene (carotenoid), 214
    lutein (carotenoid), 214
    lycopene (carotenoid), 214
  protein, 214–215
  vitamins, 208
    fat-soluble, 209–210
    water-soluble, 210–211
Nutrition Facts label, 75–76
  fat, 76
  fiber, 76
  fiber wording, 201–202
  "-free" claims, 78
  health claims, 78–79
  ingredient list, 77
  nutrient content claims, 78–79

percent Daily Value (%DV), 77–78
  servings per container, 76
  sodium, 76
  sugar, 77
  whole grains, 98
nuts. *See also* seeds
  almonds, 146–147, 149
  for dessert, 154
  health benefits, 146–147
  increasing intake, 154
  nutritional properties, 148
  peanuts, 147, 152–153
  pine nuts, 150–151
  preparation tips, 149
  storage, 149
  walnuts, 150

# O

obesity, 35
oils, smoke point, 89–90
olive oil
  baking with, 90–91
  butter substitution ratio, 91
  classifications
    extra-virgin, 86–87
    lite, 88
    pure, 87–88
    refined, 87–88
    virgin, 87
  cooking with, 89–90
  health benefits, 84
  history and production, 82
  International Olive Oil Council (IOOC), 87
  Mediterranean Diet Pyramid group, 47
  nutritional properties, 85

storing, 88–89
uses, 83
olives, 109
International Olive Oil Council (IOOC), 87
Mediterranean Diet Pyramid group, 47
omega-3 fatty acids, 187–188
seafood and, 133
omega-6 fatty acids, 188–189
Onion Apple Marmalade, 235
oranges, 114
Orange Rice Pudding, 312
Pan Seared Orange Scallops, 269
Spinach, Orange, and Feta Salad, 254
Ornish, Dean, 60
Ornish diet, 60

## P–Q

pairings, food and wine, 178
Pan-Seared Orange Scallops, 269
pantothenic acid, 211
Panzanella, 293
Parkinson's disease, 41
Parmesan Pepper Crisps, 236
pasta
Angel Hair Pasta with Pesto, Mushrooms, and Arugula, 275
Lamb Patties and Pasta, 276
Spicy Tomato Sauce with Linguine, 274
peanuts, 147, 152–153
Pear, Provolone, Asiago, and Balsamic Flatbread, 259
peas, 147
Minted Peas with Pancetta, 289
Split Pea Soup, 244

percent Daily Value (%DV), 77–78
pesto
Angel Hair Pasta with Pesto, Mushrooms, and Arugula, 275
Lamb Pesto Crostini, 233
Pesto, 223
physical activity, 26
phytonutrients, 213
anthocyanidins (flavonoid), 214
beta-carotene (carotenoid), 214
lutein (carotenoid), 214
lycopene (carotenoid), 214
Pickled Asparagus, 290
pine nuts, 150–151
pizza, 257. *See also* flatbreads
Butternut Squash and Goat Cheese Pizza, 262
Tomato Basil Pizza, 261
plant group, Mediterranean Diet Pyramid
beans, 48
fats, 47
fruits and vegetables, 47
grains, 47
herbs and spices, 48
legumes, 48
nuts, 48
olive oil, 47
olives, 47
seeds, 48
Poached Summer Fruit, 302
polenta, 100
Sweet Polenta with Sun-Dried Tomatoes, 295
polyunsaturated fats, 187
pomegranates, 111
Fruit and Cheese Plate, 305

portion sizes, 21, 64

poultry, 49, 158
  Chicken Almond Wrap, 264
  Chicken Piccata, 280
  Chicken Tzatziki Pita, 265
  Crispy Turkey Cutlets, 279
  fat, 160
  intake recommendations, 158
  nutritional properties, 159–160

processed foods, 70

Prosciutto and Roasted Vegetable Panini, 266

protein, 214–215

pure olive oil, 87

pyramid, Mediterranean Diet Pyramid, 44–46
  changes, 44
  cheese and yogurt group, 49
  fish and seafood group, 48
  meats and sweets group, 50
  plant group
    beans, nuts, legumes, and seeds, 48
    fats, 47
    fruits and vegetables, 47
    grains, 47
    herbs and spices, 48
    olive oil/olives, 47
  poultry and eggs group, 49
  wine, 50

pyridoxine (vitamin B6), 211

quinoa, 100
  Quinoa Pilaf, 297

**R**

RA (rheumatoid arthritis), 41

red meat, 70, 158

red wines, 177
  food pairings, 178

refined grains, 95
  enriched, 96
  versus whole grains, 94

refined olive oil, 87

resveratrol, wine, 175

rheumatoid arthritis (RA), 41

riboflavin (vitamin B2), 210

Roasted Beet Salad, 248

Roasted Red Pepper Tapenade, 222

romaine lettuce, 128

Rosemary Garlic Potatoes, 286

**S**

salads
  Classic Mixed Greens Salad with Balsamic Vinaigrette, 255
  Fennel and Apple Salad, 251
  Golden Couscous Salad, 249
  Marinated Artichoke Salad, 247
  Minted Cucumber Salad, 253
  Roasted Beet Salad, 248
  Shrimp and Melon Salad, 252
  Spinach, Orange, and Feta Salad, 254
  Tabbouleh Salad, 256
  Tuna Salad with Capers and Potatoes, 250

salmon, 136, 138
  Salmon Fennel Bundles, 273
  Smoked Salmon Bites, 237

sandwich options, 71
sardines, 138–139
saturated fats, 189–190
Sautéed Spinach and Mushrooms, 285
seafood, 132. *See also* fish
    Almond-Crusted Barramundi, 272
    cooking techniques, 139
    Crab Cakes, 231
    fish oil supplements, 140–141
    health benefits, 132–133
    increasing intake, 142
    mercury levels, 141
    nutritional properties, 133–134
    Pan-Seared Orange Scallops, 269
    salmon, 136–138
    Salmon Fennel Bundles, 273
    sardines, 138–139
    Seafood Stew, 268
    selection tips, 134–135
    Shrimp and Melon Salad, 252
    Smoked Salmon Bites, 237
    Sole Florentine, 271
    tuna, 137
    Tuna Salad with Capers and Potatoes, 250
Seafood Stew, 268
Sears, Barry, 61
seasoning blends, 168
seeds. *See also* nuts
    health benefits, 146–147
    increasing intake, 154
    nutritional properties, 148
    preparation tips, 149
    sesame seeds, 151
    storage, 149
selenium, 212
sesame seeds, 151

Shrimp and Melon Salad, 252
side dishes
    Barley and Vegetable Sauté, 298
    Bean and Vegetable Patties, 291
    Curried Cauliflower, 287
    Golden Chard, 294
    Lemon Kale Ribbons, 288
    Minted Peas with Pancetta, 289
    Panzanella, 293
    Pickled Asparagus, 290
    Quinoa Pilaf, 297
    Rosemary Garlic Potatoes, 286
    Sautéed Spinach and Mushrooms, 285
    Sweet Polenta with Sun-Dried Tomatoes, 295
    Two-Cheese Risotto, 283
    Zucchini and Walnuts, 282
Smoked Salmon Bites, 237
smoke point, oils, 89–91
snacks
    Baked Vegetable Omelet, 230
    Crab Cakes, 231
    Eggplant Rolls, 229
    Hummus, 228
    Lamb Pesto Crostini, 233
    Lemon Cannellini Spread, 227
    Lemon Minted Melon, 234
    Melon, Figs, and Prosciutto, 224
    Mushroom Crostini, 226
    Onion Apple Marmalade, 235
    Parmesan Pepper Crisps, 236
    Pesto, 223
    Roasted Red Pepper Tapenade, 222
    Smoked Salmon Bites, 237
    Stuffed Dates, 225
    Tomato Basil Bocconcini, 232

sodium, nutrition label, 76

Sole Florentine, 271

soluble fiber, 196

Sonoma diet, 62–63

soups. *See also* stews
    Butternut Squash Soup, 242
    Gazpacho, 245
    Lemon Lentil Soup, 241
    Mixed Bean Soup, 246
    Split Pea Soup, 244
    Tomato Basil Soup, 240
    Vegetable Orzo Soup, 243

South Beach diet, 59–60

soynuts, 147

spelt flour, 102

spices, 48, 168. *See also* herbs
    garlic, 170
    nutritional properties, 169
    seasoning blends, 168
    usage tips, 171

Spicy Tomato Sauce with Linguine, 274

spinach, 127
    Sautéed Spinach and Mushrooms, 285
    Sole Florentine, 271
    Spinach, Orange, and Feta Salad, 254

Split Pea Soup, 244

spreads
    Hummus, 228
    Lemon Cannellini Spread, 227
    Onion Apple Marmalade, 235
    Pesto, 223
    Roasted Red Pepper Tapenade, 222

spring menu plan, 323–325

squash, butternut
    Butternut Squash and Goat Cheese Pizza, 262
    Butternut Squash Soup, 242

stews. *See also* soups
    Seafood Stew, 268

storage
    legumes, 149
    nuts and seeds, 149
    olive oil, 88–89

strawberries, 113
    Berry Sorbet, 304
    Mixed Berry Torte, 303

stress, 26

Stuffed Dates, 225

sugar
    fruit, 109
    nutrition label, 77

summer menu plan, 316–318

sun-dried tomatoes, Sweet Polenta with Sun-Dried Tomatoes, 295

supplements
    fiber, 202
    fish oil, 140–141

sweeteners, 74

Sweet Polenta with Sun-Dried Tomatoes, 295

sweets and treats, 50, 74

Swiss chard, 128

## T–U

Tabbouleh Salad, 256

tannins, wine, 176

thiamin (vitamin B$_1$), 210

thyme, 171

tomatoes, 124–125
    Spicy Tomato Sauce with Linguine, 274
    Sweet Polenta with Sun-Dried Tomatoes, 295

Tomato Basil Bocconcini, 232

Tomato Basil Pizza, 261

Tomato Basil Soup, 240

trans fats, 190–191

transitioning to diet, 23–25

approach to food, changing, 71

food list, essential Mediterranean diet foods, 72–74, 94

foods to add, 71

foods to reduce, 70

replacing foods, 70

whole grains, 104–105

treats. *See* sweets and treats

triglycerides, 33–34

tuna, 137

Tuna Salad with Capers and Potatoes, 250

Two-Cheese Risotto, 283

type 1 diabetes, 39

type 2 diabetes, 38

fiber and, 198

USDA MyPlate, 51–52

**V**

Vanilla Panna Cotta, 301

Vegetable Orzo Soup, 243

vegetables, 120

artichokes, 121–122

carrots, 126

eggplant, 122–123

greens, 127

arugula, 127

kale, 127

mustard greens, 128

romaine lettuce, 128

spinach, 127

Swiss chard, 128

health benefits, 120

increased intake, 128–129

Mediterranean Diet Pyramid group, 47

mushrooms, 125

nutritional properties, 121

tomatoes, 124–125

zucchini, 123–124

Veggie Wrap, 263

virgin olive oil, 87

vitamins, 208

fat-soluble

vitamin A, 209

vitamin D, 209

vitamin E, 209

vitamin K, 210

water-soluble

biotin, 211

cobalamin (vitamin $B_{12}$), 211

folate (folic acid), 210

niacin (vitamin $B_3$), 210

pantothenic acid, 211

pyridoxine (vitamin $B_6$), 211

riboflavin (vitamin $B_2$), 210

thiamin (vitamin $B_1$), 210

vitamin C, 210

**W–X**

Walnut Cake, 311

walnuts, 150

Baklava, 308

Cinnamon Apple and Nut Phyllo Rolls, 300

Walnut Cake, 311

Zucchini and Walnuts, 282

water-soluble vitamins
    biotin, 211
    cobalamin (vitamin $B_{12}$), 211
    folate (folic acid), 210
    niacin (vitamin $B_3$), 210
    pantothenic acid, 211
    pyridoxine (vitamin $B_6$), 211
    riboflavin (vitamin $B_2$), 210
    thiamin (vitamin $B_1$), 210
    vitamin C, 210
weight management, 34, 63–65
    BMI, 36
    fiber and, 198
    obesity, 35
white kidney beans, 153
white wines, 177
    food pairings, 178
whole grains, 94
    adding, 71
    barley, hulled, 99
    cooking techniques, 103–104
    couscous, 100
    flours, 101–102
        barley, 103
        spelt, 102
        whole-rye, 103
        whole-wheat, 102
    health benefits, 96
    labeling, 97
    nutritional properties, 97
    Nutrition Facts label, 98
    polenta, 100
    quinoa, 100
    refined grains comparison, 94
    transitioning to, 104–105
    Whole Grain Stamps, 98
    whole-wheat bulgur, 99

whole-rye flour, 103
whole-wheat flour, 102
wine, 50
    flavonoids, 175
    food pairings, 178
    health benefits, 174
    moderation, 179
    nutritional properties, 175–176
    reds, 177
    resveratrol, 175
    tannins, 176
    whites, 177
winter menu plan, 321–323
wraps, 257
    Chicken Almond Wrap, 264
    Veggie Wrap, 263

## Y-Z

yogurt, 49
    nutritional properties, 165

Zone diet, 61–62
zucchini, 123–124
    Zucchini and Walnuts, 282